A History Of Nursing

...sing

The Evolution of Nursing Sy... ...om
the Earliest Times to the Fou...
of the Fi... English and Ame...
Training Schools for Nurses

By

Super...tendent of ... the Tra... School ...1;
...tructor in ... Teachers' School...s;
...ember ... American ... tion of Nurses ...of
...International ... Nursing ...t;

and

... ... New Y...
... P...   ... Nurs... and O...
... Nu...   ... Me...rof In...
... ...ation   ...l; and of ...

In T... Volumes
...ume T...

Illustrated

. . .

... York and Lo...
G... and C...pany ...
19..

A History of Nursing

The Evolution of Nursing Systems from
the Earliest Times to the Foundation
of the First English and American
Training Schools for Nurses

By

M. Adelaide Nutting, R. N.

Superintendent of Nurses, The Johns Hopkins Hospital;
Principal of Johns Hopkins Training School for Nurses;
President of the American Federation of Nurses; Member of
the International Council of Nurses;

and

Lavinia L. Dock, R. N.

Member of the Nurses' Settlement, New York; Secretary of the
American Federation of Nurses and of the International
Council of Nurses; Honorary Member of the Matrons' Council
of Great Britain and Ireland, and of the German Nurses'
Association.

In Two Volumes

Volume Two

———

Illustrated

———

G. P. Putnam's Sons
New York and London
The Knickerbocker Press
1907

The Knickerbocker Press, New York

CONTENTS

iv Contents

ILLUSTRATIONS

A HISTORY OF NURSING

CHAPTER I

KAISERSWERTH AND THE DEACONESS MOVEMENT

THE river Rhine lies broad and peaceful between its low, green banks before the little North German town of Kaiserswerth, and the majestic old ruins of the Kaiserpfalz guard the entrance from the boat-landing to the quiet streets. Their testimony to a proud and knightly past is now ignored, and no one thinks of Kaiserswerth except as the home of the famous Deaconess Motherhouse—as a sort of shrine, to which pilgrimages may be made in loving and grateful memories of the simple, self-forgetting devotion of its founders. In this quiet, remote village beat hearts whose rhythm started waves that have spread over the earth. The direct and indirect extensions of humane endeavour dating from Kaiserswerth may indeed be likened, according to the favourite simile of the German pastors, to the vast tree beginning as a tiny acorn, whose branches cover all the earth. In and around the little town itself now stand eleven noble institutions, which have grown from the Motherhouse. Extensive and spacious modern buildings fitted with every device of science for the care of the sick and the dependent stand in the beautiful large gardens of lawn, trees, and shrubbery, so characteristic of German institutions, and away beyond all of these is a fine farm. On the main street of the village, with its cobbles and quaint old-time, two-story, white-painted, low-built houses that have a hanging garden in every window, stands the Motherhouse with its simple and unpretending but extensive front, flanked at one end by the older building with its charming curved façade. Back and beyond this building through the luxuriant gardens, past the shady porches of the House of Evening Rest, where live the aged Sisters (who have served through their lives and have now come back here in the evening of their days to be taken care of), and the home for superannuated men who have served the establishment and are now having their peaceful days, stands the Kaiserswerth Museum, where the Sisters have collected their treasures from all corners of the earth. Here are a huge, stuffed crocodile from the Nile; stone slabs with Egyptian hieroglyphics and Assyrian records; cuneiform tablets, models of the Eastern temples and of the branch houses in distant lands; idols of every nation; costumes of every Oriental style; thorns from the Mount of Calvary; curious natural products; the handiwork of barbaric races and curios innumerable. On a long table in the middle of the Museum is a collection of articles picked up by the nursing deaconesses on many a field of battle; helmets, weapons, and accoutrements of war; knapsacks, flags, and cooking utensils. Then there is a case full of medals which have been bestowed either on individual Sisters for bravery in times of war and pestilence, or on the Mother-house as an institution. Again beyond and behind the Museum are more gardens, then a roadway, and then, almost buried in green, one comes upon the tiny, two-roomed cottage, the first refuge for discharged women prisoners in Germany—the spot where Friederike and Theodor Fliedner, in joy and hope, sheltered the historic Minna, their first refugee. This was the cradle of the Kaiserswerth institutions. Beyond this, again, stands an old tower, once a mill, now a water-tower, and from its broad base grows a row of little dwellings. Here was the first School for Deaconesses, and here Miss Nightingale and Agnes Jones lived during their stay at Kaiserswerth. This tiny refuge; this row of cottages and the small shady garden where "Mother" Fliedner used to sit or walk in the evening, knitting in hand, while she counselled the different ones who came to her for advice, form the heart of Kaiserswerth.[1] Here Friederike, creative, a woman of

[1] In 1886 the deaconesses bought the little garden house, which had belonged to the parish, and presented it to the Motherhouse on its fiftieth anniversary.

boundless courage and overflowing devotion, brought into existence the training of deaconesses. The Kaiserswerth deaconesses now number nearly four thousand, and under their care are more than fifty hospitals, numerous orphanages, more than forty infant schools, ten schools for the higher education of girls, with special schools, such as those for the blind, deaf and dumb, for manual work, institutions for nervous and insane patients, for the training and befriending of young women in domestic service, for the rescue and aid of fallen girls, for the recuperation of the Sisters, convalescent homes, and others.

The branch or daughter houses, some thirty in all, are found all over Germany as well as in many foreign countries. Especially interesting are those at Jerusalem, Alexandria, Cairo, Beirut, Smyrna, and Bucharest. Not only its own daughter houses, but all independent institutions for deaconesses owe their existence to Kaiserswerth, for all subsequent work wrought by deaconesses whether in France, Switzerland, or America, whether Lutheran, Methodist, or Episcopalian, has been the fruit of the Kaiserswerth tree.

Nor is this all,—the whole development of modern secular nursing, which now encircles the ent re globe, traces its genealogy through Florence Nightingale, its direct founder, to Kaiserswerth and its training school, for it was there that Miss Nightingale went to study nursing system and

method, when she was preparing, unconsciously,
it may be, for her revolutionary reforms in hospital organisation.

It was in 1822 that the young pastor Theodor
Fliedner, staff in hand, set out on a journey to
Holland and England to beg for financial rescue
for his little parish of Kaiserswerth, ruined by
the failure of a silk mill at the very moment when
he was installed there as its shepherd. He had
been offered another parish, but refused it, saying
"He wished to be a true shepherd and not a
hireling." He made at first, however, a shy and
unsuccessful beggar, until a wise brother advised
him that three things were necessary: "patience,
boldness, and a fluent tongue." With renewed
courage he went on, and with such success that
on his return he brought with him a sum of money,
the interest of which was enough to support his
little church and Sunday-school, and his association for young men. In England Queen Victoria,
then a little girl, headed the list of his subscribers.
But of far greater importance than the money
was the knowledge gained in his journey of what
the world was doing. In Holland, deservedly
famous for its many and excellent institutions
of charity and philanthropy, some of which were
the only ones that Howard had found to com-
mend, and in England, then thrilling with all the
impulses which were later to flower in private
and statutory acts of reform, he visited numbers of
schools and educational institutions, almshouses,

orphanages, hospitals, and prisons, and became informed of the methods of prison societies. "I was especially impressed," he wrote, "with the efficacy of the British Bible and Prison Societies, and returned deeply shamed that we in Germany had done so little for the prisoners."[1] In London he met Mrs. Fry and saw her work in Newgate, with which he was deeply impressed. In Holland, too, to his great joy, he had seen the Mennonite deaconesses, chosen by the church officers, living in their own homes, but busy in their parish work with the poor and the sick. He wrote of them:

This praiseworthy Christian arrangement ought to be introduced into all other evangelical churches. The apostolic church created the office of deaconess, knowing well that the ministrations of men could never form a substitute for tender womanly feeling and fine womanly tact in solacing physical and spiritual distress especially among other women. Why has the modern Church not retained this apostolic feature; must misuse destroy every good thing? To how many women and maidens would this not open a new and congenial field?[2]

Fliedner returned to Germany, and, full of zeal, founded the Rhenish-Westphalian Prison Association in 1826, the first of its kind in Germany.

[1] *Zur Erinnerung an den Besuch der Diakonissen Anstalt in Kaiserswerth.* Obtainable at the Deaconess Institute of Kaiserswerth.

[2] *Zur Erinnerung*, p. 6. Also *Theodor Fliedner, Kurzer Abriss Seines Lebens*, Georg Fliedner, Kaiserswerth Anstalt, 1892, p. 59.

He also, remembering that Klönne had written a paper on the renewal of the order of deaconesses wrote eagerly to him to hear his views. While he was thus ardent with plans and projects, foremost among which in his mind were those for discharged prisoners, whom he especially yearned to aid, Friederike Münster, who was soon to be his wife and share and double his energies, was engaged in similar efforts and filled with ideas like his own.

Friederike Münster, destined to become the mother of the revived apostolic order of deaconesses, and the immediate ancestress of modern nursing, was born in the year 1800, just twenty years before Miss Nightingale. Her birthplace was a beautiful and romantic spot, the village of Braunfels in the valley of the Lahn, where clustering cottages, set in the most exquisite frame of valley, stream, and forest, and overtopped by a stately and many-towered castle, composed a scene peculiarly German, expressive at once of the most domestic and the most idealistic traditions.

The spot had been of old associated with a famous nurse. Six hundred years earlier Elizabeth, the beloved mother of the poor, had, in pursuance of a vow, travelled barefoot to bring her little daughter to the old cloister of Altenberg (now no longer in existence) near by.

Friederike's early life was a round of those household and family duties which are so perfect a

preparation for nursing. Her father had been
a schoolmaster; later Comptroller on the estate
of Prince Solms Braunfels. As a young girl, she
had been acquainted with poverty and struggle,
but also with a life of active hospitality and
intimate association with many kinds of people,—
from those of the court circles, down to the low-
liest. The joy of usefulness irradiated Friederike's days, and when, in her twenty-fifth year,
the little brothers and sisters having grown to
self-support and her father having married a
second time she was no longer needed in the home,
she offered her voluntary services to Count Von
der Recke, who had founded an institute in
Düsselthal near Düsseldorf for the rescue of
children. What her spirit was in her service here
can be read in the prayer which she inscribed in
her diary; *Du bist die Liebe, lass mich Liebe
werden!* Two years of this work brought her
a severe illness, and whilst recuperating from it
in the home of a friend, she was introduced to
pastor Fliedner, who was then seeking for some
one to befriend the female convicts in the prison
at Düsseldorf. Friederike had been recommended
to him for her gifts of mind and heart, and she
would have devoted herself gladly to the prison
work, had not her parents been unwilling. But
when Fliedner soon after asked her in marriage
they consented, and Friederike thenceforth had
not only the convicts, but the whole parish as
well on which to lavish her energies. From first to

last she sympathised actively with her husband in the prison mission work. Her first individual effort was to start a woman's society for nursing and visiting in the homes of the poor, of whom there were many, in the little parish, and she was herself untiring in visiting, cooking for the sick, nursing and cheering them, as Elizabeth of Hungary had been before her. "In thy mother's dealings with the poor I learned what the Scripture means when it says, 'Let the poor find thy heart,'" said Fliedner[1] in later life to his daughter. She had a special gift of drawing souls to her. Her influence was oftenest a silent one, but at the right moment, she knew the right word to say.

Her next work was to establish knitting lessons for the girls. They met in the tiny garden house under the direction of Fräulein Frickenhaus and this nucleus later developed into the school for little children.[2] Paster Fliedner was continually obliged to travel from home to collect money and stimulate interest in the work of the Prison Association, and during his many absences Friederike managed the parish and carried on every undertaking. It was soon borne in upon them both that it was useless to think of helping the prisoners unless there was some place to receive them upon discharge, and Friederike urged her husband to open a refuge for them.

[1] *Jahrbuch für Christliche Unterhaltung*, Kaiserswerth, 1894, p. 10.
[2] *Ibid.*

My parish [wrote Fliedner] the smallest in the country about, seemed least fitted for such an attempt. But
none of the clergy of the neighbouring parishes would
undertake it.   My wife insisted that we should make
the beginning and I gladly agreed to it.   It was still
more difficult to find the right woman to place in
charge,—some one wise, kind, and patient enough.
But my wife succeeded, by urgent letters, in inducing
an old and dear friend, Katherine Göbel of Braunfels,
to come to us to talk it over.   Her relations were
opposed to it.   She herself fell ill, and her courage
wavered, when unexpectedly on the 17th of September,
1833, a young convict, Minna by name, just discharged from the penitentiary, came in and begged
piteously to stay.   We could not refuse, but where
to put her?   In the garden stood a tiny house, the favourite resort of the children, and we domiciled Minna
there.   The little house was only twelve feet square,
and no stairway led to its tiny garret, so Minna
ascended from the outside on a ladder to go to bed,
and the next morning climbed down the same way.

This was the seed that grew into the great tree.
From this little garden house all the institutions
of Kaiserswerth were one by one developed.
Fräulein Göbel remained; ("Minna did her more
good than iron and quinine," wrote Fliedner) but
Frau Fliedner bore the brunt of the care and responsibility of the Refuge for the first few years
of its growth, until it became a large and firmly
established asylum.

The care of the sick and how to make provision for it was the next engrossing thought of

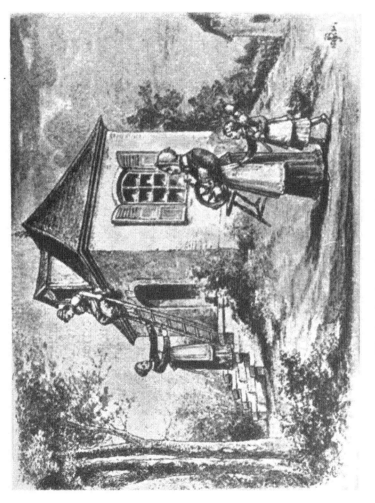

The Cradle of the Kaiserswerth Institutions
The asylum for discharged prisoners

Jahrbuch für Christliche Unterhaltung, Kaiserswerth, 1894

Friederike's mother heart.[1] Fliedner shared it
to the full.

The thought of the sick poor had long lain heavy
on our hearts [he wrote]. How often had I seen them,
forsaken; their bodily needs neglected, and their
souls quite forgotten, fading in their dull unhealthy
cabins like leaves in autumn; and how many cities,
even large ones, were without hospitals; and even
where there were hospitals,—I had seen many on my
travels through Belgium, Holland, England, and
Scotland and in our own Germany—often with
marble-trimmed exteriors, but the nursing was
wretched. Physicians complained bitterly of the
hireling service by day and night, of the drunkenness
and immorality of the attendants. And what is to
be said of the spiritual care? Little thought is given
to it. In many hospitals pastors are unknown and
chapels not thought of. Would not our young Christian women be able and willing to do Christian
nursing? Had not many such women performed
wonders of self-sacrificing love in the lazarettos and
military hospitals of the War of Freedom? The
apostolic Church had utilised this force for the benefit
of the downtrodden, and through hundreds of years
had appointed women to the diaconate. Ought
we to delay in bringing back consecrated women
into the service of the Lord? Such thoughts gave
me no rest. My wife, also, was of like mind, and of
far greater courage than myself. But was this little
Kaiserswerth, with its preponderating Catholic population; where there were not enough sick people to

[1] *Das Diakonissen Mutterhaus, und seine Töchterhäuser.*
Julius Disselhoff, Kaiserswerth, 1893, p. 7.

provide a school for instruction; where the general poverty could promise no financial aid—could this be the right place for a school for evangelical nurses? Were there not more experienced pastors than I, better fitted for so difficult an undertaking? I went to my colleagues in Düsseldorf, Elberfeld, Barmen, etc., and urged them to consider whether one of them might not undertake what must be almost necessary in their large parishes. Every one declined my proposition. "I was the right one to try it; my little parish gave me enough time for it: the quiet seclusion of Kaiserswerth would be favourable to such an undertaking. Beside, the Lord did· not intend all my travel experiences for nothing. He was able to send money to Kaiserswerth and patients and nurses as well.'" [1]

Thus the arguments—no one pointed out the fact, that no other but Fliedner knew of a woman who could begin such a work and build it up to completion, but this was the truth. This was pre-eminently a work that needed the direction of a gifted woman, and pastor Fliedner came home to his wife.

We saw at last [he says] that it was the Lord's purpose to lay this task upon our shoulders. We assumed it gladly. We looked about quietly for a house to use as a hospital. One day the largest and best house in Kaiserswerth was offered for sale. My wife had been confined only three days before; nevertheless, she persuaded me to buy the house in the name of the Lord. The price was 2300 thalers

[1] *Kurzer Abriss*, etc., pp. 59-61.

and we had no money. I bought it in faith on the 20th of April, 1836. The money was to be paid at Christmas.

When the time came to pay the money, it was all in his hands: an experience that was often repeated in later years.[1]

The hospital was not fitted up without opposition. The neighbours objected to it, and there was clerical enmity. Fliedner was threatened that the village authorities would complain of him to the government, and the physicians who had been engaged to attend the patients thought it dangerous for Fliedner to go off at that moment on a money-collecting tour, as the general excitement might bring some danger to his wife. "But she laughed at this," writes Fliedner, "and sent me gaily on my journey, for she relied on a higher power." Finally, on the 16th of October the first patient came (a Catholic maidservant) and on the 20th the first deaconess arrived.

Who was happier than our dear mother? Fifty times a day she ran back and forth between the parsonage and the hospital, advising, providing, carrying furniture, making beds and arranging the rooms, speaking a cheerful word to the patient and directing the helpers, until the inmates of the asylum grew jealous, lest in the absorption of the new work the old would be forgotten. But this did not happen.[2]

The furniture had all been donated and was of

[1] *Zur Erinnerung*, p. 7.
[2] *Jahrbuch*, p. 14.

the humblest description. A shabby table, some broken-backed chairs, worn-out knives, two-pronged forks, worm-eaten beds, and appliances to match had been sent in.

> We moved in with a mean outfit, but with boundless joy and thanksgiving. So the small and insignificant seed of the deaconess institute was planted with faith in the way of the Apostolic Church, and it has had a rich growth.

By the end of the month there were four patients in the house.

We may here draw attention to a somewhat prevalent popular error, regarding the first deaconesses, namely, that pastor Fliedner utilised the young women prisoners to establish the nursing work, and that the first members of the Sisterhood were therefore repentant sinners who had taken refuge in the asylum.[1]

This is an entire mistake. The deaconesses were never drawn from the class of prisoners, but were always carefully chosen from applicants of blameless lives. The prisoners' refuge was simply one of the many branches of loving service conducted by the Fliedners.

Gertrude Reichardt, the first Kaiserswerth deaconess, was the daughter and the sister of a physician. She was born in Ruhrort in 1788 and

[1] A magazine article, which the writers have not been able to identify, but which seems to have been rather widely read, has evidently propagated this error.

was already a woman of mature years and of much practical experience as a nurse. In her father's home she had been accustomed to assist him with dressings and operations, and during the War of Freedom she had been his constant helper. When her brother became a physician she had gained further large experience in the care of the sick among his patients. She was admirably fitted for the work of the new hospital, and the Fliedners had long known of her and for a time had tried in vain to persuade her to take up the new and experimental post of deaconess. Finally, in the early autumn they had induced her to come and see the new hospital. It looked very bare and poor and she could not decide to remain; was, in fact, about to return home when a large bundle was brought in by post, which contained a quantity of new bed-linen, clothing, and ward fittings. This simple occurrence was regarded by her as a providential sign, and she promised to come in October. Two young women promised to come and assist, though not willing to become deaconesses. Gertrude remained in the service until 1855 when she withdrew to the House of Evening Rest (*Feierabend Haus*) for the old Sisters at the age of sixty-eight years. Her experience, devotion, and character made her an ideal pioneer and a most valuable aid to Frau Fliedner in the work of training the new Sisters.[1] Friederike, how-

[1] Gertrude's life was sketched in a Church Journal, *Armen und Krankenfreund*, published at Kaiserswerth in 1869.

ever, remained the head and centre of the hospital work. Pastor Fliedner writes:

The first deaconess, whom we had intended to make the superintendent, and who was a complete mistress of the arts of caring for both body and soul of her patients, nevertheless had not the rarer but most essential talents of ruling and of administration. Consequently it was necessary for my wife to assume the position of superintendent, and the unselfish Sister yielded the ruling power with true Christian self-abnegation.[1]

In this first year six other deaconesses were received,—Beata, Johanna, Helena, Franziska, Catherina, and Carolina. Sixty patients in all were cared for in the hospital and twenty-eight in their own homes. The visited cases were all among the poor, and most of them were furnished with diets from the Motherhouse. The work was divided up in this way: one deaconess did the cooking and housekeeping, another had the laundry and linen department, one the women's ward, one the men's, with the aid of an orderly, and another the children's. They changed about systematically and in summer time one was kept busy in the garden. Theoretical and clinical instruction was given by Dr. Thönissen, who used, as a basis, Dr. Dieffenbach's manual. The deaconesses also studied pharmacy and passed the state examination on this subject. At Christmas time Flied-

[1] *Jahrbuch*, p. 14.

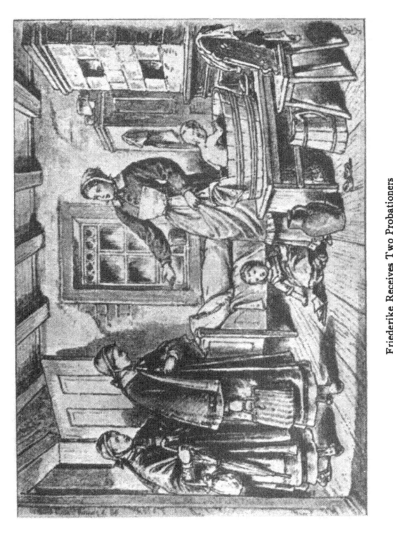

Friederike Receives Two Probationers
"Gar zwei auf einmal"

Jahrbuch für Christliche Unterhaltung, Kaiserswerth, 1894

ner invited Amalie Sieveking to take charge of the new work, in order to release his wife to her family cares, but she was unable to leave her work in Hamburg and Friederike continued as the head of the establishment. The annual report of that period speaks of her as follows: "The office of Matron (Mother, Superintendent) has been filled by the wife of the writer, who will continue until a suitable head has been trained." But this time did not come; for, though suitable ones were trained, they were urgently demanded in new fields, and Friederike kept her post as House Mother until her too early death. Wacker, judging, from the man's standpoint, the wife as an auxiliary, wrote:

Her keen glance and pure and holy spirit kept him (Fliedner) from making mistakes. With the virtues of cleanliness, order, simplicity, and economy she had a large-hearted compassion, great energy, and strong rational sense to prevent the misdirection of ministering love. She became a model to the deaconesses as well as a mother to them. Her name deserves mention as one who took an important part in the work.[1]

Thus placed in charge of an untried undertaking, the pastor's wife reflected often and earnestly upon the duties and responsibilities belonging to it—of how best to choose the Sisters; to train them and place them in new positions; of their relations

[1] *Der Diakonissen Beruf*, Emil Wacker (Gütersloh, 1888), p. 116.

to one another and to their directors. She recorded her reflections and conclusions in a small
volume, which was long the guide for those engaged in the training of deaconesses, and in all the
essentials still remains the accepted standard of
Kaiserswerth. What a pity that this volume, the
first work on the training of nurses to be written
by a woman, the fruit of her practical experience
and thought, fired by enthusiasm and directed by
a most able mind, should not have been given to
the public. It would be indeed a classic. But we
may judge of its contents by the statement of principles later presented by Schäfer. The key-note
of Friederike's teaching was a sentence inscribed
in the title-page of her note-book, "*Niemand gebe
die Seele preis um der Kunst willen*," which we
may transcribe thus: Never sacrifice the soul of
the work for its technique. Truly, if every woman made this tone her own, no other ethical
teaching would be needed.

While Friederike was supreme at home, pastor
Fliedner was untiring in his exertions abroad, travelling, speaking, rousing interest in the work, and
founding new branches. The work grew heavier,
and Friederike's letters often spoke of an almost
crushing mass of duties and demands upon her
strength. Not the least of these demands came
from the many visitors, for now the fame of
Kaiserswerth was bringing humanitarians and philanthropists from far and near to inspect the deaconesses' institute. One of the most welcome was

Mrs. Fry, who had so strongly influenced Fliedner
in his younger days.   She came in May, 1840, and
although she spoke little German, and Friederike
no English, these two enthusiasts felt little need of
words, for they were at once conscious of an inner
bond which made of looks and gestures a sufficient
language.   Elizabeth Fry's approbation of all she
saw at Kaiserswerth rejoiced Friederike's heart
and gave her fresh courage, while abroad it did
much to win new friends for the cause and allay
prejudice.   An incident of this day which is told
by Friederike's biographer is strikingly illustra-
tive of her fortitude.   Just before Mrs. Fry's arrival she had a letter telling her of the death of
pastor Fliedner's brother; but, unwilling to agitate
her husband at the moment of this eagerly expected visit, she kept the sad news to herself with
tranquil mien until the guest had left.

When it is remembered that, in addition to her
many duties, Friederike was the mother of a group
of children (she bore nine' in all, but four died at
birth), it is not surprising that sometimes even her
spirit sank under its burden.   Wrote Fliedner:

The rearing of her children brought the tender
mother much joy, and also much anxiety.   Some
of the children were delicate, and she could not devote
herself to them as she wished.   The cares of the many
poor of our parish, her share of interest in the asylum
for prisoners, in the children's school and the school
for teachers now connected with it, the post of superintendent in the young but yearly growing training-

school for deaconesses,—were no light burdens for
her to carry. Add to this the numerous visitors,
who came almost daily, and who usually stayed to
meals. No wonder that, strong as were her shoulders and great the courage, the administrative talent,
the practical knowledge and the skill with which the
Lord had endowed her, she sometimes groaned under
the burden and asked if there was not a conflict between her duties as mother and as head of the institution, and if there was not some way to reconcile
them. We talked it over from every side to see if it
were not possible to substitute for her in the work,
but we could find no way. Then she could not but
realise how especially blessed her leadership in the
work had been. In the daily, almost hourly, necessary directions and advice, the spiritual charge of so
many individuals and their training, who could be
so strong a support to the work as she? Moreover,
my wife felt that the care of the children was not
only in our hands but in the hands of God. She had
also before her the reassuring example of Countess
Zinzendorf, whose ability to lead a life crowded with
public duties, similar to her own, and yet to be an
excellent mother to her children, she had always admired. The development of the deaconess training
was new to our church, and in all the rules, in their
dress, in their discipline, there was so careful a line
to be drawn between the extreme sacrifice of freedom
of the cloister and the avoidance of a demoralising
liberty, that the keen, womanly and holy perception
of my wife was indispensable in avoiding mistakes.
The homely virtues of cleanliness, order, simplicity,
and economy, with boundless kindness for all sufferers,

so important for the Sisters in their works of mercy, who else but my wife could teach and enforce them rightly? Then the masculine energy which she possessed and the way in which she could control and subdue wrongdoers and prevent imposition—this united with her native gentleness made an extraordinary combination of character.[1]

So, for the sake of the work, Friederike continued to bear the double burden. The years 1841 and 1842 were full of family affliction. Her husband and three of her children were prostrated by severe illness, and as they slowly passed the danger line the time came when an engagement previously made to organise the nursing work in two other German cities had to be met. Fliedner, almost convalescent, was entirely unfit to go. The circumstances were urgent, for the need was very great, and Friederike, faithful to her responsibilities as head of a nursing order, put her younger sister in charge of her sick children and prepared for the journey.

"What it must have cost her to tear herself away from her loved ones only the heart of a mother can know!" She took with her four deaconesses to begin the new work. The conditions she found were horrible; they were the conditions generally prevalent in hospitals at that time, and give a realising sense of the Augean stables which were cleaned by the labours of the

[1] *Kurzer Abriss*, pp. 75-76. *Jahrbuch*, pp. 18-19.

faithful deaconesses. Friederike wrote to her husband:

At nine o'clock the director and secretary accompanied us to the hospital. I was often so nauseated at what I saw I had to run to the window — the filth and vermin were indescribable. The haunts of thieves could be no worse. A woman has been here since 1838 who is not yet cleansed from vermin. The doctors make rounds certainly not too often. They were here yesterday. A drunkard who had tried to cut his throat was proposed to me by the committee as an attendant for the sick—I declined.

The inventory is to be given us to-day. Most of the bedding will have to be dragged with prongs and tongs to the stable. We will do this on Monday. To-day the Sisters with a scrub-woman are cleaning the room into which we will move to-morrow evening, Sunday. I would like to stay here several days to relieve the dreariness for the Sisters, get the male attendant grounded in his work and have some rooms cleaned. The whole committee is coming to the hospital to-day at four o'clock, and I must meet them.

I have told the directors that if conditions are not altered we will not allow the Sisters to stay . . . for they shall not kill themselves working for nothing . . . and in such dens of immorality they could accomplish nothing.

I wish I could write a description of the glorious mountains for my beloved children, but I must hurry. I have much to do and little time to write. God bless you and the dear loyal Sisters without whom we could do nothing of all this. Oh, my beloved Hannah [the youngest of the sick children], how

fain would I be with thee, dearest life—it cannot be—
I must renounce much—the Lord give me a willing
heart—Ever thy Friederike.[1]

Friederike returned home to find that one of the
children had had a relapse and was gone from her,
and a few days later the little Hannah also died.
This double loss inspired the mother to her last
work, the founding of an asylum for orphans.
She had often thought of it, and now one day she
brought in two motherless children and made
them at home with her own remaining little ones.
From this beginning grew the many orphanages
of Kaiserswerth.

Friederike was now at the end of her labours;
she could bear and do no more, and on the 22nd of
April, 1842, after a few days' illness, she gave premature birth to a dead infant, and breathed her
last.[2]

She died the first [wrote Fliedner] of all the deaconesses: as she, the Mother, was in all things the leader
among her spiritual daughters, so she went before
them in death.   How this great void is to be filled
is known only to God.

The historical disappearance of Friederike and
the complete identification of pastor Fliedner
with all of her creative and executive work is a
characteristic example of the way in which the
woman's share of the world's work has been

[1] *Jahrbuch*, pp. 21–22.
[2] *Ibid.*, p. 24.

generally ignored.   Numerous and copious are the
books, pamphlets, essays, and magazine articles
on the Kaiserswerth revival of the deaconess
order; yet rarely is Friederike even alluded to.
All is attributed to her husband, even those details
of the actual nursing organisation and training
which he himself has expressly stated were her
own.   Pastor Fliedner is to be exonerated from
any share in this historical injustice.' His own
part in the work was sufficiently important, without taking hers, and in describing their purposes
and efforts he always said "we."   It has come
about from the unconscious vanity of subsequent
pastors who undertook in their turn similar
organisation, that the composite picture called
Fliedner has been drawn, and copied thoughtlessly
by scribes of all nations.[1]

For a year they groped on alone; the Sisters did
their best to share the burden laid down by Friederike.   To make administration easier, Fliedner

[1] The rediscovery of Friederike was due to the intuition
of Mrs. Bedford Fenwick, an English nurse and writer, who
first set on foot the inquiries which brought her real share in
the deaconess movement to light.   At the Berlin meeting
of the International Council of Women in 1904, Mrs. Fenwick
stated Friederike's eminence, which had been forgotten even
in Germany, and she first gave an English translation of her
life in the *British Journal of Nursing*, May 26, 1906, *et seq.*,
called " Friederike Fliedner, the first Superintendent of the
Deaconess Institution at Kaiserswerth," translated by Miss
L. Metta Saunders: taken from *Pastorin Friederike Fliedner:
die erste Vorsteherin der Diakonissen Anstalt.   Armen-und-
Krankenfreund*, 1871.

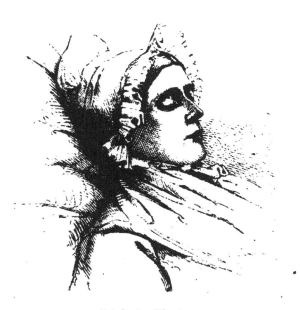

Friederike Fliedner
From *Jahrbuch für Christliche Unterhaltung*, Kaiserswerth, 1894

formed a conference of all the older Sisters, at which they took counsel together as to the conduct of the establishment. Even although the mainstay was gone, the work had to go on. The King of Prussia, Frederick William IV., was planning a deaconess house for Berlin, which Fliedner was to start. Again he went to Hamburg to see Amalie Sieveking, and, as has been already told, through her he met her friend Caroline Bertheau, who was in charge of the nursing department in the general hospital. A second time in seeking a superintendent for his work Fliedner found a wife, and again one as capable, as devoted, and as self-forgetting as the first. Caroline married him, took charge of his household and motherless children together with the whole large and rapidly growing deaconess establishment, and brought up eight children of her own as well. She survived him long, for pastor Fliedner died in October, 1864, after strenuous and increasing labours, but Frau Fliedner, truly "Mother" Fliedner, remained for almost twenty years after this the head and heart of the whole work, assisted ably by her son-in-law, Dr. Disselhoff.

On their wedding trip pastor Fliedner took her to Berlin, where the Kaiserswerth Sisters had just been placed in charge of the venereal wards of the Charité. The work was new to them and had come about as the result of a report which Fliedner had made to the Princess Marianne and the Queen, of the horrible abuses then prevalent in every department of the old city hospital. Pastor Fliedner was very anxious about this pioneer reform, and Caroline, having had experience in a similar service in Hamburg, went straight into the wards with the Sisters and worked with them until their way was smoothed out before them.

Let us pause here for a glance at the old hospital, the scene of Caroline's honeymoon.

One of the famous hospitals of the world, though not so ancient as many others, is the Charité of Berlin, long a noted centre for medical teaching. It has also had an interesting and instructive (though not admirable) nursing history, and is distinguished as one of the hospitals where nursing reforms in modern times were first attempted. If it cannot be said that these were successful at least the credit of the attempts belongs none the less to it.   Originally a pest-house, erected during the spread of the plague in 1709–1710, by King Frederick I., at his own expense, but not actually used as such because the epidemic did not reach as far as Berlin;   then a workhouse; next a lazaretto or military hospital, with some wards also for civilians, not until 1727 did it receive the name of the Charité.   Frederick William then endowed it and devoted it to educational purposes. In 1737 its internal organisation was regulated and its six divisions, the military wards, medical and surgical civil departments, syphilitic, obstetrical, and skin departments, were systematised with

the double purpose of charity and instruction.
It had then 200 beds.   The attendants were men
and women of purely secular character, and illiterate.   For every small medical ward there
was one woman attendant, and for two surgical
wards, one.

The whole edifice was rebuilt in 1785, and the
asylum for the insane added to it.

The nursing question was early considered and
the necessity for raising the standard recognised.
The experiment of improving the food and the
pay was tried; the discipline was military, and
the wards were improved in some respects.
In 1830 the *Krankenwärter Schule*, or course of
instruction for attendants, was established.[1]   As,
however, the whole nursing system was wrong
fundamentally and throughout, the results could
not be good.

For some fifty years after the first entrance of
the deaconesses into its wards, the Charité was
nursed on a plan which seems to us clumsy and
complicated.   Beside its own nurse-attendants,
it engaged groups of deaconesses for the care
of special wards.   If one Motherhouse (as was
often the case) could not supply enough, another
one was applied to, and thus in time groups of
nurses from several training institutions or Motherhouses were on duty at the same time in different
divisions of the hospital, each group being under
its own supervising Sister.   There was no one

[1] *Annalen des Charité Krankenhaus zu Berlin*, 1850.

woman head for these different groups, but they lived together as separate families, each under the final control of the institute which sent them. One can hardly imagine a more effective way of preventing unity of administration.[1]

Mother Caroline Fliedner was a character of great force and sweetness. She was described as "a joyous child full of gaiety, of strong will, and with great consideration for all around her.[2] She was of a Huguenot family that had been exiled in 1685 from France and had settled in Hamburg. She was born in 1811 and had been educated by Amalie, who delighted in training young girls to have ideals of social usefulness. She had been perusaded by her preceptress to enter the General hospital to conduct a reformation in the nursing, and had been at work there for three years. During her long administration of Kaiserswerth her great energy, practical ability, and genuine character commanded the respect, admiration, and love of all "from high to low." It was said of her by a pastor that whenever difficult problems came before the management, and she was called upon to give her opinion, she always waited long before speaking, but that when she spoke "her words were so direct, her reasons so convincing, and her solution of the difficulty so simple that

[1] At the present time the Charité is establishing a training school on modern lines, or at least making the attempt.

[2] *Mutter Fliedner: zum Gedächtniss. Kaiserswerth am Rhein*, 1892.

all instantly agreed with her." [1]   She gave up
the work in 1884, but lived ten years longer, her
mind keen and alert, her heart as warm as ever.

The annual reports during the lifetime of
pastor Fliedner are full of side-lights on the nursing
work of the Motherhouse.   The "Mother" or
Superintendent is often spoken of as directing all
the work and developing new fields.   As early as
the fourth report the need of better preparatory
education for the pupils has been felt, and the
hope is expressed that in the coming year something may be done to fill this want.   In this report
also Mrs. Fry's visit is mentioned and joy expressed
at having heard from her of the beginning of her
own "Nursing Sisterhood" on her return to England.   In the fifth, mention is made of several
pupils having been sent from France and Switzerland to be trained at Kaiserswerth.   It was from
the outset regarded by the Fliedners as most
desirable and important that room should be
made for and opportunity given to persons desiring to come for a time to study the methods of
Kaiserswerth.

In view of this well-known attitude of pastor
Fliedner and his wife toward students who might
help in spreading the new system, the story sometimes told that pastor Fliedner at first refused to
consider Miss Nightingale's application, on the

---

[1] From *Life of Pastor Fliedner*, translated from the German
by Catherine Winkworth, London, 1867, p. 85.   Authorised
by his family and published in Kaiserswerth, 1866.

ground that she was too refined and delicate, and that he required her to get down and scrub a floor before admitting her to training, seems a little apocryphal. No doubt she had to scrub floors—that was part of the work.

In the sixth report the probation time has been developed by placing a teaching Sister in special charge of the probationers, who now have a hall to themselves and are taught and prepared for their duties. The orphanage has been started, and children of respectable families are to be given a good plain education, and allowed to select their callings. It is hoped that some will be attracted to the nursing. Plans for district nursing (*Gemeindepflege*) are now projected.

The eighth report speaks of the successful planting of district nursing work in two parishes, Bielefeld and Cleve, in the previous year, and this extension is regarded with the fondest hope and joy. Several years later Cologne and Elberfeld have district nurses. In the morning they prepare nourishment for a number of poor and sick, and in the afternoon they visit and nurse. In Cleve the two district nurses have a little home hospital, and receive there several very sick patients. They have also under their charge a school of sewing and embroidery for destitute girls. At this time pastor Fliedner speaks of having to refuse to permit the district nurses to do night duty. He has now had to give up church and parish and devote himself entirely to the business

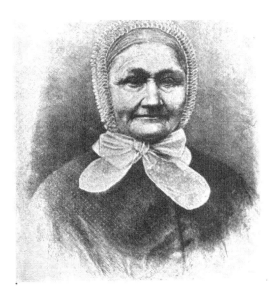

" Mother" Caroline Fliedner
From *Jahrbuch für Christliche Unterhaltung,*
Kaiserswerth, 1894

of developing the district work. In the growth of the Motherhouse there is now a *Probe-Schwester* (the "Home Sister" of the later English schools) in charge of the probationers, and two teaching Sisters who give them instruction. In 1850 mention is made in the reports of several Sisters sent to pastor Passavant in Pittsburg, in far-off America, whither Fliedner himself had journeyed with them. There had been typhus and cholera epidemics, and their record was admirable. They had hoped to establish a deaconess Motherhouse, but only one probationer came. Pastor Passavant begged for more Sisters to be sent, even offering to pay all their expenses; but Fliedner refused, saying that he had given them enough deaconesses to teach and train a new set, and they must find their own probationers. The need of the deaconesses' work in the United States was the subject of many discussions in Lutheran synods of that year. In this report also (1850) Miss Nightingale is mentioned as having come for some weeks, also a Swedish and a Russian lady. In 1856 Miss Nightingale is again mentioned. She had given the Constantinople Deaconesses' hospital thirteen beds and enough linen for forty patients. The twentieth annual report is signed by a committee. Pastor Fliedner is travelling in the East, partly to inspect the branch houses and partly, but in vain, trying to shake off the ill-health to which he finally succumbed.

The principle on which the Fliedners based their

work and that of the newly revived order of
deaconesses was that of joyful service springing
from self-sacrificing love, the old, old idea of the
salvation of the world through the might of
regenerating love—interpreted after one manner
by the doctrinaires, after another by poets, art-
ists, and musicians, and still another by thousands
of obscure hearts. Theirs was a beautiful and
a beneficent purpose. Indirectly, viewed from
the modern standpoint of the progress so far
made toward the emancipation of women, the
revival of the evangelical deaconess order was a
most important and significant movement. It
was the first step in a slow series which had to
be taken to release women from the narrow and
cramping social bondage in which, unless they
had independent means, they were held at that
period,—a period which did not educate them,
which hardly allowed them to earn their living
unless they belonged to the lowest social ranks,
and which permitted them little or no independence or initiative. Although hers was a
strict and in many respects a narrow discipline
the deaconess was far freer than her sister the nun,
and had a more natural life. Though she was
only supported and not paid, this was nevertheless
a tremendous advance over being permitted no
occupation. The deaconess movement supplied
the first great general school for improving the
practical training of Protestant women for useful
work, and was the pioneer in bringing to a highly

conservative and narrow social order the idea that every form of labour was honourable and dignified. Pastor Fliedner himself summed up the essentials of organised life as developed in Kaiserswerth as follows:

In organisation the work was a free religious association, not dependent on state or church authorities.   It takes its stand on the mother nature of the church founded by Christ.

Two errors were avoided: *i.e.* 1. Conventual vows or a contemplative ascetic character, and 2, decentralisation.   The Kaiserswerth deaconesses after five years of service were to be free to return home or to marry.   The Motherhouse is a democratic family and the deaconesses have a voice in choosing their superiors or heads.   The Motherhouse must be a protection and home for all the members, so it retains final authority over all members in outlying places and the right to call them back.

The work is regarded as in four branches with sub-branches:

A. Nursing
- Hospital
  - acute
  - chronic
  - special
- Private nursing
- Parish or district, *i.e.* visiting nursing.

B. Relief of Poor
- Orphanages
- Homes for aged and infirm
- Distribution of sewing and handwork
- Almshouses
- Asylums for the blind, etc.
- Training homes and bureaus for servants.

C. Care of Children
{
Schools for little children
Schools for girls
Training schools for teachers
Manual training schools
Special teaching for insti-
    tutions for the blind, etc.
}

D. Work among Unfortunate Women { Prisoners
                                    Magdalens }

Pastor Fliedner was a truly remarkable man;
—great in his large heart, his true, fervent, and
simple piety, his vast energy and practical efficiency. No man had more ideal helpers in his
two wives, but he deserved them, for he placed
women high, recognised their abilities, and wil-
ingly accorded them full authority in their
domain. He was one of the first to advocate the
introduction of women as teachers into the public
schools, against which there was then a strong
conservative prejudice, and he established a
normal school for girls as one of the Kaiserswerth
institutions. The striking feature of the Kaiserswerth administration was the wise and humane
treatment of their inmates as individuals. In the
intelligent use of occupation, diversion, and cheerfulness they were far ahead of their time. The
amusements and instruction of convalescent children, adults, and defectives were early thought
out with care and wisdom. The children were
taught reading, writing, accounts, singing, story-
telling, and organised play. The older patients
were taught a number of hand industries, such
as knitting, net-making, weaving, and box-making,

and had light work in the garden.   Illiterate convalescents were taught reading and writing, and singing was regarded as a universal necessity.

The formal charter of incorporation for the Kaiserswerth Deaconesses' Institution had been granted by a ministerial order on November 20, 1846, ten years after the beginning of the work, and an affiliation of Motherhouses—which were either organically related to or in full sympathy with it, and so desirous of supporting and being supported by it—was a further effort of Fliedner's organising genius. This affiliated body, called the Kaiserswerth General Conference of Motherhouses, meets triennially at Kaiserswerth and its reports show, as pastor Golder writes,

the exceedingly great scope of activity in an army of more than thirteen thousand deaconesses. There is no kind of human misery that it does not reach. They serve with loving hearts, wise discretion, and skilful hands the sick of every condition—epileptics, the imbecile, lepers, and lunatics; neglected children and abandoned infants; the crippled, aged, fallen women; incarcerated; orphans; servants out of employment; unattended children; young girls, and a number of others in need.

It is impossible not to be struck with the general resemblance between the deaconess movement and that of the Sisters of Charity, and by certain features in common in the characters of Vincent de Paul and pastor Fliedner. Different as their personalities were, both were alike in the

rare simplicity and humility of their unaffected
piety; in their complete self-forgetfulness, their un-
unflagging and active concern for human misery;
in their immense energy, in their organising and
administrative ability. These two men, like
Lambert le Bègue, knew how to call forth and
develop useful initiative in the masses around
them; how to focus and guide it. Their great
secret of management lay in a complete absence
of repressive force. They perpetually encouraged
and never discouraged the efforts of others. In
the great movements of human activity with
which their names are associated they dealt with
women and men on the same plane, showing the
former the same respect and consideration as the
latter. In a word, these eminent men were
entirely free from all narrowness or caste feeling.

The women in these two great movements,
though some had social station and education,
were alike recruited largely from the peasant
classes; alike they taught, toiled, rescued, visited,
and nursed, and in war followed their country's
flag. Though arrayed under different religious
formulas, these were essentially the same women,
animated by the same spirit and enjoying alike the
love and regard of the people. The Kaiserswerth
deaconesses, like the Sisters of Charity, were
always on the spot where there was pestilence or
misery. In 1848, when the hunger typhus deci-
mated Altdorf, they were there, and in 1849
they nursed the cholera patients in a number of

small towns. After the war of 1864 small-pox
broke out both in hospitals and in country regions.
The deaconesses found the peasants in their
cottages, often without beds, on the floor or on
piles of straw covered with rags, while the cows
and pigs inhabited a part of the dwelling, or a
group of farmhands shared the sick-room. For
nearly two years they struggled with small-pox
under such conditions, caring for more than 1000
cases in all. Then war broke out again, followed
by cholera, which swept the land in a way hitherto
unknown. Thirty-five deaconesses worked in
more than twenty localities, nursing over 1000
patients, and as the cholera died away true typhus
fever broke out in East Prussia, and eight of the
deaconesses hastened thither to the pest-houses.
Thereafter there was hardly a period when some
of the Sisters were not campaigning against
contagion, and when the alarming epidemic of
cholera raged in Hamburg, in 1892, fifteen of
their number went to the General City Hospital,
where they worked night and day, in the very
wards where their second mother, Caroline, had
served as a volunteer nurse in her youth. As in
epidemics, so in the wars of 1861, 1864, 1866, and
1870 to 1871, the deaconesses of Kaiserswerth
were conspicuously active. They served not
only in the hospitals, but on the very fields of
battle, and, accompanied by a guard of Uhlans,
they followed the Prussian army in every advance. In all, they served, in 1870, in more than

sixty military hospitals, and over 30,000 soldiers passed through their wards.

Beside its numerous integral branches, Kaiserswerth at different times organised and gave over into other hands for independent management no less than 79 different institutions, 34 of which were hospitals and 9 deaconess houses. After the successful demonstration of the Fliedners there was a general movement of active imitation, and not a year passed that new Motherhouses were not established. The hospitals which they erected set a new standard in hospital work, construction, management, and nursing. The Motherhouse did not look upon its patients as cases only, but as human individuals, each one needing kindness and consolation as well as scientific treatment. Their wards, though plain, were homelike and cheerful, and as the Sisters were called into the great city hospitals they introduced there the same atmosphere, and effected that moral renovation which has so strikingly accompanied the entrance into hospitals of women of character armed with authority, wherever they have gone, and which, though often overlooked, has perhaps been a contribution of even greater value than their more obvious, technical achievements as handmaidens of science.

An excellent exposition of the generally accepted fundamental principles in the training of deaconesses is given by Schäfer.[1]   Preëminent was the

[1] *Die Weibliche Diakonie*, vol. 3. The whole volume is given to this subject.

idea that the deaconess was not to be a narrow specialist in any one line, but was to have an all-round preparation. While her talents and inclinations were consulted in placing her in positions after her training, yet she was not to be only a nurse, or only a teacher, or only a parish worker, but ready to do anything. No form of human need in which a woman's strength could be exerted was to be excluded from her province. Her religious duty was foremost: "The most precious duty of the deaconess is to lead the ungodly into the church," and every deaconess, no matter what her work, must give testimony of her faith. She was not, however, to proselytise those of other religious beliefs. All her work should be done in the name of the Lord. Therefore she needed the continual guidance of the pastor, and the latter must not only not ignore her but must oversee and guide her. And not alone the deaconess in district nursing or parish visiting, but he must oversee every deaconess in his entire field of labour, whether in hospitals or other institutions. Equally the training school can have no objection when the pastor makes it his business to concern himself with deaconesses who are doing private duty in well-to-do families.

While the pastors did not uphold celibacy as a tenet, they urged the deaconess to make her calling a life-work, and boldly taught that marriage was not the only nor even the noblest sphere of woman, and that, as there were always more women than

men, God could not have intended marriage as
their only portion. The deaconess, as has been
mentioned, after five years of service was free to
marry or to return to her family, and she retained
the control of any property of which she might be
possessed.

It is interesting to see how much of their system and detail our modern training schools have
inherited from the Motherhouse—the probation-
ary system, and the school for preparatory training; the letters from clergyman and physician
as to character and health; the allowance of
pocket-money; the grading of work, from easy to
difficult; the chain of responsibility; the grading
of pupils from probationer to head nurse, with the
superintendent at the head; the class-work and
lectures; and every principle of discipline, etiquette, and ethics. The combination of a semi-
military form of professional discipline with social
equality, found in the Motherhouse, gave the
pattern to the early American schools even more
than did the first English schools, whose system
of class distinctions was never established in
America. From the first the probationer was
taken into the housewifely departments under
the eye of a head sister (Probe Schwester).

Kaiserswerth established a preparatory school
for its probationers in 1865. This was to supply
deficiencies in family training or in education,
but chiefly to develop their characters, and prevent them from being "institutionalised" at an

early age. Pupils were taken into the preparatory school between the fourteenth and eighteenth
years. Other Motherhouses followed this example. The time spent in preparatory work
varied in accordance with the character, education,
and age of the pupil, from three months to a
year or more. At eighteen they were admitted
as probationers. Continuous and systematic instruction was regarded as indispensable. There
was a difference of opinion as to the rougher parts
of the housework, some pastors holding that once
learned it should not be continuously performed
by the deaconesses, but that hired maids should
save their strength for more responsible work;
practically, for want of means, this was almost
never done, and all washing, ironing, and heavy
housework was usually shared by the Sisters.
(This question of housework with nursing has
been of never-ceasing interest to pastors who
write on training, and one very successful organiser, Dr. Zimmer, gives his experience as in
favour of having no maids or cleaners at all, as he
thinks the change from nursing to housework
healthful, refreshing, and good for the nurses,
and gives them an opportunity to develop all their
energy.) For training it was held that a not too
large hospital was best, and great stress was laid
on the necessity of having a spacious garden where
the Sisters could walk and rest. Cheerfulness
was regarded as an essential characteristic of the
pupil. Gloomy and despondent temperaments

(it was held) were unfit for the work, and selfishness made a life lived in common impossible. The Motherhouse was regarded as a family home; the pastor and the Oberin (lady superintendent) corresponded to the father and mother, and the deaconesses to the children. Excessive intimacies between deaconesses were considered harmful to character, and were regarded with fixed disapproval, such pupils being systematically separated. The importance of the head Sister's office was well recognised. It was important that head nurses should teach and not only do things well themselves; inasmuch as it requires more character to be able to get good work from others than to do everything one's self. A good Sister would always instruct the younger ones. The rules fixing the relationship of the deaconess to the physician were strict. She must be his assistant, not presuming herself to act as a physician but she might act independently of him in an emergency. "In all which concerns the care of the patient she is bound to obedience toward the doctor and to faithful loyalty. She must beware of any self-assertion or independence. If the doctor's orders are mistaken or harmful the Sister does not bear the responsibility." But, what is interesting, ethical difficulties are provided for: "Experienced nurses have the right to remonstrate quietly and tactfully with physicians, but not directly to oppose them." The physician on his part was to regard the hospital as a place for teaching the Sisters.   He must not only treat the patients, but remember that the training of the deaconess makes it essential that she should work in turn in all the different departments of the hospital.   Shäfer makes it clear that the physician has nothing to do with the management of the Sisters.   Their discipline, the distribution of work, and changing the pupils from one ward to another is the business of the matron.   As to the managers, it was held most important that they should never interfere in the internal management of affairs.   These must be conducted entirely by the matron and the pastor.   The managers should choose these two officers with great care, and then leave them unhampered.   As to the institutions connected with the Motherhouse (and this is also quite striking), the accepted view was not that the Motherhouse was there for the sake of the institutions, but that the latter were there for the sake of the Motherhouse, to provide suitable places to teach the Sisters.   The daily schedule of work was about as follows: The deaconesses rose at 5, and went to the wards, where they worked until 6.15 or 6.30, when the patients had their breakfast; they then had fifteen minutes for their coffee, followed by prayers for twenty-five minutes.   The physicians' rounds were at 8. At 9 there was a second breakfast for the patients and nurses, then ward-work and operations until lunch or dinner at 12 or 12.30.   There was then a resting time (if they could take it), part of which was the quiet half-hour spent in the chapel. From 2 to 3 P.M. there were lessons and study, then ward-work again, religious teaching by the pastor at 7, and ward-work until 9, then prayers and bed. The general custom for night duty was for the day nurses to divide the night service in turn. Thus of two day nurses one stayed on until midnight and the second came for the rest of the time. With this plan the turn came around to each one about once a week; but, though there was not any or but little extra rest in the day, the work was not thought hard enough to be prejudicial to health. Some Motherhouses had a regular staff of night nurses, who did one month's duty at a time. There was always a night Sister in charge. On private duty the Motherhouse requested that deaconesses should have their meals served to them alone if they did not go to the family table. They were not to eat in the kitchen. They were to have at least four or five hours uninterrupted sleep and an hour in the fresh air daily. Deaconesses who were nursing men must have an orderly or male assistant.

District work was regarded as the flower of nursing. The cardinal virtue of a district nurse was "practical wisdom" to grasp and comprehend; to sympathise, to regulate and order, to discriminate between the true and false, to penetrate to causes; to plan for regeneration. She must have intellectual mobility, combined with quiet persistence and effectiveness. Slow Sisters who are never through with their work are not good for district nursing.

Leaving aside all local and transitory features it cannot but be recognized that the early Mother-houses, following the lead of Kaiserswerth, laid down every fundamental principle of good train-ing. Many pastors wrote with great good sense on methods and principles, having learned them from Friederike and Caroline Fliedner. It is noticeable that the pastors, far more than the physicians of that time, acquiesced in the large and responsible position to be held by the woman head and the share of authority to be given her. Not the least of the services rendered to good nursing by the Mother houses was the restoration of the woman superintendent or matron, who had been eliminated by the management of civil hospitals in their system of servant-nurses under masculine officials. The extinction of the matron, still strikingly noticeable in the great hospitals of Germany, France, and Austria, made a well-bal-anced training and discipline impossible in civil hospitals; the control of the nurses, scattered among various male officials, was lost; high stand-ards were not thought of, teaching disappeared, slovenliness was the rule, immorality was fre-quent, and the patients were the sufferers.

The value of the matron as a key-stone was shown in every fresh work of the Motherhouse, and even more prominently by the reform of the

English hospitals under Miss Nightingale. The results stand in striking contrast with the deplorable conditions existing in such hospitals as the Charité, the Vienna General, and the great Paris hospitals immediately after laicisation.

It must also be noted that, as a result of accepting the authority of the matron, the German pastors were far in advance of the German physicians of that time in the recognition of Miss Nightingale's services for the elevation of nursing. Her books were translated into German, and her teachings are freely quoted by Schäfer and others.

We do not attempt to follow the great extension and duplication of the deaconess Motherhouses through the sixty years following the foundation of Kaiserswerth, as there are many excellent reference books available which give careful details of the numerous fields of work and institutions both affiliated with and independent of it.[1]

That feature of the subsequent development of the female diaconate which belongs to our subject is its relation to nursing. As time went on and competition entered undeniably into the field of the deaconess work, much of the early zeal and freshness wore off and a greater rigidity entered into the life. The economic problem was ever present, and the maintenance of this large body of workers had necessarily to be of the sparsest character. The immediate control of domestic and nursing details fell more and more

[1] See Appendix for bibliography.

(not accidentally) into the hands of the pastors, who believed they had learned enough to be able successfully to manage this part of the system. Women were taken on younger and younger, and overwork of a severe and often cruel character became common.

The necessity of earning money by sending the nurses out to hospital service often quite put an end to careful training. Women of a superior ability were less and less attracted to the calling and the ranks remained largely filled from the peasant class. The occasional devoutly religious aristocrat who entered a Motherhouse, and who thereby received much adulation from the pens of chroniclers, invariably entered upon the position of superintendent, for which she had often fitted herself but superficially, by a practical apprenticeship of a much briefer sort than that gone through by the average Sister. Thus little by little the practical ability of the women heads to teach the probationers fell below par, and the numerous members of the medical profession who were not in sympathy with the deaconess movement were able to claim with truth that the matrons were not competent to teach nursing, and thus press a disposition to dispense with them entirely. The increasing prominence of the pastors was also most obnoxious to medical men. Physicians declared their hostility to them on the grounds that they interfered with the complete subordination of the nurse to the physician;

that they told the deaconesses there were certain medical orders that could not be obeyed, such as telling patients untruths about their condition, about the safety of operation, etc. The pastors were also opposed to the use of narcotics. Certain physicians expressed themselves strongly in magazine articles and said that the pastors had no right or reason in nursing affairs, and others declared as emphatically that it was absurd to give the Oberin (matron) any place in a nursing system.[1]

Both pastors and a certain proportion of physicians were equally averse to dealing with women of force and original ability and both equally dreaded the well-educated woman. Freedom of thought became a thing definitely forbidden in the Motherhouses, as is illustrated by the personal testimony to the writers by a one-time deaconess, of having been forbidden to read the works of Schiller. This repression of the intellectual life is also amply attested by innumerable clerical writings,[2] and a certain aversion to a high educational standard is equally clearly attested in writings of physicians,[3] though these were perhaps not in the majority.

[1] See *Fürsorge auf dem Gebiete der Krankenwartung*, in *Handbuch der Krankenversorgung und Krankenpflege*, Liebe. Jacobsohn, and Meyer, vol. ii., part i., p. 174.

[2] See bibliographies in Schäfer, *Die Weibliche Diakonie*, and in Liebe, Jacobsohn, and Meyer.

[3] *Fürsorge auf dem Gebiete des Krankenpflege-Unterrichts*, See Liebe, Jacobsohn, and Meyer op. cit, vol. ii., part i., pp. 174-328.

Strangely characteristic of those who apply
repression, they yet felt dissatisfied with their
own results and seriously discussed them without
perceiving their causal relations. Very significant are the titles of papers read by the pastors
of deaconess institutes in later years, such as:

Why do so few Pastors' Daughters devote themselves to the Calling of the Deaconess?

How shall we gain more Sisters for the Deaconess
Calling?

Means of Increasing the Numbers of Deaconesses
and of Overcoming Prejudice against the Office.

What is done and What can be done to Preserve
the Sisters' Physical Strength?

How are the Deaconesses to be Kept in the right
frame of Joy in their Work and Guarded from Apathy
and Dulness?

Of certain Present or Threatening Defects of the
Deaconess Institutions.

How shall the Sisters Protect Themselves from the
Dangers of the Morphine Habit?

What Dangers to the Deaconess' Calling are inci-
dental to Institution Life and How shall we Meet
Them?

What is Necessary on the part of the Directors to
Preserve the Health of the Sisters and Guard them
against Premature Invalidism.[1]

The narrowness and arbitrary limitations introduced little by little into the deaconess' life could
not fail to strike vigorous and reason-loving minds

[1] Schäfer, *op. cit.*, vol. i., *Anmerkungen*, гp. 315–320.

unpleasantly, and the whole inner atmosphere and character of the more recent training and discipline have been set forth in the pages of a very remarkable book,[1] which, in the form of a simple narrative framed on nothing more exciting than the story of an average group of persons, gives a picture of the deaconess life drawn by a master hand and with as much depth of human feeling as of intellectual perception. Gabriele, the daughter of a well-to-do family, and who was endowed richly with qualities of head and of heart, went, following a sane and balanced yet insistent wish to give service, to a deaconess house and entered upon the training. She found that what was arbitrarily demanded of her, above and beyond the natural claims of nursing to self-sacrifice, was nothing less than the negation of her whole personality, the sacrifice of her natural relations with the outer world, the renunciation of mental recreation and of all higher education; in short, the atrophy of her individual self.

All the minutest details of the daily life are sketched in with a delicate touch and sympathy, and the round of the days in training home and hospital wards could only have been described by one who had lived it all. The character sketches are vivid and speaking; each one seems drawn from the life. The matron, of bounteous motherly goodness, but a little removed from the

[1] *Frei zum Dienst, by Luise Algenstædt* (L. Annshagen). Ernest Bredt, Leipzig, 1904.

close immediate touch with the individual pupils; the assistants and Sisters; the probationers, who always tried to eat two rolls in the short breakfast time allowed them; the pastor, chief of all instruction given the probationers, who gave his own daughters every social and family pleasure in his power, and would not have dreamed of letting them become deaconesses; the patients, even the porter at the door—all are lifelike.

As Gabriele looked around the table at her first meal, she saw the assembled Sisters looking very much alike in their uniforms:

Peaceful countenances—a little subdued perhaps and tired, yet a readiness for jest and cheerfulness was there. Faces of good intelligence, showing a little indifference to the impression made by them on others, perhaps a little indifference in general towards all persons who were not sick. Or was this only absorption in work, and overstrain, which was more evident as they sat down? Most of them were pale and looked as if they needed air, while others were fresh and pretty, not unbecomingly clad in the close cap. Close, smooth, scanty hair combed down from broad partings—the continuous rubbing with the cap border wore it so— [1]

How did most of the applicants come?

The Margaret School was the preparatory institution for the Motherhouse. Fourteen-year-old girls came to it from the common schools and were then during four years prepared for the deaconess

[1] *Op. cit.*, p. 72,

calling. The world and humankind and the great
dynamic forces outside were unknown to them, and
there was for them no sacrifice of social ties. Instead, for most of them their importance in the social
scale rose when they donned the deaconess dress.
The Sisters' cap was their goal through all their
young years, and when they received it they were
so delighted that they would not have understood
a suggestion that they had anything more to wish
for. Good, earnest, cheerful maidens were they,
full of loyalty and zeal for their work, full of reverence
for the house. Scarcely one of them would, in the
world, have been called an educated young woman.[1]

Gabriele had at the outset attributed the scanty
pin-money to the necessity for economy, and, herself financially independent, had never faced the
economic question, until it was brought to her
one day by hearing the teaching Sister speak
belittlingly of those who nursed for their living.
"Our Sisters," said she, "work solely for the love
of Christ—not for a salary."
Gabriele thought a moment:

Does money make a difference? [said she] Do you
mean that the love of mankind and a salary are
irreconcilable? . . . Can money prevent one from
working in a spirit of love? Teachers, physicians,
pastors, all take money—and no one reproaches them
for it. Even without the payment of money one
might still work without love. . . . [2]

[1] *Op. cit.*, p. 77.
[2] *Op. cit.*, p. 92. On this point Miss Nightingale said: "It
appears to be the most futile of all distinctions to classify as

The pastor's classes were painful occasions, for the pastor did not know how to teach, and only succeeded in intimidating his already shy and unready pupils. At his questions the probationers shrank into themselves and appeared even more mediocre than they really were. Then so wearied were they always that, in spite of themselves, their eyes closed in sleep and their heads fell whenever the attention of the teacher was turned from them for a moment, until a sarcastic exclamation wakened them, embarrassed and self-conscious. Gabriele was concerned and depressed by these half-hours.

Could the pastor believe in making them humble through humiliations? the poor things were already, with their work, their sick, and their discipline, continuously exercised in humility,—did they need crushing to learn to place all their hope in divine mercy? Could it be possible that what was aimed at was the destruction of individuality, instead of the sanctification and development of the in-

---

between 'paid' and 'unpaid' art; so between paid and unpaid nursing—to make into a test a circumstance as adventitious as whether the hair is black or brown, *viz.*, whether people have private means or not, whether they are obliged or not to work at their art or their nursing for a livelihood. Probably no person ever did that well which he did only for money; certainly no person ever did that well which he did not work at as hard as if he did it solely for money. If by amateurs in art or nursing are meant those who take it up for play, it is not art at all, it is not nursing at all. You never yet made an artist by paying him well; but an artist ought to be well paid."—Introd. to *Life of Agnes Jones*.

dividual for the service of God by every gift and force and by the use of all the means of help and culture that abound in the world?

She was terrified at the boldness of her own thoughts. Yet the "womanly simplicity" on which pastor Löhe had written a whole book seemed to her like nothing but—*stupidity*.

Finally came the day when her relation with the Motherhouse came to an end. It was the hour for pastor Eck's Bible class, and the meek young women sat before him, struggling with their fatigue. A hint of ironic expression on the pastor's ruddy countenance conveyed a thought, without words, that made them dimly conscious of being foolish, stupid, uninformed. To-day he spoke especially of the requirements of the deaconess calling. "Examine yourselves [said he] to see whether you bring with you a flexible spirit, out of which a yet higher may be moulded; set natures, that resist modification, fit ill to the service."

Gabriele wondered whether by "modification" he meant the crushing of personality and the grinding in the wheel of toil, and whether that was a means of attaining complete domination. Of learning he said that it dared never be sought for its own sake, as it then nourished pride; that "the greatest happiness of the work lay in obedience," and he then drew a picture of the ideal deaconess. She sparkled with the diamonds of every imaginable virtue, including loftiness of thought, down to the smallest and finest. That was what deaconesses must and should be; then followed what they must not be:

"Be not only humble—no—love humiliation, and take no offence therefrom. Can you quote a verse, Sister Lisbeth?"

"For God resisteth the proud, and giveth grace to the humble." "Where is it found?" She gave the place. If any one approached to this ideal, it was Sister Lisbeth, and yet she always seemed to inspire a certain feeling of vexation in the pastor.

"But it is also possible to fall into a pride of humility, some have boasted of their humility—beware of this. Egotism is sinful, and even the craving for enjoyment is so. Naturally I speak of spiritual enjoyment, for you have separated yourselves from that of the world. . . . Friendships and family ties conceal dangers also—I have warned you against these, and in this connection I may mention letter-writing. Seek not after novelties and complain not. . . . Read the paragraph on page 38, 'On Dressing'."

Sister Lisbeth stood up and read in reverential tones:

"As a Christian sanctifies everything through prayer and the word of God, why shall not a deaconess make dressing also a time of holiness? To this end I recommend the following prayers. In the bath: 'Wash me well from my misdeeds and cleanse me from my sins.' In putting on the clothing: 'Our righteousness is like a soiled garment. But he who conquers shall be clothed in white raiment.' In tying on the apron: 'Who will serve me, let him follow me.' In putting on the cap: 'Thou, Lord, blessest the righteous and crownest him with mercy.'"

Gabriele looked at the thin, unworldly face of the grey-haired probationer, and then at the morning dress of the pastor, and wondered, doubting, whether he followed a like programme. He continued:

"What I say now I do not make a matter of conscience,—it is only my advice. Order is also wholesome for the soul. Once a day a deaconess should humbly examine herself—preferably toward evening. Once—better in the course of the forenoon—bring God a thank-offering for His mercies; once—perhaps about three o'clock—reflect on the hour of death. It is also advisable often to practise a prayerful exercise of faith and hatred of sin. . . . Finally I recommend satisfying reading; not only the word of God, and not by any means the flood of Christian tales which enfeeble one and suggest a love of pleasure, but the reading of our old ascetics.

"Exercise yourselves daily in obedience, in humility, and in submission both of body and soul. Our blessed father Löhe said: 'You shall practise an obedience that shames the authorities. Your joy shall be more and more in lowliness, in unpretentiousness, and in meekness.'"

He then turned to Sister Gabriele and asked her for an appropriate verse, and she, overborne by a rising tide of rebellion and dissent, forgetting herself and all around, arose and in a strange voice said: "Woe unto you, Scribes and Pharisees, hypocrites!" . . . "For they bind heavy burdens and grievous to be borne, and lay them on men's shoulders; but they themselves will not move them with one of their fingers"; and again: "Woe unto you . . . for ye lade men with burdens grievous to be borne, and ye yourselves touch not the burdens with one of your fingers." They are found in Matthew and Luke.

It was like the breaking of a bomb, and pale horror sat upon the faces of the frightened Sisters.

After this scene Gabriele's further continuance in the sisterhood was naturally not to be thought of, even had she herself not eagerly welcomed the regained freedom. Later, in the pastor's study, he required her to explain herself.

"Now you shall tell me what you meant by your extraordinary words. Literally, they seem to mean that I do not myself do what I demand from others?" She nodded. "But I did not mean you especially, but the principle."

"Indeed. So you spoke with intention and hold to your words. . . . What, exactly, did you mean by speaking so audaciously before the class? Well?"

"I meant the double standard by which you, but not you only, measure yourself and the Sisterhood."

"Then I must first point out to you, that the authority is derived from God, and is supported by the Scriptures. Leaders and doers—both—are necessary in every sphere of work; . . . where you have labour of hand or foot I have that of the brain. My responsibility is much greater than yours. My work is quite different—therefore my preparation and my mode of life must be different. You cannot compare the two."

"That is just what I mean—that difference. . . . You speak now of work, but in class you speak of renunciation, of self-denial, of resignation. We are to be holier than you—the clergy."

The pastor sprang up and resented this independent speech, and reminded Gabriele of the authority of the captain of a ship.

"But that is different," said she, "for he has gone through every stage of the sailor's work. He knows exactly what he commands. But you, Pastor Eck, have never had any experience of what you make binding on us. . . .

"You demand the very highest of us, even to our most secret thoughts and most intimate feelings— an unnatural strength—and at the same time you close the source of this strength to us. Strength is life. You demand from us, in the same breath, both a highly concentrated life, and the denial of life. You ask what is impossible." . . .

"The source of strength is the holy Gospel." . . . said Pastor Eck.

" Truly, I have never been so little able to read it, as here. If it is true that 'man lives not by bread alone, but also by the word,' it is also true that he lives not by the word alone, but by bread—both are essential. . . . Our heavenly Father gives us many pleasures, and it is His will that we shall ask for them.

Much is bestowed upon us for the animation and elevation of our feelings and our intellect—for we also work with both of these, not only with hand and foot—for refreshment and exercise, for enrichment and development, such as you prize and know how to use, such as you consider your matter-of-course right, even necessity. The pleasures of nature, of art, the cultivation of the intellect, noble literature, family, friendship, and congenial society—these are the additional springs of strength that we also need to enjoy in moderation. Without them our calling is a continuous out-giving without in-taking. But we must give up all that—your will and the overwork crushes it. And, instead, obedience shall be the highest joy of our calling, and to be despised a pleasure. Do you not call that laying unendurable burdens?"

Pastor Eck seemed somewhat impressed; but defended himself by the argument that most of the Sisters did not feel in this way; that Gabriele possessed a strong mind, which they had not; that the majority of women desired to be led and were not capable of original thinking and doing; that in their ardent love of God they were not conscious of self-sacrifice—but Gabriele interrupted him:

"Of *being* sacrificed. . . . They all suffer—all the Sisters" said she, "from the mental starvation that is directly apportioned to them. If there are perhaps those who do not, it is because their subjection is complete, or—because there was nothing in them to starve. We have the protection of the sixth commandment— Thou shalt not kill. Oh, I know very well hunger is a means of discipline—a means of gaining mastery over the mind."[1]

Gabriele left the deaconess work and studied medicine.

The story is no imaginary one, but taken from the life. The intellectual poverty (and not that only, for poverty night be remedied,) and the restrictions on freedom of thought in the deaconess' calling go hand in hand with the economic dependency and the social bareness of the life, and all are out of touch with the progress of the present century.

Those women who first renounced the claims of the Motherhouses on grounds similar to Gabriele's, and who then endeavoured to make a self-supporting occupation of their calling as nurses, had a hard and bitter struggle against prejudice, but nevertheless the exodus of the least submissive and meek began and still continues. The basis of all resentment against them was that women who had for centuries worked and slaved for a bare livelihood should now cease to be satisfied with so doing. Not easily would charitable institutions and the Church give up their unpaid workers, and the assertion of a right to the earnings of one's labour was characterised as godless, sordid, and debasing.

As the deaconess organisation was in its first development a great step forward, it has proved

[1] *Op. cit.*, pp. 274–286.

to be not the final, but one of a number of steps or phases of social and of nursing progress. It is still active and strong, holds a definite and important place in church and mission work, conducts a vast deal of beneficent institutional work, and transplants its branches further.

It seems probable that, like the Sister of Charity, the deaconess will gradually count for less and less in nursing proper, while she will continue to be skilled, valuable, and active on other lines of service.

In Germany, the home of the Motherhouse, further and more recent lines of nursing progress have been successively marked by the Red Cross associations; by the large city schools for nurses, arranged upon the English pattern; by the Diakonie Verein; and lastly by the organisation of " Free " Sisters which, with the opening of modern training schools in the large new hospitals, speaks the latest word in nursing evolution from monasticism to voluntary self-government after training, and a progressive educational standard.[1]

[1] The modern nursing movement in Germany, as well as that of other European countries, will be taken up in another volume.

CHAPTER II

PRE-NIGHTINGALE TIMES

FROM the time of the dissolution of the monasteries under Henry VIII. there had been occasional protests over the lack of any career for unmarried women. Fuller, the historian, would have been glad if such feminine foundations had continued—"good shee-schools" but without vows. The subject had received much attention in the early part of the nineteenth century. More than thirty years before Kaiserswerth was founded, Dr. Gooch, a physician and philanthropist, had been greatly impressed by what he had seen of the nursing of the Béguines and Augustinian Sisters in the hospitals of the Netherlands, and by what he heard from the physicians there of their excellent qualities and devotion. He corresponded with Southey on the subject, and Southey discussed it in the *Colloquies:* "Where is the woman who shall be the Clara or the Teresa of Protestant England, labouring for the certain benefit of her sex with their ardour, but without their delusion or fatal superstition, which have entailed such misery upon thousands!"[1] Southey had hopes [2] (says Mrs. Jameson) that Mrs. Opie would do for the hospitals what Mrs. Fry had done for the prisons. He also looked to the Quakers as being more likely than the Church of England to found an order of Protestant Sisters of Charity. Sir Thomas More and Montesinos discuss a Gynæceum —a college rather than a convent, for the education and training of women for useful lives.

Why, then, have you no Béguines, no Sisters of Charity? Why, in the most needful, the most merciful form that charity can take, have you not yet followed the example of the French and the Netherlands? No Vincent de Paul has been heard in your pulpits; no Louise le Gras has appeared among the daughters of Great Britain! Piety has found its way into your prisons; your hospitals are imploring it in vain; nothing is wanting in them but religious charity; and oh! what a want is that! and how different would be the moral effect which these medical schools produce upon the pupils educated there, if this lamentable deficiency were supplied. I know not whether they or the patients suffer most from its absence. . . . A school of medicine ought to be also a school of Christian humanity. . . . It is not to the hospitals alone that this blessed spirit of charity might be directed; while it reformed those establishments by its presence, it would lessen the pressure upon them by seeking out the sick, and attending them in their own habitations.[3]

[1] *Colloquies*, p. 214, vol. ii.
[2] *Sisters of Charity* (London, 1855), p. 92.
[3] *Colloquies*, ii., p. 228.

An anonymous article, "Protestant Sisters of Charity" (believed to have been written by Dr. Gooch), had appeared in *Blackwood's Magazine* in December, 1825, and a year, later a pamphlet appeared under the same title containing a "Letter" addressed to the Bishop of London. Both of these articles urged the formation of an order of women devoted to nursing and good works, on the pattern of the Sisters of Charity, and some efforts were made to induce the Established Church to experiment with this plan, but without success.[1] There was then no inkling of an idea that refined and conscientious nursing could be thought of outside of the bands of a religious sisterhood, and so lacking was that time in a rational humanity, that the idea would without a doubt have sounded preposterous. The writer in *Blackwood's* said: "They [the nurses] should be animated with religion; science and mere humanity cannot be relied on. . . . Let all serious Christians join, and found an order of women like the Sisters of Charity in Catholic countries." Other letters followed, and there was a revival of the history of the Béguines and Sisters of Charity. Dr. Gooch also urged his plan for the reformation of nursing upon his professional brethren, in the *London Medical Gazette*, over the signature "A Country Surgeon."[2] In this paper he described some nursing experiences of his own in hospital

---

[1] Appendix of *Colloquies*, ii., p. 349.
[2] Quoted in *Colloquies*, Appendix, vol. ii., p. 343.

practice.   He wrote in an urbane, persuasive style, evidently possessed a nature of great sympathy and tenderness, and had acquired nursing skill of a high order.   He would select (he said) two or three women at a time and place them in a hospital under some clear-headed, practical physician who should take them from bed to bed, explaining to them the signs by which he is guided in his remedies; why he gives opium, and why he draws blood; . . . he would assist their memories by frequent examinations, and when they had acquired a readiness in detecting all ordinary diseases, in selecting the guiding symptoms, and in the use of a short list of remedies, he would place them in the midst of some country district, maintain them partly from charitable funds and partly from the parish, and he believed that a few cures would be followed by medical reputation and that the villages would bless the day of their arrival.

But this was not the way that Dr. Gooch had acquired his own skill in *nursing*, though he may have learned his *medicine* by some such method, nor does he seem to have thought of this, when he tells how he learned to manage a patient with a frightful bedsore.   It seems actually to have been his intention to create an order of medical practitioners, for he says further:

It may be objected that women with such an education would form a bad substitute for a scientific medical attendant.   Be it remembered, however, that the choice is not between such women and professional or perfect physicians and surgeons, but between such women and the ordinary run of country apothecaries, the latter labouring under the additional disadvantage of wanting time for the application of what skill they have.

In his article in *Blackwood's* he says again:

Let them receive not a technical and scientific but a practical *medical* education: let books be framed for them, containing the essential rules of *practise;* [1] let them be distributed in country parishes and be maintained by the parish allowance which now goes to the parish surgeon, who should be resorted to only in difficult cases; let them be examined every half-year by competent physicians, about the state of their medical knowledge, and I fearlessly predict that my friend [the country clergyman] will no longer complain that his sick flock suffers from medical neglect.

Thus medical reformers and philanthropists advocated the creation of a nursing staff taught after the system of medical students, yet no one thought to ask, if this manner of teaching made nurses, why were not the medical students nurses?

There were others, no longer known by name, who had a more correct idea of the solution of the problem.   A writer in the *Christian Observer*, in an article published in 1820, said:

---

[1] The italics are ours.

I am not, however, aware that a school for nurses forms a regular part of hospital discipline, though it appears well worthy of doing so, and would be an incalculable benefit to the community. I would propose that in every infirmary any respectable female who wished to learn the art of nursing should be apprenticed, if I may so express it, for a certain term, say six or twelve months, and receive a course of theoretical and practical instruction in her intended profession, and if found competent, should be entitled to a certificate of her ability and moral deportment.

Among the anonymous answers to the "Inquiry" already spoken of were several that went to the point. Said one:

The best way to effect your object would be to form an institution in which women would be trained to become nurses. None of the institutions now existing answer this purpose, as they train for private families only. The institution should be for hospitals only . . . and sufficiently near to some hospital for the women to learn the art of nursing.

Another wrote:

It has occurred to me that a training institution for nurses might be a practicable and useful improvement. It might be a model hospital, where the business of nursing might be taught, and religious training added.

To these opinions was added that of Dr. Chatto, of St. Bartholomew's Hospital, who, in 1835, writing in the *London Medical Gazette*, made a plea for better nursing and urged that the large hospitals were well adapted as training fields and that they should be utilised for providing good nurses. He criticised the bad methods of the time severely and attributed the general intemperance of nurses to their desire to stimulate themselves when exhausted.

Both touching and extraordinary was a proposition set forth in 1847 by Sir Edward Parry of the Royal Navy and superintendent of Haslar hospital.[1] He had learned of the success of the Kaiserswerth experiment in training deaconesses, and after delineating in noble language the ideal nurse, womanly and gentle, he describes his and his officers' wish that the naval hospital service might be improved by following the Kaiserswerth example. He cannot doubt (he adds) that many of his countrywomen will be ready to devote themselves to the "work and labour of love" and suggests as his plan:

1. To endeavour to engage in the first instance the services of three or four Christian women, between the ages of thirty and fifty, who, upon the principles and conditions adopted at Kaiserswerth, are willing to devote themselves to this work at Haslar Hospital.

2. These persons, when engaged, to be trained for six months at the German hospital at Dalston, according to the system pursued at Kaiserswerth (but he forgot that at Kaiserswerth the probation

[1] *Hospitals and Sisterhoods*, 1855, pp. 38–41.

time alone was often more than six months), or if circumstances permit, to be placed at Kaiserswerth for their training.

3. Their training being completed, the nurses to be admitted to Haslar Hospital, where they will receive no pecuniary allowance, but a comfortable home, neat, and respectable lothing, and a sufficient maintenance. Their duties will be arduous and self-denying, and they will meet with much to exercise their Christian patience and forbearance, but they will receive encouragement and support from the captain-superintendent and the other officers.

A call for contributions followed, in the hope that a successful experiment might be imitated throughout the kingdom. It was signed William Edward Parry, Captain-Superintendent, Haslar Hospital, 1847. Later he wrote (sadly, one cannot doubt): "For this plan we did not get one offer to do this service—though hundreds of my paper were circulated far and wide." Good, brave, and simple-hearted sailor, with a genuine vision reflecting only nobly on his own character, his was the same error, ever old and ever new, of thinking that a work wrought out of life-long effort and the souls of rare characters like the Fliedners, or Louise le Gras and Vincent de Paul, can be copied at will and reproduced anywhere on demand in the short space of six months.

The first practical demonstration of training nurses in England did, however, own a spiritual bond with Kaiserswerth. It was that given by Mrs. Fry.

Elizabeth Gurney,[1] born on May 21, 1780, and early married to Joseph Fry, possessed a nature of rare beauty and goodness, which impressed itself with extraordinary strength upon her contemporaries. She belonged to an eminently liberal and progressive Quaker family and circle —reformers one and all—and she, in her beautiful and gracious presence, typified mercy, benignity, and practical wisdom. She began her reform work coincidently with her married life by following home a beggar woman carrying a half-frozen child. The woman, wishing to beg but not to be visited, tried in vain to evade the brave young woman, who succeeded in tracing her and in unearthing a shocking trade in starved infants. In her country home she laboured incessantly in the cottages of the poor—hers was friendly visiting work in its most loving and intelligent form. She was an ardent believer in vaccination, and performed the operation skilfully herself, making frequent rounds of inspection for this purpose in villages near by, with the result (unusual at that day) that smallpox was almost non-existent in the regions round. Mrs. Fry's special life-work, like that of Howard, was the amelioration of the lot of prisoners and the humanisation of prison conditions. She began in 1813 her famed work in the Newgate prison,

[1] *The Life of Elizabeth Fry*, by Susanna Corder, 1884; and *A Memoir of the Life of Elizabeth Fry*, in 2 vols. By her Daughter, 1847.

led to it by the reports of Quaker friends who had been in the habit of visiting there. Conditions were so distressing that it might have been thought that Howard's life had been spent in vain. The description of the female side of Newgate pictures a hell—which indeed it was:

Three hundred women, with their children, in the same room, in rags and dirt, destitute of sufficient clothing (no provision being made for this), sleeping without bedding on the floor, at one end of which the boards were raised to form a sort of pillow, . . . here they lived, cooked, and washed. Howard and his humane exertions appeared to have been forgotten. Dungeons, damp, close, and narrow cells often formed the common prisons of offenders of either sex and of all grades of crime. The danger of escape was guarded against by heavy iron fetters, dirt and disease abounded; these evils were magnified by the crowded state of the prisons. . . .

The death penalty was still fixed for trifling offences. A note from Mrs. Fry's journal reads:

Beside this poor young woman there are also six men to be hanged, one of whom has a wife near her confinement, who is also condemned, and seven young children. Since the awful report came down he has been quite mad from horror of mind and has bitten the turnkey. A strait-jacket could not keep him within bounds.[1]

In this place Mrs. Fry and her friends estab-

[1] *Life* of Mrs. Fry, by S. Corder, p. 243.

lished a school for the children and started sewing classes, providing material for work and food for the women. They helped them to earn and save, and befriended them upon release. Every day for years there was some one of this circle in the prison, and the change effected, little short of miraculous, attracted the attention of philanthropists in all countries. In 1818 Mrs. Fry was called to give testimony as to the prisons before the House of Commons.

On his visits to England pastor Fliedner had learned of this work and had met Mrs. Fry, of whom he wrote: "Of all my contemporaries none has exercised a like influence on my heart and life. . . . In January, 1824, I had the privilege of witnessing the effects - of her wonder-working visits among the miserable prisoners of Newgate." In 1840, on a trip to the continent, Mrs. Fry had visited Kaiserswerth, to the great joy of the pastor and his wife. He wrote: "My happiness may be imagined when she came in person to see and rejoice over the growing establishment of Kaiserswerth. She saw the whole house, going into every room, and minutely examining every detail." Mrs. Fry's habitual acquaintance with sickness among the poor and her hours at their bedsides had long impressed the need and importance of nursing on her thoughts. Now, what she heard and saw at Kaiserswerth made her most desirous of beginning something of the kind at home. Her own work made it impossible for her to give much time to the project, but through her sister and a daughter it was taken up and brought to fruition.[1] In 1840 an Institute of Nursing was established in Devonshire Square, Bishopsgate, and the pupil nurses were first called " Protestant Sisters of Charity." The name gave rise to suspicion and sectarian prejudice and was later changed to that of " Nursing Sisters."[2] The nurses were domiciled in the Home, where, on the plan of Kaiserswerth, they were carefully supervised and mothered. Their hospital training was received at Guy's Hospital, and was of the sort which has characterised the beginnings of the training in nursing in almost every country, namely, what one might call hospital visiting, for these pupils had no organic relation to the hospital, but went there daily for a short term of several months (later lengthened in accordance with the rising standard), to work under the untrained nurses of the wards, and to be taught by the physicians. It is not evident that they had any theoretical instruction or classes. The Sisters were most carefully chosen, and we may well believe that they made up in earnestness for the desultory character of their training. They were prepared only as attendants for private nursing, and made little, if any, impression in hospital work. In the fact that they did, however, have some experience in a general hospital, they were ahead of the school in Philadelphia, in the United States, which at that same

[1] Corder's *Life*, p. 565.   [2] *Ibid.*, p. 565.

time was developing under the care of a group of Quakers of that city for private nursing: otherwise the general lines on which the two groups were arranged, the home training and serious spirit, the earnest purpose and practical good sense of the founders, give these two early experiments a good deal of similarity. We do not know that there was any relation between the English and the American early nursing schools of the Quakers, but as Mrs. Fry had a brother in Philadelphia, it is not improbable.

Naturally, no imitation of churchly orders would arise under the management of the Friends. The extent to which Mrs. Fry was in advance of her time was shown by the coldness in the attitude taken by religious writers toward the principles on which the Nursing Sisters were founded. While others insisted on the necessity for holding nurses in the strict bands of religious discipline, Mrs. Fry started hers without bond or forms of ceremonial, though the spirit which animated their Home was a devoutly pious one. Hers was a secular order, and she intended to create a method by which a reasonable maintenance for the nurses would be combined with an efficient and often gratuitous care of the sick. The Sisters were to be maintained by the institution and were not permitted to receive any money or gifts. They were to work in the spirit of the Sisters of Charity, yet, after all, theirs was a lay sisterhood

and their training was only for nursing.[1]   For
this reason Pusey, who was at this time interesting himself in projects of nursing reform, did not
entirely approve of them, as their mode of life
contemplated only so much self-denial as was
necessary for a nurse's work[2] (even so much
may have been rather more than the good divine
quite realised).   Miss Stanley, who in speaking
of them said: "The English Protestant Sisters
of Charity were only paid nurses belonging to a
society established by Mrs. Fry," added, "The
further and higher idea she did not live to establish." [3]   Even pastor Fliedner was ultimately
disappointed in them, for he told Agnes Jones,
in 1860, of his regret, after the consultations he
had had with Mrs. Fry about her nursing work,
to find it such a limited one; he thought her
nurses' sphere restricted, in comparison to what it
might be, and regretted also that no attempt
was made to improve them by mental culture.[4]

Mrs. Fry did not live long enough to see more
than the beginning of her nursing reformation.
She died in 1845, and her *Life*, as it was written,
makes only slight mention of the Nursing Institute and throws no light upon its details.
Nor does the hospital history mention Mrs.

---

[1] *Memoirs of Agnes E. Jones*, 1885, by her Sister, p. 383.
[2] *Life of E. B. Pusey*, by Canon Liddon, 1894, vol. iii., chapter on " Early Days of Anglican Sisterhoods.".
[3] *Hospitals and Sisterhoods*, p. 59.
[4] *Memoirs of Agnes E. Jones*, p. 135.

Fry's nurses.[1] By 1857 ninety nurses had been trained there, all of whom were engaged in private duty. The Institute is still in existence as a very successful and well-managed training institution for private nurses.

The next wave of effort rose in the Established Church and brought into existence much interesting and historically significant nursing organisation and training, for the early Anglican sisterhoods experimented in many forms of social service, including visiting nursing; they entered hospitals, gave a demonstration of refined and educated gentlewomen taking up the despised duties of the nurse, and some of their members were pioneers not only in the humbler but also in the higher fields of hospital management and ward guidance. They had some well prepared women ready to go to the Crimea with Miss Nightingale, and from one of their groups came the Sister who later successfully organised the Bellevue school of nursing in the United States.

Dr. Pusey wrote to Keble in 1839 of his conviction that it was necessary to have Sisters of Charity and employ them as nurses in hospitals and lunatic asylums "in which last Christian nursing is so sadly missed." He also corresponded with a physician, Dr. Greenhill, on the same subject, and, through him, obtained a copy of the rules of the Augustinian Sisters and the Sisters

[1] *Biographical History of Guy's Hospital*, Wilks and Bettany, London, 1892.

of Charity of Vincent de Paul. The first sisterhood in the English Church arose under Pusey's guidance in 1845. It was called the Park Village Community, and, under the care of a committee, was housed in Regent's Park. Pusey had gone abroad in 1841 to study French sisterhoods and nursing orders. But the leanings of his mind drew him from the more active orders of Augustinians and Sœurs to the rule of St. Francis de Sales' Order of the Visitation, from which, as we have seen, active nursing work had been displaced by ascetic regulations, and it was a modification of this rule, providing for about four hours daily of visiting among the poor, which was finally adopted for the Park Village Community. There was no training in nursing provided for, not even a course of walking the hospitals, but there was friendly visiting of the poor and sick, at home and in hospitals and workhouses, burying the dead, Ragged School work, etc. The members were called Sisters of Mercy. Gladstone was among the important sympathisers with the movement.

In 1848, Miss Sellon began a similar work at Devonport, by gathering a group of devoted women together for service among the poor. The Bishop of Exeter approved their labours and permitted them to form an order of Sisters of Mercy under the wing of the Church. Miss Sellon and her Sisters were active in Bethnal Green and Plymouth, and later in the east end of London. Although they had no regular training as nurses,

they took every opportunity of giving service in
sickness, and in 1849, during an epidemic of
cholera in Plymouth, they were courageous and
untiring in seeking out the sufferers, visiting and
aiding them. That they then attempted nursing in
the strict sense is doubtful, but they did not spare
themselves in meeting all kinds of emergencies
and in efforts to relieve distress. That they later
developed a somewhat systematic preparation for
the care of the sick is evident from the fact that
the Superior and a number of Sisters accompanied
Miss Nightingale to the Crimea. About this time,
they had a hospital at Bristol and a Nursing
Sisters' Home connected with the church of
St. Barnabas, Pimlico, where a few patients were
received and from which nurses went out to nurse
the poor in their homes.[1] In 1866 the cholera
raged in London, and Pusey helped to found a
cholera hospital there. By this time there had
been a fusion between the Park Village and Miss
Sellon's communities, and Pusey offered the
services of Miss Sellon and her Sisters to take
charge of the hospital, which they did, for they
had worked as volunteers through a number of
epidemics, and were fearless and energetic.

As this Sisterhood had developed extremely
high church tendencies, it had many enemies;
and attacks were made upon it in print, which
still survive, sounding, it must be felt, absurdly

---

[1] *Hospitals and Sisterhoods*, p. 52.

hysterical and sensational.[1] It is perhaps true, however, that some of the ceremonials instituted by Miss Sellon and Dr. Pusey lent themselves easily to the ridicule of the irreverent. Nevertheless the exquisitely refining influence of the Sisters' atmosphere should not be forgotten by critics, for this must remain as their most precious contribution to the social life around them. The love of beauty, with the consistent determination to bring it into the lives of the people, and a sensitive consideration for the feelings of the poor, were abiding principles with Miss Sellon, and so sordid and hideous appears to have been the lot of the poor by whom she was surrounded that this should ever be remembered of her gratefully.

The community of St. John's House, founded in 1848, was the first purely nursing order in the Anglican Church, and has had an important and interesting part in the development of English nursing. Dr. Todd, of King's College hospital, was conspicuous in the preliminary movement, as was also Mrs. William Morrice.[2] In a letter privately circulated in 1847, Dr. Todd originally projected an establishment for training nurses in connection with King's College hospital, and

[1] See *Sisterhoods in the Church of England*, by Margaret Goodman, London, 1864.

[2] A pamphlet entitled: "A Brief Account of the Design, Origin, and Progress of the Training Institution for Nurses for Hospitals, Families, and the Poor," published by Richard Clay, in a report dated Nov., 1850, gives Mrs. Morrice as the Lady Superintendent at that date.

under the auspices of Bishop Blomfield and in concert with other friends he took a leading part in drawing up the fundamental rules and in framing the arrangements under which St. John's House was set on foot in the following year.

Dr. Bowman, also of King's College hospital, was likewise very active in working for nursing reform, and one of the earliest steps in the foundation of St. John's House appears to have been a circular letter, of which no copy survives, written by Dr. Bowman to eminent medical men. The first public action, which was apparently the result of this letter, was the gathering of a very impressive array of bishops and clergy, lords, and members of the royal family on the 13th of July, 1848. At this meeting the following proposal was considered:

It is proposed to establish a corporate or collegiate institution, the objects of which would be to maintain in a community women who are members of the Church of England, who should receive such instruction and undergo such training as might best fit them to act as nurses and visitors to the sick and poor. It is proposed to connect the institution with some hospital or hospitals, in which the women under training, or those who had been already educated, might find the opportunity of exercising their calling or of acquiring experience. It is absolutely necessary to the success of the design and the real amelioration of the class of persons for whose benefit it is intended, that the proposed establishment should be a religious one, and that all connected with it should regard the work in which they are embarked as a religious work.[1]

The society thus formed under the most distinguished auspices later issued a pamphlet dealing more fully with the proposed plans. A committee of sixteen clergymen and physicians, among whom were many noted men but with whom no woman was associated, was formed to arrange the details.

Lord Nelson was warmly interested in this plan, and wrote soon after the meeting to Dr. Wordsworth:

MY DEAR DR. WORDSWORTH:

We shall publish in the papers as soon as possible a meeting of the Council, having first found out the most convenient day for the Bishop of London and the principal members to attend.

We must then pass the formal resolutions as to quorums, etc., and fix four quarterly meetings or monthly ones, etc.; decide how to begin work; state what funds will be sufficient to warrant a beginning; appoint a place for applicants; consider the important rules, especially the dietary and board money, which a great many think too high . . . fix on our locality, etc. All this should be done before the effect of our meeting cools, remembering always that if we do

[1] As St. John's House has taken an important part in nursing history we have quoted freely from the articles "St. John's House in the Past" in the *St. John's House News*, beginning in October, 1902, and continued to date. The Sister Superior in granting this permission desires it to be noted that these records are but fragmentary.

not get a start soon we shall be sadly thrown back by the absence from town of many members. I think the Council ought to appoint some five a Committee to meet at all times and to report to their monthly or quarterly meeting, and I should be delighted to be one of the workers, or if my absence from town should render me unfit, I should be happy to assist by written suggestions, sending out circulars, etc.

Do see if you can stir up people for our first Council meeting, for I am sure time is most precious to us just now, lest people's ardour cool after reading our speeches, and check their charitable feelings by the remark "but nothing has come of it."

Believe me,
Yours sincerely
NELSON.

Some few months after the date of this meeting, during which time the organisation and raising of funds was carried on with much zeal, the "Training Institution for Nurses in Hospitals, Families, and for the Poor" began its work, finding its first home in 36 Fitzroy Square, in the district of St. John the Evangelist, in St. Pancras, from which it took its name of St. John's House. (This was in the year 1848.) At this early period it derived most important help from the devotion of Miss Elizabeth Frere,[1] who for the first six months personally superintended and developed all internal arrangements for the

[1] See also a pamphlet published by Harrison and Sons, called: "A Short Account of the History and Work of the House and Sisterhood of St. John the Evangelist," p. 3.

house. Although Mrs. Fry had been first in the field with her Institute for Private Nurses in Bishopsgate (founded in 1840), St. John's House was the first attempt of an Institute for Nurses on definite Church lines, and it may claim a distinct position of having a religious foundation. All the nurses were members of the Church of England, and were under the supervision of the "Master" of the House, who was to be a Clergyman in Priest's orders, and was to give definite religious instruction to the nurses and to conduct their services. The first Master was the Rev. F. W. Twist. Miss Frere acted as first Lady Superintendent.

The writer of the articles quoted from thinks the first probationers were sent to the Middlesex Hospital for training.[1] An old letter in the *Nursing Record* said they were sent to the Westminster.[2] It would seem probable that a small group of probationers might have been taken by each of these hospitals.

The Bishop of London acted as President of the Society. The Master was to be either married, or a widower, and the Lady Superintendent was to regulate, with the concurrence of the Master, the domestic arrangements and the appointments of nurses.

There were to be three classes of members:

1. Probationers: these must be at least

[1] *St. John's House League News*, April, 1903, p. 80.
[2] *The Nursing Record*, London, May 30, 1889; letter signed K. H.

eighteen years old and able to read or write (it is evident from this proviso that this class was not of a high social grade); they were to be under training two years, receiving board, lodging, and laundry, and paying fifteen pounds a year. At the end of the two years they might, if approved, enter the second class, called

2. Nurses: To this class suitable women might also be admitted without probation (these would probably be from the class of educated or gentlewomen) and all nurses must remain at least five years. They would receive board, lodging, and wages, and at the end of five years, if competent and deserving, a certificate.

3. Sisters: these might either be residents in the Home, paying fifty pounds a year, or they might live with their families and friends. They must remain at least two years, and were expected to be examples to the other two classes, sharing in the religious and professional instruction and the work in families and hospitals. The connection with King's College hospital, which lasted until 1885, dates from 1849, at which time the first probationers were sent to this hospital, so closely connected with the history of St. John's House. The Council meetings were often held in the hospital hall, and Dr. Todd, whose statue stands there now, was always there to give advice and help. The whole charge of the wards was not given to the Institute at first, but, as with Mrs. Fry's nurses, the probationers and nurses

were permitted to spend some time daily in the wards in the care of the sick.[1]

It may be of interest to know what the arrangements for the day, etc., were in those early times. A copy of the Time-table of the Master's day in 1849 reads:

" 7:30. Prayers in Chapel or
" 8.00. Service in St. John's Church.
" 10.00. Interview with the Lady Superintendent, when all details about the House, Nurses, etc., were discussed and settled. Instruction to individual nurses.
" 12.00. Instruction for Sisters, Tuesday, Thursday, Saturday, on the Parables of our Lord.
" 1.00. Dine with inmates (at least three times a week). Shew house to visitors.
" 3.00. Instruction for Probationers, Tuesday, Thursday, Saturday, on the Book of Common Prayer, or private interviews with nurses, etc.
" 4.00. House Committee (Mondays.)
" Office hours: 10.00 to 1.35—3 to 5."

The Master appears to have had charge of many household matters for he " saw Treloar's man to measure hall and staircase for cocoanut matting"; " arranged with Clay's man about painting Chapel window"; " interviewed Sarah . . . whom I admonished." He sent out the accounts, saw applicants for admission, and in his diary are terse comments on some of them:

" Oct. 10.—Saw M—— E—— candidate for the situation of nurse; well recommended . . . but appears

---

[1] *The British Magazine* gave the scheme of training in July, 1848.

too diminutive in person to discharge the duties of nurse efficiently; sent to consult Dr. Todd, who is of opinion she may come for a fortnight on trial. . . ."

" Dec. 6.—E——— H——— applied as nurse, . . . but appears self-conceited and ill-tempered. No room for such at present. . . .

It was later found best that the Lady Superintendent should be responsible for many of the details which had first been undertaken by the Master, but which lay more in the province of the lady of the house. . . . [1]

When the crisis of the Crimean war came, St. John's House made the first offer of service. The Master (the Reverend C. P. Shepherd) wrote a proposal to the Lord President of the Institution (Bishop Blomfield), that certain nurses from St. John's House should proceed to Scutari, and that he should himself accompany them, "not only to be their guardian, but also to act as Chaplain generally in the Hospital." We quote part of the correspondence:

From the Bishop of London to the Master of St. John's House

FULHAM, 24th Oct., 1854.

MY DEAR SIR:

I quite approve of both parts of your proposal, and I should think the Council would also. I have written to Mr. Sidney Herbert to ascertain what the Government will do in the matter.

I am, yours truly,

C. J., London.

[1] *St. John's House League News*, Nov., 1903, pp. 126–127.

From the Secretary of War to the Bishop of London

WAR OFFICE, Oct. 17th, 1854.

MY DEAR LORD:

Miss Nightingale has consented to go out to Scutari to undertake the whole management of the female nursing. Her great hospital experience and skill and courage in surgical treatment, together with her administrative capacity, peculiarly fit her for this undertaking, and in a Military Hospital, where subordination is everything, without some recognised head with ample authority, there would be no chance of success. She is in communication with the Nurses of St. John's House, and, I have no doubt, will take them with her. . . .

Pray believe me, yours sincerely,

SIDNEY HERBERT.

Letters were written to the *Times* and subscriptions asked for the "St. John's House Fund for the Sick and Wounded English in the East," also volunteers for the work, who were to be trained by St. John's House before leaving for the seat of war.

After various negotiations with the government and Miss Florence Nightingale, it was finally arranged that St. John's House should furnish a certain number of its nurses, to be placed under the sole and exclusive charge of Miss Nightingale, and to proceed with her without delay to the East. At a meeting of the Council in October, 1854, the Secretary of War (Mr. Sidney Herbert), the Chaplain-General to the Forces, and Miss Nightingale attended at St. John's House in order to facilitate arrangements. It was resolved that in the great public emergency the institution would, at considerable pecuniary loss, spare six of its nurses to proceed to serve under Miss Nightingale in the British hospitals in the East, and that they should be entirely under her jurisdiction. The original plans being thus altered, and the work being done under Government instead of by the institution, the services of the Master were not required.

On October 23d the six nurses—Rebecca Lawfield, Emma Fagg, Ann Higgins, Elizabeth Drake, Mary Ann Coyle, Mary Ann Bournett—having received a parting charge and benediction from their bishop, started for Scutari, and were accompanied by the Master as far as Paris. The Lady Superintendent (Miss Mary Jones) was to select and prepare additional nurses to follow this first detachment as soon as possible. Twenty went out the next year.

Four, alas! out of the first party of volunteers returned shortly from Scutari, not being prepared to bear and accept the discipline and privations of the life out there. The remainder served their country with great devotion, as the following entry in the Minute Books for 1855 testified:

"The Lady Superior has also received an anonymous donation of £100 for the Institution from 'A Sister of an Officer Fallen in the Crimea.' The donor also wishes this sum added to the fund for the purpose of building a suitable residence for St. John's House, and expresses a hope that the House may be able to make arrangements for taking charge of the sick in King's College Hospital."

Nurse Elizabeth Drake died of fever at Balaclava, serving at her post faithfully to the last. Miss

Nightingale writes of her in the highest terms, saying in a letter dated August 16, 1855: "I have lost in her the best of all the women here. . . . I feel like a criminal in having robbed you of one so truly to be loved and honoured. It seemed as if it pleased God to remove from the work those who have been most useful to it. His Will be done!" Miss Nightingale also erected a small marble cross to her memory in the cemetery at Scutari, inscribed with her name, the date, and her profession.[1]

The providing of nurses for the Crimea was the indirect cause of a great expansion in the work of St. John's House, for the need of systematic training in a hospital was then fully and widely acknowledged. It now also became evident that the machinery of organisation was unwieldy and delayed progress, as there were no less than five different authorities and no one definite head. The Master's report of 1855 instanced the slow growth of the institute as a result of divided authority. The Lady Superior explained it by the want of a sufficient and well-defined field of labour, and the lack of sufficient hospital facilities. So far, the nurses had only been going for a few hours daily to learn what they could under the paid nurses of the hospitals. In 1853, Miss Stanley had referred to their results in the following words:

There has been great comfort afforded to the rich by these nurses, but hitherto the original promises

[1] *St. John's House League News*, April, 1904, pp. 126–128.

have not been fulfilled. For hospitals it [the institution] has not provided at all; for families insufficiently, and for the poor very imperfectly. It has so far trained seventeen nurses, but it is now greatly in need of funds and without considerable augmentation of its funds it cannot go on.[1]

About this time propositions were made to St. John's House by King's College hospital, which had been founded as a centre for teaching as well as for the relief of the sick poor,

as to whether an arrangement could be entered into by which the entire nursing of the hospital could be undertaken by St. John's House. Terms of agreement were at last made between the committees of King's College Hospital and St. John's House, and on March 31, 1856, the Sisters and nurses took over the work, in order to introduce a higher class of nurses and a better system of nursing into the wards of the hospital, and to carry out more fully than hitherto one main object of the St. John's Institution—that of training and providing nurses for the sick in hospitals as well as for private families and the poor.

Many are the stories told of the day the Sisters took possession; nearly all the old staff, who resented the change, waited bonneted and cloaked in the hall for their arrival, and then left at once, leaving them "to find out the bad cases for themselves"; and by the end of the day the new-comers, who had arrived in clean and dainty uniforms, were more like a set of sweeps or char-women, in such an appalling state

1 *Hospitals and Sisterhoods*, p. 46,

of disorder had they found their wards. Very soon a marked improvement began, and we find the committee warmly thanking the Sisters and nurses for their devotion to their duties.[1]

A letter in the *Times* [2] describes the organisation and system of the new hospital training from the time of its foundation in 1856. The staff consisted of a lady superior, Sisters, associate Sisters, lady pupils, nurses, assistant nurses, probationers, and candidates on trial. The Sisters were ladies of refinement who gave their services gratuitously and bore the cost of their own maintenance. They entered for three months' trial, and then became lady pupils, assistant Sister, or Sister. The probationers were usually of the servant class and were paid. The time of probation was three months. They then became assistant nurses for nine months, and were thereafter called nurses. The time of training (one year) was all spent in the hospital. After that the nurses were employed in hospital or in private duty. St. John's House took charge of the entire household department of King's College hospital, the kitchen, the store-rooms, linen-rooms, and laundry; it retained entire control over all the nursing staff, and by its contract with the hospital the directors or officers of the latter were not to interfere so long as the nursing was well done. The wards were thoroughly staffed

[1] *St. John's House League News*, Oct., 1904, p. 184.
[2] Feb. 14, 1874.

and the work was faultlessly done, as innumerable witnesses testified. The patients were tenderly nursed, their surroundings kept exquisitely clean and orderly, and an atmosphere of refinement, sweet cheerfulness, and serenity characterised the wards. Miss Nightingale once said of the nursing there that it was the most "homelike" she had ever seen.[1]

The house came to have traditions of good nursing which gave it an atmosphere greatly cherished by the members. The patients were always put before everything, and the little niceties and refinements of personal care were steadily impressed upon the probationers. The nurses looked forward to spending the whole of their nursing days on the staff, and were jealous of the honour and standards of the house. Many of them spent twenty, twenty-five, and thirty years in private nursing, and then retired on a pension. But the present generation is less stationary and may receive a larger salary in lieu of the pension.

In 1861 the Lady Superintendent expresses her opinion, in the Report, of the desirability for the completeness of St. John's House that the nurses should have opportunity for training in midwifery, and in the following year this special branch of work, for which ever since St. John's House has been famed, was taken up.

In 1874 a struggle took place between the

[1] Quoted by Lord Hatherly in a letter to the *Times*, Feb. 28, 1874.

administrative authorities of the hospital and
St. John's House, which was written up freely
in the *Times* of that year,[1] and in the *British
Medical Journal* of the same date.[2]

The contest, which was in brief an attempt on
the side of the hospital officials to obtain an
aggressive and unfair power over the nursing
staff, which would have impaired discipline and
degraded the standards of nursing, and, on the
side of St. John's House, to defend and protect
its standards, need not be entered into. It arose
entirely from ignorance of what good nursing
work was, on the side of certain· hospital officials. It is of interest, however, to note the loyal
support given to the House by the medical staff
of the hospital, and by the *Medical Journal*.
The latter said editorially: "One thing is
abundantly evident, and that is, that no fault
can be found with the manner in which the
nursing has been performed."

The hospital staff spontaneously remonstrated
with the committee, saying : "Any change which
would remove the nursing from the care of the
Sisters of St. John's House is greatly to be deprecated and would be calamitous to the hospital
and to the interests of the patients."

The difficulty was finally adjusted by arbitra-

[1] See *Times*, Feb. 14, 18, 20, 28, Apr. 27, May 4, 15, 29,
June 19. 1874.

[2] See *Journal* of 1874, pp. 208, 243. 245, 283, 493, 591, 654,
619, 592.

tion and the resignation of some of the officials who had fomented the trouble, and St. John's House remained in charge of the nursing until 1885, when, under an entirely friendly agreement, the hospital established its own training school.

St. John's House also carried on the nursing for the Charing Cross Hospital, from 1866 to 1889, of the Metropolitan Hospital from 1888 to 1896, and of several lesser hospitals. In 1883, as the result of an unfortunate controversy, a serious schism occurred, and, a majority of the Sisters having separated from the House, the Council called the community of All Saints to take charge of its work.[1] This connection lasted for ten years, when, All Saints having urgent calls from its foreign missions, it withdrew from much of its English work, and the community of St. Peter assumed the management of St. John's House, which it has kept until the present day.

St. John's House is in many respects one of the most interesting and attractive nursing founda-tions in England. It has drawn to its service an admirably endowed set of women, and has been distinguished by an extreme liberality and intelligence of view in social questions. As a re-fining factor in nursing its influence is hardly to be overestimated.

As we are now attempting only an outline of the early history of the Anglican nursing sisterhoods,

[1] The seceding Sisters took the name Nursing Sisters of St. John the Divine, and established themselves in Lewisham.

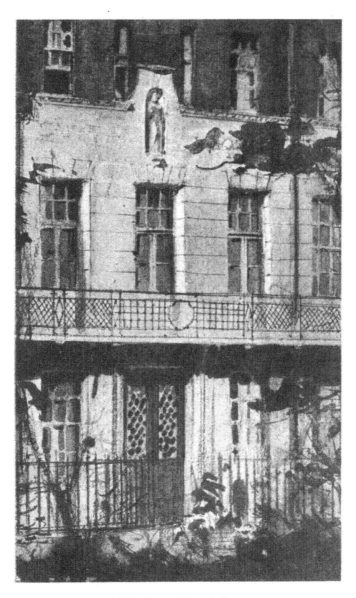

St. John's House, Queen's Square

the important part which St. John's House has taken in modern educational questions, and its progressive attitude on social problems must be left for later consideration.[1]

The Sisterhood of All Saints is peculiarly entitled to the interest and regard of American nurses, for it was to this community that Sister Helen, who organised Bellevue Training School, belonged.

All Saints has had a distinctive nursing history. Its first Superior was Miss Byron; its founder and Chaplain was the Rev. Upton Richards, Vicar of All Saints, Margaret Street, London. Its existence dates from 1851, and the first work it undertook for the care of the sick was the establishment of St. Elizabeth's Home for Incurable Women and Children, in Mortimer Street. From this arose the more definite and systematic relation to hospital nursing which came to characterise this order. In 1857 the community undertook regular nursing duties in University College hospital, several wards being put entirely under its care, and so successful was its administration that in 1862 the entire charge of the whole hospital was given to the Sisters. This relation between hospital and sisterhood continued until 1899, when the hospital established its own secular school of nursing. Three Sisters held in turn, during the

[1] We are indebted to Miss Margaret Breay, Hon. Secretary of the Matrons' Council of Great Britain and Ireland, for many details of St. John's House history.

whole time, over thirty years, the position of Sister-in-Chief in the hospital: they were Sister Elizabeth, Sister Gertrude Anna, and Sister Cecilia.

The relation with St. John's House, which dated from 1883 and continued until 1893, brought an enlarged field of hospital nursing to the community of All Saints—the Metropolitan hospital, St. Saviour's, and the Maternity at Battersea all for a time coming under its care. Increasing demands from foreign countries led the community to relinquish some of its English posts, but it still cares for a large convalescent hospital at Eastbourne for men, women, and children, and a children's hospital in the same place which was built in memory of the Mother Foundress. The Sisters are now active in Bombay, where nursing is a prominent feature of the branch house. Two or three hospitals are under their management there, and during the plague of 1899 they supplied the nursing in eight hospitals, some of which, however, were temporary structures.[1]

Another sisterhood which made nursing a special interest, and still does so, was St. Margaret's, founded by the Rev. Dr. Neale in 1854. A rarely fresh and mediæval fervour seems to have characterised this little community under the leadership of Dr. Neale, who was another St. Francis, poetic and artistic, more scholarly also than St. Francis probably was. Its story has

[1] From private sources.

been told in a very engaging and unaffected style by one of the Sisters.[1]

A short experience of hospital work was regarded as sufficient preparation for the demands made upon the Sisters; they did not include any private work among the rich in their nursing plans, but devoted themselves to the service of the poor. Sincere and unselfish devotion, with zeal to perform the most menial duties of scrubbing and cleaning in their patients' homes, constituted the chief outfit in the nursing armoury of the Sisters. Dr. Neale's idea was that still found to-day among the clergy—nursing was not regarded as a specialty, but as an accessory to general mission work. The Sisters were often sent to remain with a patient. "If a Sister was nursing in some lonely out-of-the way hamlet he (Dr. Neale) would always find time and go to see her at least once during her period of nursing," runs the memoir spoken of.[2] And a letter written by Dr. Neale to an applicant, fixing a day for her to be met by one of the band, said, "All the others [the Sisters] are out nursing." The Sisters went sometimes to one, sometimes to another hospital to gain their experience. Sectarian animosity sometimes made it hard for them to get even this little training. One letter, dated December 13, 1859, said: "Will you tell A. L. that if she

[1] *Memories of a Sister of St. Saviour's Priory.* London. A. R. Mowbray Co., 1904.

[2] Page 30.

wants to go to the hospital she must go before she is a Sister, for Sister Martha cannot get admission into one on account of her cross, and Dr. Neale will not let her put it off." [1]

A frightful scene of superstitious hatred was enacted one time at a funeral of one of the Sisters, when mob brutality burst forth, and a couple of the Sisters were almost torn in pieces and had to be taken under escort of the police to a place of safety.

In many years' work in Soho, St. Giles, and Haggerston the Sisters, in spite of their elementary training, fearlessly braved small-pox, typhoid, and cholera. Several of them helped to nurse in Miss Sellon's temporary hospital in Spitalfields, she and Dr. Pusey having taken a large warehouse and fitted it up for the purpose, receiving there men, women, and children. Sisters of Holy Trinity also assisted there, while, in true mediæval fashion, the Cowley Brothers under Father Grafton helped in the men's wards and in the kitchen.

Small-pox was a frequent scourge, and the Sisters relate a number of inconceivably pathetic instances of its horrors: one story tells how they themselves, by night, carried the little coffin of a child, which no one else would touch, to the morgue; and another of four children in one bed, two of whom were dead of small-pox and two living, but all in so much the same state that the undertaker who had come to remove the dead

[1] *Memories of a Sister of St. Saviour's Priory*, p. 29.

bodies hesitated, when the living children cried,
"Oh, Mother, Mother, don't let us go too."

In 1871 the Sisters were so overwhelmed with
calls to small-pox patients that they appealed for
aid in the *Times* of Feb. 20. Besides visiting, four
Sisters worked continuously in an emergency hospital for small-pox on the Hackney Road.[1]

In later years, after the Jubilee Nurses were
established and a branch was placed in Nichols
Square, the Sisters wrote: "How we ever managed
to help our poor sick people before those invaluable
nurses came I cannot think. We did the little
we could ourselves, just in our own parish, but it
was but a tiny drop in the ocean of sickness and
misery. Now it rejoices the heart of every one to
see the bright, cheery, kindly face of the nurse
going about on her errands of helpfulness and
accomplishing on a very large scale, with trained
skilfulness, what we used to attempt on a very
small scale with anxious unskilfulness." [1]

We have now followed, at least in outline, the
early efforts and achievements in English nursing
reform. It is clear that, admirable as was the
spirit animating them, high as were the ideals,
and great the energy and courage of these early
reformers and pioneers, yet, indisputably, their
nursing organisations, modelled as they all were,
more or less consciously and of set design, on the
forms of the past (thus being, in fact, imitations,

[1] *Memories of a Sister of St. Saviour's Priory*, p. 123–124.
[2] *Ibid.*, p. 304.

or survivals of a former order of things), did not contain within themselves the principle of growth or adaptation to new social forms. Society was about to take on a new phase—the industrial—a phase unlovely in itself, but beyond which fairer domains of social justice might be descried; medicine was about to become a new and commanding science: based on research and allied with a glorious figure—sanitation, that had well-nigh disappeared for over 2000 years from the earth—the medical art was now preparing to proclaim the doctrines of prevention rather than the assuagement of disease. Even religion, that for so many centuries had decided the forms and extent of the nurse's ministrations, was on the eve of turning from a sole contemplation of the next world, to this one, to become less abstract and more practical. The creative energy that was to transform the nursing of England and of a new continent was even then ready to break forth. Miss Nightingale was preparing, not to imitate the forms of the past, but to shape a new order; not to reproduce the Sisters of Charity or the deaconesses, but to re-create the ancient work of nursing on a plan fitted for and adapted to the oncoming changes of the future.

CHAPTER III

FLORENCE NIGHTINGALE, the revered foundress of modern trained nursing, the heroine of the Crimea and the guiding spirit in a long series of reforms in military and civil hospital administration and public hygiene, was born in May, 1820, and is still living. Her chief contribution to the inheritance of the race has been that, besides demonstrating in action the full perfection of the allied arts of nursing and sanitation, she has left in her writings a philosophy, as it were, of nursing, together with an intellectual demonstration of the scientific and natural basis of hygiene and its practical application, and has laid down once and for all their essential underlying principles with a clarity, a logic, an originality, and a depth of reflection that mark the genius and place her works among the classics.

A complete and authoritative history of Miss Nightingale is naturally not to be expected until she or some authorised member of her family shall decide to give it to the world. All through her long life she has shown great reticence as to her own achievements, and has displayed a self-detachment as great as her deeds—amounting even to an aversion to being written about. But public services as distinguished as hers could not be left untold, and a number of biographies, more or less fragmentary, and biographical chapters in histories of the Crimean War have been written of her. It is indeed doubtful whether any woman's story has been repeated oftener, or with greater homage, admiration, and gratitude. Yet every one of the existing accounts of Miss Nightingale falls far short of being proportioned to her place in the sphere of social progress. It is true that certain chapters in Crimean War histories which are devoted to her work have the most genuine ring, as of personal knowledge, but they touch only that one epoch of her long and consistently useful life. Of the earlier biographies[1] aiming at a general account of Miss Nightingale, it is not evident that any of the writers was able to draw from sources other than the daily press and records open to every one, while of later ones it may be assumed that they contain only second-hand material, rewritten in a new setting. Hence it has been inevitable that a somewhat conventionalised saintly type, not unlike that of the mediæval legends, has come to be accepted as the orthodox figure of Miss Nightingale, so that it is not always clear how much of the human and real personality of this great

[1]See bibliography in appendix.

woman is shown. This, indeed, the writers believe, is only to be fairly estimated by a close and thorough study of her writings.

The most serious and adequate accounts of Miss Nightingale's army nursing work have been given by men, notably by Kinglake, who more than any other recognised and delineated accurately the intellectual quality of her achievements in the Crimea; but few indeed are they who read Kinglake to-day, and his graphic and fascinating portrayal of the Lady-in-Chief is hidden in the oblivion which now obscures the Crimean War. Few persons have wielded influence so extensive as hers, and no other has had so definite and weighty a share in shaping and advising in hospital and nursing affairs; and yet so quietly and unassumingly has this influence been exercised from her invalid's couch, that few of those directly benefited by her counsels have known their source. Her writings, too, containing as they do incomparable statements of principles, enunciated with consummate mental supremacy, have, unfortunately, been largely hidden away in Blue Books, reports, proceedings, and encyclopedias. With the exception of the *Notes on Nursing; What it Is and What it is Not,* which finds a place in all well-selected libraries, they are not readily accessible to the general public, and are all but unknown to the younger women who are following the nurse's calling. We must hope that some day we may know the full inner history of her long years of experience and observation in the many hospitals of Europe; of her training at Kaiserswerth; of the vast military hospital system in the Crimea to which she applied her controlling mind and hand; of her confidential reports, communications, suggestions to the War Office, and important share in the reorganisations that followed the war; of those early days in nursing reform when all work was pioneer work, and every new step an experiment and a revolution; of the innumerable conferences, the unceasing current of advice, suggestion, and inspiration, that flowed in all directions from her sick-room.

A work has recently appeared[1] which contains certain hitherto unpublished material concerning the Crimean epoch, but in so fragmentary a form that it adds little or nothing to the already existing records of importance that refer to that period; moreover, it is knit in a context so biassed and narrow, and interpreted in a spirit so small and acrimonious, that it is more calculated to mislead than to enlighten.

The writers realise well their limitations in being unable to present any new and authoritative material relating to Miss Nightingale and her life: what they have tried to do is to gather together those records and bits of scattered personal testimony which seem the most valuable and to

[1] *Sidney Herbert, Lord Herbert of Lea, A Memoir*, by Lord Stanmore. In 2 volumes. John Murray, London; E. P. Dutton & Co., New York, 1906.

interpret them, so far as lies in their power, by virtue of a common calling.

A generous fate seems to have presided at Miss Nightingale's birth, for every advantage of family, social position, culture, and wealth was hers. But most grateful must her followers feel to her father, whose passion for education so far outran the standards of his day that he was indifferent to sport—that idol of his contemporaries —and cool toward local charities and alms-givings, but ardent in his support of schools for the rural population. To this enlightened father we owe it that Miss Nightingale was educated with a breadth, scope, and thoroughness uncommon not only then, but now. Her mother, a woman of beautiful and gracious personality, herself the daughter of a notably liberal and philanthropic father, endowed her with every kindly and gentle gift, and taught her social accomplishments; but her father trained and disciplined her mind, fortified it with an ample stock of Greek and Latin, mathematics, and natural science, made her proficient in German, French, and Italian, and took her through ancient and modern literature. In the delightful *Memoirs of Caroline Fox* is found this anecdote:

June 12th [1857] Warrenton Smythe talked with great delight of Florence Nightingale. Long ago, before she went to Kaiserswerth, he and Sir Henry de la Bèche dined at her father's and Florence Nightingale sat between them. She began by drawing Sir Henry out on geology and charmed him by the boldness and breadth of her views, which were not common then.   She accidentally proceeded into regions of Latin and Greek and then our geologist had to get out of it.

She was fresh from Egypt and began talking with W. Smythe about the inscriptions, etc., where he thought he could do pretty well; but when she began quoting Lepsius, which she had been studying in the original, he was in the same case as Sir Henry.

When the ladies left the room, the latter said to him, "A capital young lady that, if she hadn't floored me with her Latin and Greek.[1]

It has been said of her: "The peculiarity in the case of herself and her relatives seems to be their having been reared in an atmosphere of sincerity and freedom—of reality, in fact—which is more difficult to obtain than might be thought."[2]

Much as Miss Nightingale owed to her family inheritance, she was even more a product of her times.   The nineteenth, often called the woman's century, was one of unexampled richness in strong personalities, insistent, inquiring minds, protest, dissent, research, discovery, and reform. The span of Miss Nightingale's days was the time of Owen and Shaftesbury; of Huxley and Darwin; of John Stuart Mill (whom she ardently admired), Mrs. Fry, Harriet Martineau, Mrs. Jameson and

[1] *Memories of Old Friends*.   Extracts from the Journal and Letters of Caroline Fox, 1883, p. 336.   By permission of the publishers, J. B. Lippincott Co., Philadelphia.

[2] *Life of Florence Nightingale*, by Ingleby Scott, in *Notes on Nursing*.   William Carter, Boston, 1860, p. 1.

Louisa Twining, George Eliot, Margaret Fuller, and the Brownings. It was the time when a whole galaxy of strong notable women began working for causes, reforms, and progress; writing, striving, and demanding to speak for emancipation and justice. As early as 1816 an article written by Catherine Coppe had appeared in the *Pamphleteer* called "On the Desirability and Utility of Ladies Visiting the Female Wards of Hospitals and Lunatic Asylums." It was a dignified appeal, very gentle, unaggressive, and touching. The writer spoke of the "debate still at issue respecting the official appointment of females to visit the apartments of those of their own sex;" of the great evil of political appointees in such institutions. She touched bravely on the jealousy of men in fearing an enlarged influence and sphere of activity for women, but mentioned two institutions, York County hospital and a lunatic asylum, where the practice of having female visitors had been established, the former in 1814 and the latter in 1815. While Miss Nightingale was investigating hospital and nursing conditions, ruling in the Crimea, and founding St. Thomas's Training School for Nurses, Mary Carpenter was toiling in Ragged Schools, Mrs. Jameson was lecturing on the "Social Employments of Women," and the "Community of Labour," and urging the opening of the great institutions of misery and poverty as schools for the training of kind-hearted, helpful women, whose energy was then wasted

for want of a vocation, and declaring the bitter
need of the inmates of hospitals, prisons, asylums,
workhouses, and reformatories, in all of which,
under the routine machine-like control of men,
the poor, the sick, and the delinquent were
suffering for the care of compassionate and
motherly women.

It was the time of the establishment of the
National Association for the Promotion of Social
Science, at whose meetings some of Miss Nightingale's epoch-making papers which, according to
Lord Brougham, were the most important ever
presented to it, were read; of the first women
pioneers in university education, medicine, and
the suffrage movement. John Stuart Mill was
writing on "Liberty" and the "Subjection of
Women," and a little later Arnold Toynbee
went to live in the East Side of London. No less
significant for the future of nursing was the fact
that, contemporaneously with the woman who
was to revolutionise this ancient calling, lived the
scientist who was to herald the change of the
whole course of medicine. Lister was studying
in the medical school while Miss Nightingale was
training herself at Kaiserswerth. Three years
after the declaration of peace following the Crimean war, when Miss Nightingale had laid her
plans for St. Thomas's Training School and all was
in readiness for it to open, Lister published his
Early Stages of Inflammation; and in 1875,
as one hospital after another was adopting the

system marked out by the skilled hands and controlling mind of Miss Nightingale for the care of patients, Lister brought out his *Theory of Fermentative Changes* which marked a new epoch in medicine and surgery. What the union of science with skilled nursing was to do for hospitals can be realised by reading some of the titles of the papers read before medical meetings just before that time: "Epidemic Erysipelas in Hospitals," "Relation between Diphtheria and Gangrene and Hospital Plague," "Alleged Greater Mortality of Fevers in Hospitals than in Homes of the Poor," "Poison Saturation of Old Hospitals." Nor, in fact, do many modern nurses know even by name the scourges which were familiar entities to the attendants in hospitals in that day.

Miss Nightingale may be regarded as a most impressive example of a human being in whom inherent genius and natural inclination were allowed the fullest development and expression. In her the true nurse seems to have been born, as well as made. Her earliest tastes inclined that way, and few of her biographers have omitted the story of Shep, the wounded collie dog. It is said that when she was a very young girl one of Pastor Fliedner's reports fell into her hands and made a deep impression on her, even making her vocation clear to her.[1] Julia Ward Howe has given an interesting glimpse of this

[1] *Life of Pastor Fliedner,* Winkworth, London, 1867. p. 128.

early desire to study nursing in the year 1844, when she and Dr. Howe were abroad. Miss Nightingale was then twenty-four years old.

Mrs. Bracebridge, in speaking to me of Florence Nightingale as a young person likely to make an exceptional record, told me that her mother rather feared this, and would have preferred the usual conventional life for her daughter. The father was a pronounced Liberal, and a Unitarian. While we were still at Atherstone, we received an invitation to pass a few days with the Nightingale family at Embley, and betook ourselves thither. We found a fine mansion of Elizabethan architecture, and a cordial reception. The family consisted of father and mother and two daughters, both born during their parents' residence in Italy, and respectively christened Parthenope and Florence, one having first seen the light in the city whose name she bore, the other in Naples.

Of the two Parthenope was the elder; she was not handsome, but was *piquante* and entertaining. Florence, the younger sister, was rather elegant than beautiful; she was tall and graceful of figure, her countenance mobile and expressive, her conversation most interesting. Having heard much of Dr. Howe as a philanthropist, she resolved to consult him upon a matter which she already had at heart. She accordingly requested him one day to meet her on the following morning, before the hour of the family breakfast. He did so, and she opened the way to the desired conference by saying, "Dr. Howe, if I should determine to study nursing, and to devote my life to that profession, do you think it would be a dreadful thing?"

"By no means," replied my husband, "I think that it would be a very good thing."

So much and no more of the conversation Dr. Howe repeated to me. We soon heard that Miss Florence was devoting herself to the study of her predilection; and when, years after this time, the Crimean War broke out, we were among the few who were not astonished at the undertaking which made her name world-famous.[1]

A similar glimpse, but of an occurrence that happened after Miss Nightingale had been at Kaiserswerth, is given by Dr. Elizabeth Blackwell, another revered figure among pioneer women, who became well acquainted with Miss Nightingale. She speaks of her as a young lady at home chafing under the restrictions that crippled her active energy, and recalls the many hours that they spent together in discussing the problems of the present and the hopes of the future. Of one of these visits, she writes in a letter to her sister, April 17, 1851:

Walked much with Florence in the delicious air . . . at Embley Park. As we walked on the lawn in front of the noble drawing-room she said: "Do you know what I always think when I look at that row of windows? I think how I should turn it into a hospital, and just how I should place the beds."[2]

[1] *Reminiscences of Julia Ward Howe.* Houghton & Mifflin, Boston, 1900. pp. 137–138.

[2] *Pioneer Work in Opening the Medical Profession to Women,* Dr. Elizabeth Blackwell. Longmans, Green, & Co., London, 1895. p. 185.

Possessing the natural gift, no one ever cultivated it more thoroughly than she. Just how much time she spent in studying hospital conditions we do not know exactly, but certainly a period of several years was devoted to a careful and systematic examination of hospitals in England, Scotland, Ireland, France, Belgium, Germany, and Italy, and to the study of nursing history, before Miss Nightingale went to Kaiserwerth to be trained as a nurse. Her own words are well worth remembering:

I would say to all young ladies who are called to any particular vocation, qualify yourselves for it as a man does for his work. Don't think you can understand it otherwise. Submit yourselves to the rules of business as men do, by which alone you can make God's business succeed, for He has never said that He will give His success to sketchy and unfinished work.[1]

Another time she wrote:

Three fourths of the whole mischief of women's lives arises from their excepting themselves from the rules of training considered needful for men.[2]

Miss Nightingale went to Kaiserswerth for three months'[3] training in 1849, and again for a shorter time (some weeks), Pastor Fliedner wrote, in 1850. Only scanty records of her stay there

[1] From an article on Kaiserswerth.

[2] From "Una," introduction to *Memorials of Agnes Elizabeth Jones*, by her sister. London, 1885. p. xxxii.

[3] From anonymous biography in *Notes on Nursing*, edition 1860.

are to be found, but personal recollections of aged Sisters have testified to the distinguished ability of the English lady. Sidney Herbert, who was later destined, as Secretary at War, to put her in charge of the Crimean military hospitals, visited her here as an old friend, saw her at work, and heard the encomiums of the Fliedners upon her work. Of Kaiserswerth, Miss Nightingale said afterwards:

I was twice in training there myself. Of course, since then hospital and district nursing have made giant strides—indeed, district nursing has been invented; but never have I met with a higher tone, a purer devotion, than there. There was no neglect. It was the more remarkable because many of the deaconesses had been only peasants; none were gentlewomen when I was there. The food was poor. No luxury but cleanliness. [1]

She next spent some time with the Sisters of St. Vincent de Paul in Paris, studying French surgery, which was famous, and the admirable method of institutional administration and management of the Sisters. It was his knowledge of her long, rigorous, and adequate training, and of the executive ability she had shown later in bringing order out of chaos in the Harley St. Home for Sick Governesses, as well as personal admiration for her as an old and intimate friend, that prompted Sidney Herbert, when the storm of war broke in the East, and the appalling break-down in the

[1] In a letter preserved in the British Museum.

hospital service became known, to write to her from the War Office urging her to go to the rescue, with the words: "There is but one person in England that I know of who would be capable of organising such a scheme."

The Crimean War had broken out in March, 1854, and with the news of the first battles had come grievous accounts of neglect and misman-agement in the medical department; Russell, the special correspondent of the *Times*, wrote on Sept. 26, 1854:

It is with feelings of surprise and anger that the public will learn that no sufficient preparations have been made for the wounded. Not only are there not sufficient surgeons—that, it might be urged, was unavoidable; not only are there no dressers and nurses —that might be a defect of system for which no one is to blame; but what will be said when it is known that there is not even linen to make bandages for the wounded—after the troops have been six months in the country, there is no preparation for the com-monest surgical operation? Not only are the men kept, in some cases, for a week without the hand of a medical man coming near their wounds; not only are they left to expire in agony, unheeded and shaken off, though catching desperately at the surgeon whenever he makes his rounds through the fetid ship, but now, when they are placed in this spacious building [the Barrack Hospital at Scutari], it is found that the commonest appliances of a British workhouse sick wards are wanting.[1]

[1] *The Times*, Oct. 12, 1854.

Two days later he wrote:

It is impossible for any one to see the melancholy sights of the last few days without feelings of surprise and indignation at the deficiencies of our medical system. The manner in which the sick and wounded have been treated is worthy only of the savages of Dahomey. Numbers arrived at Scutari without having been touched by a surgeon since they fell, pierced by Russian bullets, on the slopes of Alma. The ship was literally covered with prostrate forms, so as to be almost unmanageable. The officers could not get below to find their sextants, and the run was made at hazards.

The worst cases were placed on the upper deck, which, in a day or two, became a mass of putridity. The neglected gunshot wounds bred maggots, which crawled in every direction, infecting the food of the unhappy beings on board. The putrid animal matter caused such a stench that the officers and crew were nearly overcome, and the captain is now ill from the effects of the five days of misery. All the blankets, to the number of 1500, have been thrown overboard as useless. There are no dressers or nurses . . . Their [the French] medical arrangements are extremely good . . . they have also the help of the Sisters of Charity[1] who have accompanied the expedition in incredible numbers. We have nothing. The men must attend to each other or receive no relief at all.[2]

[1] The Russian soldiers were also attended by Sisters of Mercy. Mme. Bakounina, their head, was called the Russian Florence Nightingale. She and her staff used to go out in long boots, and carry in the wounded.

[2] *Times*, Oct. 13, 1854.

Shortly before he had written:

The sick appeared to be attended by the sick, and the dying by the dying.

Indignation and pity swept through England, and the papers were full of letters and calls for assistance. A ringing appeal for nurses, signed by "Medicus," in the *Times*,[1] said: "Why are there no female nurses? Away with this nonsense [rules of service]! there *must* be female nurses." This demand was echoed on all sides, and when Russell's impassioned appeal to the women of England was read, military red tape was swept away in an outburst of public emotion.

Are there no devoted women among us [he cried], able and willing to go forth and minister to the sick and suffering soldiers of the East in the hospitals at Scutari? Are none of the daughters of England, at this extreme hour of need, ready for such a work of mercy? France has sent forth her Sisters of Mercy unsparingly, and they are even now by the bedsides of the wounded and the dying, giving what woman's hand alone can give of comfort and relief in such awful scenes of suffering. Our soldiers have fought beside the troops of France, certainly with no inferior courage and devotedness, in one of the most sanguinary and terrific battles ever recorded. Must we fall so far below the French in self-sacrifice and devotedness in a work which Christ so signally blesses as done unto himself?—"I was sick, and ye visited Me"?[2]

[1] Oct. 14.
[2] *Times*, Oct. 14.

The response was instantaneous. The offer made by St. John's House has been mentioned. The Catholic bishop of Southwark offered to send Sisters; there were volunteers from medical students and, as in later wars, enthusiastic but undisciplined society women deluged the War Office with applications. The first practical steps seem to have been taken by Lady Maria Forrester, the daughter of an Irish nobleman, who engaged three nurses, promised to pay their expenses, and asked Miss Nightingale, on the 11th of October, if she would take them to the Crimea. Miss Nightingale consented, and wrote her historic letter asking if Mr. Herbert, then Secretary at War, would endorse and authorise their going.[1] She also asked Mrs. Herbert (her personal friend) to send word to Lady Stratford, the wife of the British Ambassador at Constantinople, that Miss Nightingale was not just a lady, but was a hospital nurse with experience.[2]

The coincidence of this letter crossing one from Mr. Herbert, begging her to go to the Crimea, is well known. He offered her the support and backing of the government, and assured her that she alone was capable of saving the situation, saying:

Would you listen to the request to go out and

[1] *Eastern Hospitals and English Nurses*, by a Lady Volunteer. Hurst & Blackett, London, 1856. 2nd edition, vol. i., pp. 4-5.
[2] *Memoirs of Sidney Herbert*, vol. i., p. 336.

supervise the whole thing? Upon your decision will depend the ultimate success or failure of the plan. Your own personal qualities, your knowledge, your power of administration, and among greater things your rank and position in society give you advantages in such a work which no other person possesses.[1]

One week after that time Miss Nightingale had her group of nurses ready to start. She gives the list as follows: 10 Roman Catholic nuns, of two different orders, one cloistered, one not; 8 Sisters of Mercy of the Church of England, of two different houses; 6 nurses from St. John's Institute; 14 nurses actually serving in different hospitals; Mrs. Bracebridge, who undertook the domestic management; Miss Nightingale, superintendent.[2] Some of the Anglican Sisters came from Miss Sellon's sisterhood.[3]

The first place to which Miss Nightingale turned to look for nurses was the institute founded by Mrs. Fry,—but the spirit of Mrs. Fry must have been for the time being absent, for the directors were not willing to accede to the very necessary

[1] Pincoffs says that this letter, which appeared in the *Daily News* of Oct. 25th, was given out by an indiscreet friend. See *Experience of a Civilian in Eastern Military Hospitals.* Peter Pincoffs, M.D. Williams & Norgate, London, 1857. p. 73. Pollard gives it in full. See *Florence Nightingale,* by Eliza F. Pollard. S.W. Partridge Co., London, 1902. pp. 74–78.

[2] In *Notes on the British Army,* p. 154.

[3] *The Times* of Oct. 30 mentions a Miss Erskine, daughter of a Welsh nobleman as a "certificated nurse" who had gone with Miss Nightingale.

condition that the nurses should be solely under Miss Nightingale's authority, and, for the time being, removed from that of their own home establishment. St. John's House had at first also objected to this, but then waived their objection. Miss Nightingale left England for the Crimea on October 21, 1854, arriving there on Nov. 4, and remained there for nearly two years, or until August 8, 1856, the date of her return to England.

Grateful recognition must ever be given to Sidney Herbert, for the daring and firmness with which he carried out the then unheard-of experiment of introducing gentlewomen as nurses into the military hospitals. Kinglake says:

He quietly yet boldly stepped out beyond his set bounds, and not only became in this hospital business the volunteer delegate of the Duke of Newcastle, but even ventured to act without always asking the overworked department of war to go through the form of supporting him by order from the Secretary of State.[1]

The official position which the government had given Miss Nightingale was Superintendent of the Nursing Staff in the East, and the title by which she eventually became known was that of the " Lady-in-Chief."

A little book of somewhat questionable relia-

[1] *The Invasion of the Crimea*, 1880, vol. vi., chapter xi., p. 409.

bility[1] quotes from the report issued by Miss Nightingale after the war to the donors of voluntary subscriptions, thus: that her "superin. tendence extended over the female nursing establishment of the Barrack and General hospitals at Scutari, of those at Koulalee, and of five general hospitals in the Crimea." It seems probable, from Sidney Herbert's letters that her supervision of the last-mentioned hospitals was, at first, more like that of a sanitary chief or general director, and not directly that of an organiser of nursing, although her authority as nursing head was finally recognised in all.

The first and chief scene of her labours was the great Barrack hospital at Scutari, which had been lent to the British Government by the Turks. It is an enormous square building, three stories high and whose corridors have a total length of four miles, and is now restored to its original use as a military barrack. The *Times* correspondent wrote of her arriving with her ladies, all dressed quietly in black, and of the hope inspired by the sight in those who watched them wend their way up from the shore. The conditions in and around the hospital were such as to defy description, though Russell, perhaps somewhat chastened by the military officials,

[1] *Autobiography of a Balaclava Nurse*, by Mrs. Elizabeth Davis, 2 vols., London, 1857. Questionable because the writer was an illiterate and egotistical person of narrow intelligence, one of the paid nurses, who had been a cook.

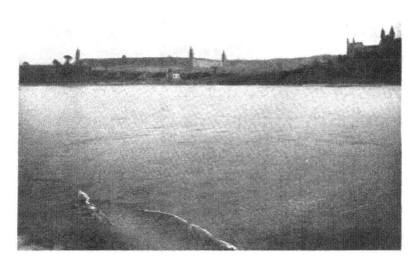

Photographed for the American Journal of Nursing
The Barrack Hospital at Scutari

now wrote rather whitewashing letters, saying
that the men were "not uncomfortable" and the
wards were "clean."[1]   But after the battle of
Alma the wounded had poured into the hospital,
their wounds still undressed, their fractures not
set, and they were half starved.   It was said that

There were no vessels for water, or utensils of any
kind; no soap, towels, or hospital clothes; the men
lying in their uniforms, stiff with gore and covered
with filth to a degree and of a kind no one could
write about; their persons covered with vermin,
which crawled about the floors and walls of
the dreadful den of dirt, pestilence, and death to
which they were consigned.   The medical men toiled
with unwearied assiduity, but their numbers were
inadequate.

This was the scene on which Miss Nightingale
entered, and, at the very time of her arrival,
the wounded were again pouring into the hospital
by the hundred.   The Rev. Sydney Osborne has
left a graphic account of the conditions with
which Miss Nightingale had to grapple on her
arrival and of the colossal indifference of the
military officials:

I arrived at Constantinople on the eighth of
November: on that or the following day we heard of
the battle of Inkerman, a transport ship having
arrived with a large number of the wounded.   The
same day that I arrived, I crossed the Bosphorus to
Scutari, and went to the general hospital, and there
presented a letter from Mr. Herbert to the superior

[1] *The Times*, Nov, 18 and 23, 1854.

medical officer, Dr. Menzies; he took me round some of the wards of that building, and to my repeated offers, either from my own or other funds, of assistance in any way in which it could be afforded I received the answer "they had everything—nothing was wanted." . . . I was not for one moment deceived by the declaration of Dr. Menzies that nothing was wanted; I have had, as my friends all know, for many years an intimate acquaintance with most matters relating to medical and surgical practice; I think I can say with truth I have followed the study of medicine and surgery for twenty years of my life, with an attention equal to that of many who do so as a matter of professional duty—a hospital and its requirements were no new thing to me.

It would only tire the general reader if I were to go, day by day, into the occurrences which, following in quick succession, soon proved to me, not only that these vast hospitals were absolutely without the commonest provision for the exigencies they had to meet, but that there was in and about the whole sphere of action an utter want of that accord amongst the authorities in each department, which alone could secure any really vigorous effort to meet the demands which the carrying on of the war was sure to make upon them. It is quite true that, as ship after ship brought down their respective cargoes of wounded and sick, the medical and other officers, with Miss Nightingale and her corps of nurses, did work from morning till night and through the night, in trying to meet the pressure upon their scanty resources; but the whole thing was a mere matter of excited, almost frenzied energy, for where so much that was necessary was absent it followed that all that zeal and labour could effect was, by various temporary expedients, to do that which when done was wholly inadequate to what was really required. I saw all the Balaclava and Inkerman wounded had to go through; I had it from the lips of the chief actors in the scene what the preparations were which awaited the wounded of "Alma." I know what the chaplain and officers had to do then; the "Sisters" had not arrived—there was no Miss Nightingale with that wonderful power to command help, the quickness to see where it would most avail. I can say with truth I am glad I have not that tale to tell. And yet I could not find that anything had been asked from Lord Redcliffe even up to the time I saw the hospital myself. Why should he have been asked for help? The chief authority was clearly under the delusion that "nothing was wanted." . . . I have never seen any accounts yet that have in their united information really given the whole truth as it might be given. I cannot conceive, as I now calmly look back on the first three weeks after the arrival of the wounded from Inkerman, how it could have been possible to have avoided a state of things too disastrous to contemplate had not Miss Nightingale been there, and had the means placed at her disposal by Mr. Macdonald [a special commissioner sent with large funds by the *Times*.] I could enumerate through a very long list article after article of absolute necessity, as a part of hospital stores, which was either not in existence, or so stored as to defy access to it. It was not merely that with the exception of a ward here and there there was no appearance of the order which one would have expected in a military hospital, supported at an almost fabulous expense;

but there was an utter absence of the commonest preparation, to carry out the very first and simplest demands in a place set apart to receive the sick and wounded of a large army. . . . I here deliberately record my conviction that not only was the Home Government grossly deceived by the information it received from the East, but that it must have been most grossly betrayed at home by those to whose several departments the proper management of the details of those hospitals was entrusted. Had Miss Nightingale and her staff taken up their post in the best regulated hospital conceivable, with four thousand patients, their task would have taxed to the utmost their every energy. Here was an utter want of all regulation; it was a mere unseemly scramble; the staff was altogether deficient in strength, the commissariat and purveying departments as weak in power as in capacity; there was no real head, and there existed on all sides a state of feeling which was inclined to resent all non-military interference; whilst at the same time it was shamefully obvious that there was no one feature of military order. Jealous of each other, jealous of every one else, with some few bright exceptions there was little encouragement from any of the officials for any one out of mere benevolence to lend any aid. The fact is, the stout denial of the shameful condition of the hospitals, made to the authorities at home, could not be made on the spot; the officials therefore walked about self-convicted. As a warm friend of the government, sent out under the direct sanction of the War Office, I am satisfied it was the wish of Miss Nightingale to make the best of everything. She at once found the real truth and cheerfully and gratefully availed herself of that help from irregular sources which to this moment has been her chief support.[1]

No one at home had a conception of the total absence of all supplies in the hospital. Sidney Herbert, knowing that tons of hospital appliances and thousands of sheets had been sent out, and confident of having foreseen every emergency, had assured Miss Nightingale that she would find everything necessary to work with. But what had actually happened was that the medical stores, for various reasons, had gone to wrong ports or were buried under shell and cannon in the hold of vessels, while the Home Office had never been apprised of their non-arrival or non-delivery.

Within ten days after she had landed Miss Nightingale had a kitchen fitted up for special diets, which supplied nourishment for nearly 1000 men,[2] and her next work was to fit up a laundry in a private house which she rented for the purpose. Lavish funds and stores had been placed at her disposal personally, and in addition the *Times* had raised a fund to be administered on the spot by Mr. Macdonald. During the first three months Miss Nightingale provided 10,000 shirts for the men, and other necessities in proportion, out of her own supplies.

[1] *Scutari and its Hospitals*, by the Hon. and Rev. Sydney Godolphine Osborn. London, 1855. pp. 2-25.
[2] *The Story of Florence Nightingale*, by Wintle. London, no date. p. 69.

All that official authority could do to make her position an effective one Sidney Herbert did. The nurses had not been asked for or wanted by the military heads at Scutari, and although, as was to be understood, Miss Nightingale and her nurses were to work "in strict subordination to the medical officers,"[1] it seems quite evident that this was meant to apply to the medical orders only. Had she been reduced to the necessity of obeying "regulations" all reformation would have been impossible. That she had large, and in some directions unhampered, powers to regenerate, to improve, and to advise seems plain. Kinglake says that the letters sent from the War Office to Scutari, though tactfully sparing the feelings of those in authority, made it quite plain that Miss Nightingale had the government behind her, and adds:

Most happily this gifted minister [Herbert] had formed a strong belief in the advantages our military hospitals would gain by accepting womanly aid, . . . and . . . whilst requesting the principal medical officer at Scutari to point out to these new auxiliaries how best they could make themselves useful, Mr. Sidney Herbert enjoined him to receive with attention and deference the counsels of the Lady-in-Chief.[2]

Probably at no time in the history of war nursing has an irresistible public opinion forced upon an unwilling military hierarchy a lady-in-

[1] Letter by Sidney Herbert, *Times*, Oct. 24.
[2] *Op. cit.*, vol. vi., chap. xi., p.

chief with such extensive authority, such dis-
cretionary powers, and well understood, though
confidential, relations with the War Office. The
fact that this was the first time in the history of
civilised nations (or, so far as we know, of the
world) that a nurse had been put into such a
position makes it especially interesting to hear
what those who were personal witnesses of her
actions in this post of unexampled difficulty have
to say of her. The Rev. Mr. Osborne has left
this description of her:

Miss Nightingale in appearance is just what you
would expect in any other well-bred woman who
may have seen perhaps rather more than thirty years
of life; her manner and countenance are prepossess-
ing, and this without the possession of positive beauty:
it is a face not easily forgotten, pleasing in its smile,
with an eye betokening great self-possession, and giving, when she wishes, a quiet look of firm determination
to every feature. Her general demeanour is quiet and
rather reserved; still I am much mistaken if she is not
gifted with a very lively sense of the ridiculous. In
conversation, she speaks on matters of business with
a grave earnestness one would not expect from her
appearance. She has evidently a mind disciplined
to restrain under the principles of the action of the
moment every feeling which would interfere with it.
She has trained herself to command and learned the
value of conciliation towards others, and constraint
over herself. I can conceive her to be a strict disciplinarian; she throws herself into a work as its
head—as such she knows well how much success

must depend upon literal obedience to her every
order. She seems to understand business thoroughly,
though to me she had the failure common to many
"heads," a too great love of management in the small
details which had better perhaps have been left to
others. Her nerve is wonderful; I have been with
her at very severe operations; she was more than
equal to the trial. She has an utter disregard of
contagion; I have known her spend hours over men
dying of cholera, or fever. The more awful to every
sense any particular case, especially if it was that of a
dying man, her slight form would be seen bending
over him, administering to his ease in every way
in her power, and seldom quitting his side until death
released him.[1]

Soyer, the French *chef*, who offered his services
in the hospitals of the Crimea, and whose entertaining book is full of homely daily allusions to
Miss Nightingale as he saw her going about her
work, describes her with French vivacity thus:

She is rather high in stature, fair in complexion, and
slim in person; her physiognomy is most pleasing;
her eyes, of a bluish tint, speak volumes, and are
always sparkling with intelligence; her mouth is small
and well formed, while her lips act in unison, and
make known the impression of her heart—one seems
the reflex of the other. Her visage, as regards expression, is very remarkable and one can almost
anticipate by it what she is about to say: alternately
with matters of the most grave import, a gentle smile
passes radiantly over her countenance, thus proving

[1] *Scutari and its Hospitals*, pp. 25-26.

her evenness of temper. At other times, when
wit or a pleasantry prevails, the heroine is lost in
the happy, good-natured smile which pervades her
face, and you recognise only the charming woman.
Her dress is generally of a greyish or black tint; she
wears a simple white cap, and often a rough apron.
In a word, her whole appearance is religiously simple
and unsophisticated. In conversation no member
of the fair sex can be more amiable and gentle than
Miss Nightingale. Removed from her arduous and
cavalier-like duties, which require the nerve of a
Hercules—and she possesses it when required—she is
Rachel on the stage in both tragedy and comedy.[1]

Macdonald, the *Times* commissioner, after his
return to England said of her:

Wherever there is disease in its most dangerous
form, and the hand of the spoiler distressingly nigh,
there is that incomparable woman sure to be seen;
her benignant presence is an influence for good comfort, even among the struggles of expiring nature.
She is a "ministering angel," without any exaggeration, in these hospitals, and as her slender form glides
quietly along each corridor every poor fellow's face
softens with gratitude at the sight of her. When all
the medical officers have retired for the night, and
silence and darkness have settled down upon those
miles of prostrate sick, she may be observed alone,
with a little lamp in her hand, making her solitary
rounds. The popular instinct was not mistaken,
which, when she had set out from England on her
mission of mercy, hailed her as a heroine; I trust she

[1] *Soyer's Culinary Campaign*, Alexis Soyer. G. Routledge,
London, 1857. pp. 153-154.

may not earn her title to a higher though sadder appellation. No one who has observed her fragile figure and delicate health can avoid misgivings lest these should fail. With the heart of a true woman, and the manners of a lady, accomplished and refined beyond most of her sex, she combines a surprising calmness of judgment and promptitude and decision of character. [1]

Ingleby Scott draws attention to two qualities of mind which no doubt might have affronted egotistical natures:

She was never resorted to for sentiment. Sentimentalists never had a chance with her. Besides that her character was too strong, and its qualities too real, for any sympathy with shallowness and egotism, she had two characteristics which might well daunt the sentimentalists—her reserve, and her capacity for ridicule . . . ; and there is perhaps nothing uttered by her, from her evidence before the Sanitary Commission for the Army to her recently-published *Notes on Nursing*, which does not disclose powers of irony which self-regardant persons may well dread. . . . The intense and exquisite humanity to the sick, underlying the glorious common-sense about affairs, and the stern insight into the weaknesses and perversions of the healthy . . . lay open a good deal of the secret of this wonderful woman's life and power. . . . We see how her minute economy and attention to the smallest details are reconcilable with the magnitude of her administration, and the comprehensiveness of her plans for hospital establish-

[1] Wintle, *op. cit.*, p. 97.

ments, and for the reduction of the national rate of mortality. As the lives of the sick hang on small things, she is as earnest about the quality of a cup of arrowroot, and the opening and shutting of doors, as about the institution of a service between the commissariat and the regimental, which shall insure an army against being starved when within reach of food. In the mind of a true nurse nothing is too great or too small to be attended to with all diligence; and therefore we have seen Florence Nightingale doing and insisting upon the right about shirts and towels, spoon-meats, and the boiling of rice, and largely aiding in reducing the mortality of the army from nineteen in the thousand to eight, in times of peace. . . . Except for the purpose of direct utility she never speaks of herself or even discloses any of her opinions, views, or feelings. This reserve is a great distinction in these days of self-exposure and descanting on personal experience.[1]

Even more discerning and graphic is Kinglake, who sets off his study of Miss Nightingale, to whom he devotes an entire chapter, with a recurring refrain of ironic "motif" against the "males." All the women, he says, were devoted; but

there was one of them—the Lady-in-Chief—who not only came armed with the special experience needed, but also was clearly transcendent in that subtle quality which gives to one human being a power of command over others. Of slender, delicate form, engaging, highly bred, in council a rapt, careful listener as long as others were speaking, and strongly

[1] Ingleby Scott, *op. cit.*, pp. 1–3.

though gently persuasive whenever speaking—the Lady-in-Chief gave her heart to this enterprise in a spirit of absolute devotion, but her sway was not quite of the kind that many in England imagined. . . . None knew better than she did that if kind, devoted attention will suffice to comfort one sufferer, it is powerless to benefit those who number thousands, unless reinforced by method, organisation, by discipline; . . . far from being a spurner of rules, she had so deep a sense of their worth as to be seemingly much more in danger of being too strict than too lax.

Her detractors said that "the soundness of judgment disclosed by the Lady-in-Chief upon questions needing rapid decision, and the apt, ready knowledge with which she always seemed armed, might be traced to the power she had over men in authority"; the theory being, it seems, that because they felt her ascendent, these officials were always longing to give her the very choicest and best of their facts and ideas.   But a simpler explanation of the abundant mental resource, at which people wondered, might be found in the keen discrimination enabling her to judge at the instant whether any of the words addressed to her should be treasured or set at naught.

And besides that her perfect knowledge of hospital business and how to conduct it:

However originating, the gift without which she could never have achieved what she did was her faculty of conquering dominion over the minds of men; and this, after all, was the force which lifted her from out the ranks of those who were only "able" to the height reached by those who are called "great." . . . The will of the males was always to go on performing

their accustomed duties—if need be, even to death
—in that groove-going state of life. . . . The will of
the woman, while stronger, flew also more straight
to the end; for what she almost fiercely sought was
. . . not to make good mere equations between official
codes of duty and official acts of obedience, but,
overcoming all obstacles, to succour, to save our
prostrate soldiery, and turn into a well-ordered
hospital the hell—the appalling hell—of the vast
barrack wards and corridors. Nature seemed, as
it were, to ordain that in such a conjuncture the all-
essential power which our cramped, over-disciplined
males had chosen to leave unexerted should pass to
one who could seize it, should pass to one who could
wield it,—should pass to the Lady-in-Chief.[1]

Mr. Macdonald, the *Times* commissioner, finding
that "nothing was wanted" by the army officials,
now turned to Miss Nightingale and worked in
conjunction with her. She had with her her
friends Mr. and Mrs. Bracebridge, the latter of
whom undertook the housekeeping, and an assistant whom we may well believe to have been
invaluable was a young man who came out from
London to "fag" for her, writing letters, running

[1] Kinglake, *op. cit.*, vol. vi., pp. 419–424. Interesting
notes are also to be found in the French histories of the
war: "This frail young woman, who was seen going on
horseback from one hospital to another, embraced in her
solicitude the sick of three armies." *La Guerre de Crimée*,
M. L. Baudens, 1858, p. 104. "There, to care for them,
a young woman, beautiful, rich, intelligent, of infinite
merit and rare distinction, Miss Florence Nightingale, had
left family, friends, and home." *Histoire de la Guerre de
Crimée*, Camille Rousset, 1877, vol. ii., p. 13.

errands, and making himself generally useful. [1]
On arrival they took up their quarters in the famous tower and the nurses were appointed to
their divisions.

Let us now follow the narrative of one of the
nurses as told by herself:

We landed at the wharf, and climbing the steep
hill found ourselves at the main guard or principal
entrance to Scutari Barrack hospital. The hospital
is an immense square building; three long corridors
run completely round it, and it is three stories high.
Numberless apartments open out of all these corridors,
which are called wards. At each corner of the building is a tower. The main guard divides A corridor;
turning to the left, after passing through one or two
divisions from which the guard rooms open, we came
to the sick.

To avoid the cold air of the long corridor, wooden
partitions were put up, and the spaces between these
were called divisions. We made our way through
the double row of sick to the tower at the corner
(Miss Nightingale's quarters); the smell in this corridor of sick was quite overpowering. . . .

On arriving in Miss Nightingale's quarters we
entered the large kitchen or hall, from which all the
other rooms opened. There were four rooms on the
lower story, occupied as follows: Mr. and Mrs. Bracebridge in one; Miss Nightingale in another; the five
nuns in the third; fourteen nurses and one lady in the
last. A staircase led up the tower to two other rooms;
the first occupied by the Sisters from Miss Sellon's
and other ladies, the second by the nurses belonging

[1] Kinglake, *op. cit.*

to St. John's training institution. The kitchen was used as Miss Nightingale's extra-diet kitchen. From this room were distributed quantities of arrowroot, sago, rice puddings, jelly, beef-tea, and lemonade, upon requisitions made by the surgeons. This caused great comings to and fro; numbers of orderlies were waiting at the door with requisitions. One of the nuns or a lady received them, and saw they were signed and countersigned, and then served them.

We used, among ourselves, to call this kitchen the tower of Babel, from the variety of languages spoken in it and the confusion. In fact, in the middle of the day everything and everybody seemed to be there: boxes, parcels, bundles of sheets, shirts, and old linen and flannels, tubs of butter, sugar, bread, kettles, saucepans, heaps of books, and of all kinds of rubbish, besides the diets which were being dispensed; then the people, ladies, nuns, nurses, orderlies, Turks, Greeks, French, and Italian servants, officers and others waiting to see Miss Nightingale; all passing to and fro, all intent upon their own business, and all speaking their own language.[1]

Mr. Osborne has also left a lively description of the nurses' tower:

Whatever of neglect may attach elsewhere, none can be imputed here. From this tower flowed that well-directed stream of untiring benevolence and charitable exertion which has been deservedly the

[1] *Eastern Hospitals and English Nurses*, by a Lady Volunteer. London, 1856, vol. i., pp. 66–69. This lady was one of the second party.

theme of so much praise. Here there has been no
idleness, no standing still, no waiting for orders
from home, no quibbling with any requisition made
upon those who so cheerfully administered the stores
at their disposal.

Entering the door into the "Sisters" tower, you
at once found yourself a spectator of a busy and
most interesting scene. . . . In the further corner,
on the right-hand side, was the entrance to the sitting-
room occupied by Miss Nightingale and her friends
the Bracebridges. I shall ever recall with the live-
liest satisfaction the many visits I paid to this apart-
ment. Here were held those councils over which
Miss Nightingale so ably presided, at which were
discussed the measures necessary to meet the daily
varying exigencies of the hospitals. From hence
were given the orders which regulated the female
staff, working under this most gifted head. This
too was the office from which were sent those many
letters to the government, to friends and supporters
at home, which told such awful tales of the sufferings
of the sick and wounded, their utter want of so many
necessities. Here might be seen the *Times* almoner,
taking down in his note-book from day to day the
list of things he was pressed to obtain which might all
with a little activity have been provided as easily by
the authorities of the hospital.

To attempt the narration of the business trans-
acted in this room would be a task beyond my powers.
It was of a nature comprehending somewhat of the
detail of every recognised "department"; it embraced
the consideration of every failure of duty on the part
of "authorities" at home and on the spot; it aimed
at the attainment of order and humanity by limited

Photographed by R. James, Montreal

Miss Nightingale Making her Night Rounds

Barrett, 1861

means, to be directed against the widest possible field of disorganisation.[1]

Let us continue the narrative of the Lady Volunteer:

Two days after my arrival, Miss Nightingale sent for me to go with her round the hospital. (Miss Nightingale generally visited her special cases at night.) We went round the whole of the second story, into many of the wards and into one of the upper corridors. It seemed an endless walk, and it was one not easily forgotten. As we slowly passed along the silence was profound; very seldom did a moan or cry from those multitudes of deeply suffering ones fall on our ears. A dim light burned here and there. Miss Nightingale carried her lantern, which she would set down before she bent over any of the patients. I much admired Miss Nightingale's manner to the men—it was so tender and kind.

All the corridors were thickly lined with beds laid on low trestles raised a few inches from the ground. In the wards a divan runs round the room, and on this were laid the straw beds, and the sufferers on them. The hospital was crowded to its fullest extent. The building has since been reckoned to hold with comfort seventeen hundred men; it then held between three and four thousand. Miss Nightingale assigned me my work—it was half A corridor, the whole of B, half C, the whole of I (on the third story), and all the wards leading out of these respective corridors; in each corridor there were fifteen of these, except in No. I, where there were only six. This work I was to share with another lady and one

¹ *Scutari and its Hospitals*, pp. 23–24.

nurse. The number of patients under our charge was, as far as I could reckon, about fifteen hundred.

Miss Nightingale told us only to attend to those in the divisions of those surgeons who wished for our services. She said the staff surgeon of the division was willing we should work under him, and she charged us never to do anything for the patients without the leave of the doctors. . . .

It seems simply impossible to describe Scutari hospital at this time. Far abler pens have tried and all in some measure failed; for what an eye-witness saw was past description. Even those who read the harrowing accounts in the *Times* and elsewhere could not have imagined the full horror of the reality. As we passed the corridors we asked ourselves if it was a terrible dream. When we woke in the morning, our hearts sank down at the thought of the woe we must witness that day. At night we lay down wearied beyond expression; but not so much from physical fatigue, though that was great, as from the sickness of heart from living amidst that mass of hopeless suffering. On all sides prevailed the utmost confusion; whose fault it was I cannot tell—clear heads have tried to discover in vain: probably the blame should have been shared by all the departments of the hospital. . . .

We could not get the assistant surgeons to write out the number of the requisitions which were necessary in order to procure these materials. At last some of us persuaded one or two of our surgeons to write a requisition for dry stores; that is, for tins of preserved beef-tea, and for lemons and sugar to make lemonade. . . . One difficulty only remained, *i. e.*, hot water. It was of course necessary to make the beef-tea, and also for the lemonade, as the water was so unwholesome it could not be used without boiling. We contrived to boil water in small quantities on the stoves in the corridors and wards. It was a slow process, but still we succeeded. . . .

Our plan of thus helping the men was put a stop to by an order from Dr. Cumming, the inspector-general, that no cooking was to be done in the wards, and thus our only means of assisting the men was ended.

We seldom dressed the wounds, as there were dressers who performed this office, and the greater number of patients were cases of fever and dysentery, who needed constant attention and nourishment, frequently administered, in small quantities, and this we were now not suffered to give. All the diets not issued from Miss Nightingale's kitchen were of such a bad quality, and so wretchedly cooked, that the men often could not eat them. After a man had been put on half or even full diet, the surgeons were often obliged to return him to spoon diet from his not being able to eat the meat.

It was very hard work after Dr. Cumming's order had been issued to pace the corridor and hear perhaps the low voice of a fever patient, "Give me a drink for the love of God!" and have none to give—for water we dared not give to any; or to see the look of disappointment on the faces of those to whom we had been accustomed to give the beef-tea. The assistant surgeons were very sorry, they said, for the alteration but they had no power to help it—their duty was only to obey. On one occasion an assistant surgeon told us that Dr. Cumming had threatened to arrest him for having allowed a man too many extras on the diet roll. Amid all the confusion and distress of Scutari hospital, military discipline was never lost sight of, and an infringement of one of its smallest observances was worse than letting twenty men die from neglect. . . . The want of clean linen was bitterly felt at that time in Scutari. How it was issued from the stores was a mystery no one could ever unravel. If things were sent to be washed they never returned, and there was not the slightest order or regularity in the issue of linen, either sheets or shirts. Towels and pocket-handkerchiefs were both considered unnecessary luxuries for the soldiers, and could be obtained only from Miss Nightingale's free-gift store, and, generally speaking, only from them could flannel shirts be had. . . .

Confusion, indeed, so prevailed in all quarters at that unhappy time that though quantities of things were sent to Scutari but few ever reached the sufferers for whom they were destined. Every ship that came in brought to Miss Nightingale large packages of every imaginable article of wearing apparel. . . . It was a common thing to find men with sheets and shirts unchanged for weeks. I have opened a collar of a patient's shirt and found it literally lined with vermin. It was common to find men covered with sores from lying in one position on the hard straw beds and coarse sheets, and there were no pillows to put under them. . . .

A great deal of sickness prevailed among ourselves; two nurses at this time were lying ill with fever, one not expected to live; two of the five nuns were in the same state—they both lay for days at the point of death, but ultimately recovered. During the whole of their illness they remained in the room where the three other Sisters slept and ate. There was no infirmary to remove the sick ladies to. The sick nurses were taken to a room outside the hospital. Of course among ladies and nurses not ill with fever many were laid up for a day or two at a time from over-fatigue and want of proper food.

Our life was a laborious one: we had to sweep our own rooms, make our beds, wash up our dishes, etc.; and fetch our meals from the kitchen below. We went to our wards at nine, returned at two, went up at three (unless we went out for a walk, which we had permission to do at this hour), returned at half-past five to tea, then to the wards again till half-past nine, and often again for an hour to our special cases. . . . We suffered greatly for want of proper food. Our diet consisted of the coarse sour bread of the country, tea without milk, butter so rancid we could not touch it, and very bad meat and porter; and at night a glass of wine or brandy. . . .

The quantity of vermin in the wards was past conception; the men's clothes and beds swarmed with them, so did every room in the hospital. Our clothes had their full share, and the misery they caused us was very great; we never slept more than an hour at a time because of them.[1]

By Christmas-time cleanliness, order, suitable food and clothing had transformed the wards of the General and the Barrack hospitals; but, though easy-going critics now pronounced them to be in perfect condition, Miss Nightingale was burdened with the heaviest anxiety, for the state of the

[1] *Eastern Hospitals*, etc., vol. i., pp. 69–94.

buildings as regards arrangements for the disposal of sewage was so hideous that it can only be
described in technicalities.   There was, in fact,
no drainage, no plumbing; there were almost no
sanitary conveniences.   It had all been known in
time to have been remedied.   It was not remedied,
and the patients sent to the hospitals were sent to
death traps.   Miss Nightingale states: _"The
deaths on cases treated were no less than 315 per
1000, or nearly one in three." [1]

It was the knowledge of this criminal neglect,
this official murder, that compelled Miss Nightingale to war single-handed, except for Sidney Herbert's support, against the bureaucracy of the
army medical, sanitary, and engineering staffs.
It was her urgent reports and her itemised statements and demands, says Kinglake, that finally
brought about the undertaking of extensive
sanitary engineering works, which were completed
in June, 1855, when the death rate fell to "22 per
1000 on cases treated" (Miss Nightingale's words),
and he hints strongly that even in the very word-
ing of the directions which came out from the
War Office, and especially in the mandates to
speed and celerity, there was a minuteness of
detail which suggested the personal share of the
Lady-in-Chief therein.

[1] *Notes on Matters affecting the Health, Efficiency, and
Hospital Administration of the British Army*, by Florence
Nightingale. Presented by Request to the Secretary of
State for War. Harrison & Sons, London, 1858. Preface,
sec. 1, p. xxvi.

This tragic winter of 1854–55 saw what Kinglake calls an interesting trial of brain power and speed between the woman at work and the "males" in power. At the same time that the nurses sailed Parliament appointed a commission to go out to the Crimea and investigate the conditions. With the greatest celerity in transportation, and allowing for no delays, it could only have reported back to Parliament in thirteen weeks, whereas by Christmas Miss Nightingale had a fairly good system running. The commission set forth with no powers to do aught but report, but acting on a letter from Miss Nightingale Sidney Herbert wrote to them to take steps on the spot to have deficiencies corrected. They only received this order in time to begin making recommendations on the 22nd or 23rd of January—and this for the troops only; their report from Scutari was forwarded about the 23rd of February, reaching London about the 29th of March, in time for the ministers to get their orders out for the late spring, three or four months (says Kinglake) after Sir George Brown (at the outset hostile to Miss Nightingale) saw perfection in the hospital wards, and ascribed it to womanly energies.

Thus sorrily lagged the males [he concludes] in their undesigned trial of speed and power with what proved to be not only the swifter, not only the more agile mind, but also the higher capacity for executive business, and even the more intent will.[1]

[1] Kinglake, *op. cit.*, vol. vi., pp. 443–445.

After her return from the Crimea Miss Nightingale gave testimony before a royal commission, in which she outlined a working plan of organisation for military hospitals and briefly pointed out the radical defects then obtaining as follows: [1]

In the military general hospitals, as they are now constituted, the governing power is wanting which by its superior authority can compel the co-ordinate departments within the hospital to the complete co-ordination necessary for success. [She compares the naval hospitals, where there is one head, and continues:] One executive, responsible head, it seems to me, is what is wanted in a general hospital, call him governor, commandant, or what you will, and let it be his sole command.

The departments should not be many:

1. A governor, solely responsible for everything except medical treatment.

2. A principal medical officer, and his staff, relieved of all administrative duties and strictly professional.

3. A steward who should fulfil the duties of purveyor, commissary, and barrackmaster, and supply everything, subject to the governor.

4. A treasurer, who should be banker and paymaster.

5. A superintendent of hospital attendants, who should undertake the direction of cooking, washing,

[1] *The Sanitary Condition of the Army*; A Report of the Commission appointed to inquire into the Regulations affecting the Sanitary Conditions of the Army, the organisation of Military Hospitals, the treatment of the Sick and Wounded. Presented to both houses of Parliament by command of her Majesty. London, 1858. *Westminster Review*, Jan., 1859.

care of hospital furniture, and government of orderlies. All of these officers to be appointed at home by the War Department. According to this plan the government would culminate the functions of quarter-master-general and adjutant-general and, under the advice of a sanitary officer attached to him for that purpose, would be solely responsible for carrying out the works advised and for engaging the requisite labour. With regard to the mode of supply let the steward furnish the hospital according to a fixed scale previously agreed upon.

With regard to food let the steward make contracts subject to the governor's approval, and with power to buy in the markets at the contractor's expense if the contractor fails. A scheme of diets should be constructed, according to the most approved authorities, in order to save the cumbrous machinery of extra diet rolls. Equivalents might be laid down, so as to afford the necessary choice, dependent on the nature of the climate, the season of the year, the state of the market, the produce of the country, etc.

This schedule shows in brief, and her remarkable monograph on the British army in detail, the lamentable absence of all intelligent foresight which made the Crimean calamities so spectacular. Common-sense was stifled in routine and regulations; these, in turn, were fossilised by professional jealousy, timorousness, and selfishness. This shines out clearly from all the testimony given later before the commission, and is thrown into even stronger relief by apologists, while the experiences of later wars have reduplicated all

of Miss Nightingale's accusations, and verified
her warnings.

Her letter of Jan. 8th, to Sidney Herbert [1]
shows a masterly grasp of the whole cause and
root of the disorganisation, and is of peculiar
interest both as a study of her graphic, vivid, and
concise mode of expression and of her mental
keenness. It is indeed a "terrible letter," for the
truth was terrible. Its sentences are like flashes
of lightning. Stanmore from his library com-
plains that it is exaggerated and mischievous,
thus provoking the inference that he had forgotten to refer to even so much of the official testimony as Miss Nightingale quotes in the *Notes.*
One of its opening paragraphs sets forth very
strikingly the moral cowardice and supineness of
the men in charge:

The Commission has done nothing. . . . Cumming has done nothing. Lord William Paulet has
done nothing. Lord Stratford, absorbed in politics,
does not know the circumstances. Lord William
Paulet knows them but partially. Menzies knows
them and will not tell them. Wreford knows them
and is stupefied. The medical officers, if they were
to betray them, would have it reported personally
and professionally to their (dis)advantage. . . .

. . . You will say that I ought to have reported
these things before. But I did not wish to be made
a spy. I thought it better if the remedy could be
brought quietly, and I thought the Commission was

[1] *Memoirs of Sidney Herbert*, vol. i., pp. 393–396.

to bring it. But matters are worse than they were two months ago. . . .[1]

After the war was over and Miss Nightingale had returned to England the question of how to remedy the evils of which she had become cognisant absorbed her mind and energy for a long time. She took a keen interest in the appointment of the Royal Commission to investigate the Sanitary State of the Army, of which Sidney Herbert was appointed chairman, and, perceiving well that powerful interests would endeavour to delay and mutilate the Commissioners' findings, she urged Sidney Herbert not to accept the chairmanship without receiving a definite pledge that the recommendations of the Commission should be acted upon. She wrote to him:

All that Lord Panmure has hitherto done (and it is just six months since I came home) has been to gain time, and this Commission, I hold it, granting it only as he does *now*, is also merely to gain time.

He has broken his most solemn promises to Dr. Sutherland, to me, and to the Crimean Commission, and three months from this day I publish my experience of the Crimean campaign, and my suggestions for improvement, unless there has been a fair and tangible pledge by that time for reform.[2]

In this connection it is of interest to note Queen Victoria's comment on Miss Nightingale, after the war, in a personal letter to the Duke of Cambridge:

[1] *Memoirs*, vol. i., p. 393.
[2] *Ibid.*, vol. ii., p. 123.

We have made Miss Nightingale's acquaintance [she wrote] and are delighted and very much struck by her great gentleness and simplicity, and wonderful, clear, and comprehensive head. I wish we had her at the War Office.

We return now to Scutari, where the nursing service experienced one of the haphazard methods of the War Office. It had been arranged for that reinforcements of nurses should be sent out if needed, but only on Miss Nightingale's "autograph request." [1] The Lady Volunteer writes of the later nursing staff:

Their selection was left in the hands of Mrs. Sidney Herbert, Miss Stanley, sister of Dean Stanley, and Miss Jones, Superintendent of St. John's House. As a test of qualifications of the applicants, it was agreed that, with few exceptions, all should go through training at some of the London hospitals, and to facilitate this, St. John's House and St. Saviour's home were opened to receive probationers, and latterly a third institution was established for the same purpose under the patronage of the Earl of Shaftesbury. [2]

In some unexplained way, a second party of forty-six was sent out in charge of Miss Stanley in December, 1855, not only without Miss Nightingale's "autograph request," but even without her knowledge, until they were on the way.   But

[1] Her own words in *Notes on the British Army*, p. 154, showing Stanmore to be inaccurate in his account of this incident.

[2] *Op. cit.*, vol. i., pp. 9–10.

this was not all. Not only were the nurses de-
spatched without inquiring whether they could be
quartered and assigned to duty, but, to complete
the blunder, they were consigned to Dr. Cumming (who, as many indications would appear to
show, was by no means friendly), and *not* to the
Lady-in-Chief.[1]

It is unnecessary to point out the unsystematic
character of this proceeding, and, remembering the
regular correspondence between Miss Nightingale
and Mr. Herbert, it seems quite inexplicable,
unless it was that the problems of the nursing
department were lost in the titanic proportions .
of the general mismanagement.

No one at this distance can estimate properly
the dangers and difficulties surrounding Miss
Nightingale and her nurses in this at that time
new and untried position, nor may it be wondered at that this action disturbed and annoyed her.

As Miss Nightingale's own story of those days
has never been told, nor her letters published, the
few extracts from them presented with carp-
ing criticism by Sidney Herbert's biographer in
relation to this incident cannot be considered
as affording definite or final information, nor,
without the ability to show her side of the story,
does it even seem worth while to discuss them.

Miss Stanley and her nurses were halted at
Therapia, puzzled enough at the delay. They

[1] *Memoirs of Sidney Herbert*, vol. i., p. 372.

were told to take up their abode in an empty house, which, however, Miss Stanley succeeded, before nightfall, in furnishing. It had been her intention to return immediately to England after landing the nurses, but now, seeing that difficulties were before them, she decided to remain with them. Three days afterward she went to Scutari to see Miss Nightingale, whom she writes of as "dear Flo."

I went through a door [she wrote home], and there sat dear Flo writing on a small unpainted deal table. I never saw her looking better. She had on her black merino, trimmed with black velvet, clean linen collar and cuffs, apron, white cap with a black handkerchief tied over it. . . . I was quite satisfied with my welcome. . . . [1]

Although Miss Stanley then learned the whole state of things, it has not been made known to the public. Her letter shows perplexity and concern. The inference is clear that, in order to resist the undermining of her legitimate authority, and, possibly, to expose intrigue, Miss Nightingale was fearless enough to declare her determination to resign rather than remain under conditions which would fetter her.

The crisis passed. Sidney Herbert would not hear of resignation; loyally (and properly) took upon himself the blame of the unannounced party of nurses, and after a month's delay they were distributed among the various hospitals.

[1] *Memoirs*, vol. i., p. 374.

Miss Stanley remained with them for six months, and, though of delicate health and without any experience in nursing, gave invaluable service in supervising and chaperoning them, and in overcoming prejudice and opposition.

This second party consisted of fifteen Roman Catholic nuns, nine lady volunteers, and twenty-two nurses. Miss Nightingale has left the following allusion to the nursing staff.

It [the party] was followed by numerous additions during the year 1855, and the female nursing establishment was only broken up with the return of the army in July 1856, the Superintendent leaving finally on July 28, 1856. During this period a great number had returned home from sickness and other causes. Nine died.[1]

That the responsibility of the nursing staff was a heavy one may be learned from the Lady Volunteer, who writes on this point:

There was one great trouble which we began to feel at this time—namely, the conduct of the hired nurses. We had indeed been tried by this from the beginning, and several, as I have mentioned, were sent home for bad conduct; but still the distress around them and the frequent sickness among their own numbers kept some sort of check among them, and after some had been dismissed for bad conduct, and others from sickness, only two remained when the new party arrived on April 9th.

The hospital costume in which Miss Stanley's

---

[1] *Notes on the British Army*, p. 155.

party left England was worn alike by ladies and
nurses, which was intended to mark the equality
system, but soon after beginning hospital work we
found it impossible to continue wearing the same
dress as the nurses, and therefore discontinued it. . . .

The ladies soon found it necessary for their own
comfort and for the good of their work that in every
possible way the distinction should be drawn. None
but those who knew it can imagine the wearing
anxiety and the bitter humiliation the charge of the
hired nurses brought upon us, for it should be remembered that we stood as a small body of English
women in a foreign country, and that we were so far
a community that the act of one disgraced all. . . .
On April the 21st, a second party of three ladies and
seven nurses joined us. . . .

A few weeks only had elapsed since the departure
of the two women I have mentioned, when disgraceful
misconduct caused the dismissal of a third. Ere a
passage could be had for her another was obliged to
go, from her habits of intoxication, and she had been
one most highly recommended. . . .

Our trials were not ended. A similar case of bad
conduct obliged the dismissal of one whom we had
looked upon as one of our best nurses. Another
was found intoxicated in the wards; these two went;
and so till, out of twenty-one, in less than eight
months we had eleven left. To our profound aston-
ishment we found that our sending home so many
gave great umbrage to the authorities. . . . They
thought fit to send a reproof, demanding more par-
ticulars of the cases. . . .

They were respectfully reminded that our superintendent's duties did not include the reformation of

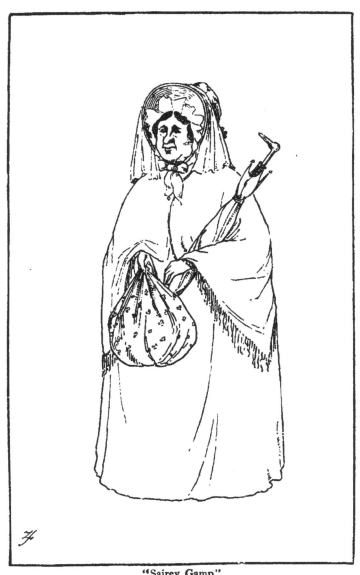

"Sairey Gamp"
A nurse of sixty years ago

By permission from Wellcome's *Professional Nurse's Diary*. Borroughs, Wellcome &
Co., 1907-8

women of loose character and immoral habits, nor did we imagine the authorities would require details which were often too terrible to dwell on.

Of the remaining nine two were very unsatisfactory.

Six were respectful and industrious, and under a lady's supervision did very well, but not a single one except Mrs. Woodward could be trusted alone.

The light conduct of another of the hired nurses, even at this time of distress, obliged her dismissal.

. . . After some days she recovered, was sent home, and I believe is now a nurse in a London hospital.[1]

What with the inexperience of the ladies and the unreliability of the paid nurses, the nursing was chiefly confided to the hands of the Sisters of Mercy, whose rigorous training stood them in good stead, and whose talents for system and management were of primary importance. They were indefatigably seconded by the lady volunteers, and bore the brunt of difficulties in the General hospital of Scutari, and in that at Koulalee, whose lady superintendent, after Miss Stanley left, was Miss Emily Hutton. This hospital came to be considered a model. The Lady Volunteer writes:

The Mother had four Sisters, two ladies, and two nurses to assist her. She had long experience in hospital work, and possessed a skill and judgment in nursing attained by few. This hospital from first to last was admirably managed. When the means of improvement were placed in her hands, they were

---

[1] *Op. cit.*, vol. ii., pp. 13–20.

judiciously used, and the hospital so improved that it became the admiration of all who visited it, and the pride of the ladies and nurses who worked in it; we used to call it "the model hospital of the East."

Miss Nightingale has left eloquent and heartfelt tributes to the Sisters, for many of whom she entertained affection and regard.

The army orderlies, as every nurse may imagine, were at first a most trying class, but they appear to have developed under the influence of the ladies, better than the paid nurses. Miss Nightingale inspired them, as she did the soldiers, with a chivalrous devotion, and there were no bounds to the services they would do for her. She herself said of them:

And here, homely and sickening as is the subject [she had been describing the revolting duties that she had been compelled to require them to perform, and, indeed, to assist them in], I must pay my tribute to the instinctive delicacy, the ready attention of orderlies and patients during all that dreadful period: for my sake, they performed offices of this kind which they neither would for the sake of discipline, nor for that of the importance of their own health. . . . And never one word nor one look which a gentleman would not have used; and while paying this humble tribute to humble courtesy, the tears come into my eyes, as I think how, amidst scenes of horrible filth, of loathsome disease and death, there arose above it all the innate dignity, gentleness and chivalry of the men (for never, surely, was chivalry so strikingly exemplified) shining in the midst of what must be considered as the lowest sinks of human misery, and preventing, instinctively, the use of one expression which could distress a gentlewoman.[1]

In the other hospitals the same was said. The Lady Volunteer wrote:

Without their [the ladies'] superintendence, they [the orderlies] were an idle, useless set of men, callous to the suffering of those around them, not trying to learn their business, which was of course new to them, and regardless of carrying out the doctor's orders, when they could do so without getting into disgrace; but under the Sisters' and ladies' hands they became an excellent set of nurses, forming that class of men-nurses of course essential in a military hospital.

. . . The orderlies at Balaclava had been a troublesome set, unaccustomed to habits of cleanliness and order; reforms were now introduced and carried out; encouragement from the Sisters and their gentle manners did much more good in teaching the orderlies than all the blame they had previously received. Just at this time, the corps of civil orderlies, reported to be already trained to undertake nursing, arrived from England. They landed at Scutari and were soon dispersed among the other hospitals. They all wore a uniform dress of blue smocks, and were pronounced by the soldiers to be "a set of butchers."

Not the least of Miss Nightingale's brilliant achievements in the Crimea was the social and relief work she did there, which Pincoffs among earlier biographers has given in more detail than

[1] From *Notes on the British Army*, pp. 93–94.

others but to which we can only make the briefest
reference: the care of the wives who had followed
their husbands, and of the little new-born children; the establishment of reading-rooms, amusements and lectures for the men; of a café at
Inkerman to draw the men away from the can-
teen; of the enormous personally conducted
correspondence with the wives and families at
home, and of the extemporised money order office
in her rooms at Scutari, where she took in the
men's pay for transmission home, sending thus
to the families in England about £1000 every
month.   This work of hers was later taken over
by the government.

In May Miss Nightingale made a tour of inspection of the hospitals of Balaclava, and while
there suffered an acute attack of Crimean fever.
She was nursed through it by Mrs. Roberts and
returned to Scutari, weak but undiscouraged,
about a month after leaving it.   The many in-
tensely interesting details of her tours among the
hospitals, of which a number are related by Soyer,
her later return there and her life in the little hut,
while superintending the arrangements of the
army of occupation, as well as the later events in
the hospitals at Scutari, must be passed over,
and the reader referred to the pages of her
biographies.

We shall now quote from Miss Nightingale's
own summary of the work of the nursing staff:

. . . Quarters and rations were assigned to them

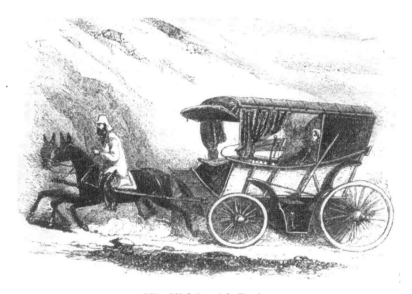

Miss Nightingale's Carriage

"The extraordinary exertions Miss Nightingale imposed upon herself after receiving this carriage would have been perfectly incredible, if not witnessed by many. I can vouch for the fact, having frequently accompanied her to the hospitals as well as to the monastery. The return from these places at night was a very dangerous experiment, as the road led across a very uneven country. It was still more perilous when snow was upon the ground. I have seen that lady stand for hours at the top of a bleak rocky mountain near the hospitals, giving her instructions, while the snow was falling heavily. All one could say to her on the subject was so kindly received, that you concluded you had persuaded her to take more care of herself. Yet she always went on in the same way, having probably forgotten good advice in her anxiety for the comfort of the sick.

"I often warned her of the danger she incurred in returning so late at night, with no other escort than the driver. She answered by a smile, which seemed to say, 'You may be right, but I have faith.'"—SOYER, *op. cit.* pp. 418, 419

within the Barrack hospital, at Scutari, . . . and Miss Nightingale was furnished with Instructions.

It was not until March, 1856, that Miss Nightingale was put individually into General Orders. But no General Order has ever existed defining the duties of the nurses, in the various hospitals to which they were respectively attached.

This will indicate how ill-defined the position of the nurses was, and how easily their control and discipline might have been usurped by the military officials had not Miss Nightingale been strong and able enough to insist on retaining her power.

In the civil hospitals of Smyrna and Renkioi the number was fixed before leaving home, together with that of those serving in other departments. With regard to Miss Nightingale's first party, the number admitted into the Barrack and General hospitals, Scutari, was fixed by arrangement with the respective principal medical officer of those hospitals.

But, nevertheless, the number admitted into each division depended upon the medical officer of that division, who sometimes accepted them, sometimes refused them, sometimes accepted them after they had been refused; while the duties they were permitted to perform varied according to the will of each individual medical officer, and each one successively, and according to the amount of occupation of medical officers and orderlies, and according to the estimation in which each individual nurse was held by each individual medical officer.

With regard to extra diets, medical comforts, and

"free gifts" nothing was given by the nurses, except by the order of the superintendent, which order was consequent upon the requisition of a medical officer and that only, with some few exceptions.   .   .   .

The principle introduced by Dr. Meyer in the civil hospital at Smyrna—and afterwards carried out in that of Renkioi—was, that a certain number of ladies should have the superintendence of a certain number of paid nurses. This did not interfere with the action of the male orderlies, except by reducing their labour and their number. In each case the females were distinctly under the direction of the medical officers and had more or less charge of the extra diets. . . .

Immediately upon the arrival of the nurses at Scutari in November, extra diets were prepared by them for the patients, in the stoves which they had brought with them. . . . In the Crimea, extra-diet kitchens were organised in the General hospital, in February, 1855; and at the Castle hospital, Balaclava, in April 1855; *i.e.* as soon as female attendance was incorporated into each respectively. . . .

A portion of the materials for the extra diets at the Barrack hospital, Scutari, and also in the Crimea, was found by Miss Nightingale's funds; on some occasions because the supplies in the purveyor's store had run short; on others, because they were of bad quality; on others, again, because the purveyor declined to furnish the articles of food (although on the diet rolls of the medical officers), which Miss Nightingale then purchased in the open market.

The second purveyor-in-chief, in May, 1855, placed the whole of the linen and small stores for the wards, arranged under divisions, under the care of the nurses as far as regarded the Barrack hospital, Scutari. In November, 1855, they assumed the same charge, on a somewhat different footing, in the General hospital; but in the Crimea it was arranged that the mass of linen should be sent down to Scutari to be washed. Where women form part of a hospital establishment the charge of the linen should evidently devolve upon them.

In conclusion, it should be recorded that the three periods when the Female Department gave the greatest proofs of their utility were: first, on the arrival of the wounded from Inkerman, at Scutari, Nov. 9, 1854, and during the subsequent months when the army suffered most from sickness up to April 1855. After that time, a great many officials of every department were added to the hospitals at Scutari, a great decrease of sick and wounded took place there, owing to the improved health of the army and the development of hospitals in the Crimea, and a considerable accession of stores had arrived. The second period of their usefulness was during the heavy summer work of nursing the wounded in the Castle hospital, Balaclava, 1855, and the third, when, in the spring of 1856, in consequence of great sickness among the Land Transport Corps, there was a pressure upon the two general hospitals for that corps organised near Karani in the Crimea by the excellent Principal Medical Officer, Dr. Taylor.

Any one who has well considered the subject of nurses and hospitals . . . will probably come to the conclusion that, when the nursing is applied not to civil but to military hospitals, the mode of nursing by orderlies, who perform also the drudgery of hospital servants, should by no means be done away with.

To take anything from the authority of the medical officers, or to reduce their responsibility, would never be contemplated by any one con/inced of the paramount importance of the promptitude of action resulting from unity of government. It remains, therefore, that female nursing, while entirely subordinated to the medical authority, should not be charged with the mere drudgery in the necessary cleansing and labour of a military hospital, but should be made capable of performing what may be termed "skilled" nursing, by a course of previous instruction, and should add to the niceties of female attendance, which have been found so grateful to the patient in all civil hospitals and in domestic life, a moral influence which has now been proved, beyond all doubt, to be highly beneficial to the soldier.

Although, from the great difficulties presented by the diversity of character of those who went out first and of those who subsequently followed during the whole of the campaign, a stumbling block was added to the many difficulties at the very threshold of the undertaking, yet nevertheless the withdrawal from the work of those who, from time to time, showed themselves incompetent, and the recognised system of discipline introduced, brought the corps of female nurses into such a condition as to enable them to continue the work throughout the campaign. . . .

Discipline, founded on actual efficiency in the service, and without respect of persons, was immediately adopted, and this necessarily occasioned the sending home of those who proved incompetent. . . .

A primary principle of discipline was, that no interference with the regulation of the hospital, or

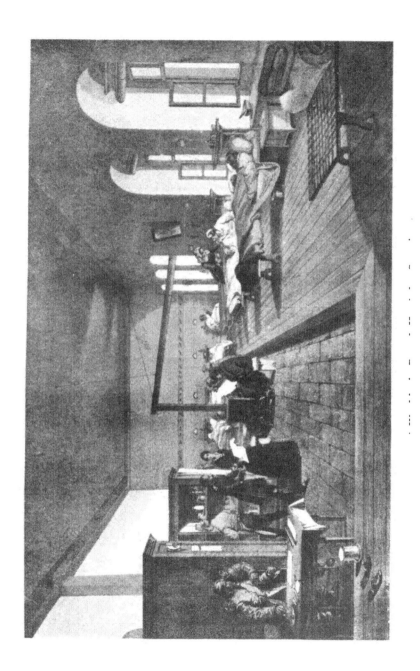

with the legitimate orders of the medical officers, should take place. . . .

Upon the foregoing principles the nurses in some cases performed larger duties, in assisting the surgeons, than in others, according to the orders of the particular medical officer. The system of requisition by a medical officer was also accepted and acted upon by Miss Nightingale, who answered the requisition of surgeons, both for extra diets, medical comforts, and necessaries. [1]

After peace was declared, Miss Nightingale saw all the hospitals of the Crimea closed one by one; stopped at Scutari and closed the Barrack hospital—with what emotions one may imagine—and returned to England, reaching home in August, 1856.

That Miss Nightingale could hold such a positon as hers in the Crimea without incurring enmity is naturally not to be expected. As a matter of history, she did encounter every variety of antagonism which might be expected to-day in such work, and another beside, fortunately less common now than then — the antagonism of sectarian intolerance. In reading the history of social movements in the first half of the last century, it is strikingly evident that doctrinal jealousies and animosities were often fatal obstacles to the improvement of pitiful or even shocking social conditions; and it was with only

[1] *Notes on the British Army*, pp. 152–163. (In these reports Miss Nightingale always speaks of herself in the third person.)

too much reason that Sidney Herbert had stated, in a public letter, that the hospitals should not be used as "the arena of hostile efforts directed by rival creeds one against the other.[1]   Miss Nightingale with her whole family belonged to that serener circle which rose above narrow sectarian prejudice.   Her heart went out equally to Mrs. Fry the Quaker, Pastor Fliedner the Lutheran, and the Catholic Sisters of Mercy, but the buzzing of intolerance must sometimes have risen to her ears.   Lady Byron once wrote: "I hope you have traced the course of Florence Nightingale.   She has placed women in the right position, as head of the *humane* department. . . . The enmity towards her appears from various testimonials to be increased, but she smiles at it all—an angel smile."   Dean Stanley in a letter said: "In this nurse business there is no question that the rabid Protestant party have shown by far the greatest incapacity for tolerating anything beyond their own infinitely little minds"; and he then related how his sister was stopped one day in the hospital by the chaplain, who complained of having found a copy of Keble's *Christian Year* in the wards.   The next Sunday, in the presence of Miss Stanley and her nurses, this chaplain preached against herself and them as "creeping in unawares." [2]   Mr. Osborne wrote of Miss Nightingale: "I have heard and read with indignation

[1] *The Times,* Oct. 24, 1854.
[2] *Life and Letters of Dean Stanley,* vol. i., p. 492.

the remarks hazarded upon her religious character.
I found her myself to be in every word and action
a Christian; I thought this quite enough. It
would have been in my opinion the most cruel
impertinence to scrutinise her words and acts to
discover to which of the many bodies of true
Christians she belonged." The Sisters of Mercy
have recorded the warning letters they received
from the War Office, inspired, as they felt, by some
of the Protestant clergy, and reminding them that
they were only nurses, and that St. Paul had said
women were not to teach or preach. But "millions of tracts" most offensive to Catholics were
distributed among the Catholic soldiers, and the
Sisters found them in every supply of clothing
sent out of England.[1]

Sister Mary Aloysius, who possessed a great
fund of humour, described vivaciously the merri-
ment caused in the nursing staff by ponderously
solemn warnings against popery in the English
papers.

As a result of one tirade, the Sisters named Miss
Nightingale "Your Holiness" and she in turn
called one of them always "the Cardinal." [2]

Besides religious suspicion it seems probable
that the racial enmity of Celt for English inspired
some unfriendly acts; such was perhaps the source
of certain medical antagonisms and of the petty

[1] *A Sister of Mercy's Memories of the Crimea*, Sister Mary
Aloysius, Burns & Oates, London, 1904, p. 41.
[2] *Ibid.*, p. 89.

refusal of hospital officials at Balaclava to allow Miss Nightingale to put up a tent which she had made to shelter the convalescents from the glaring sun; and the same motive is irresistibly suggested by the otherwise inexplicable animosity of a volume published in recent years.[1]

Trouble with some too zealous Sisters is also hinted at in Sidney Herbert's letters.[2] It was a period when religious enthusiasts of all beliefs were keen to proselytise. Whether the Sisters actually broke rules in this respect or not, their own chronicles show that the interest was close to their hearts, and in the midst of hardships and toil they found time to prophesy that Lady Herbert and Miss Stanley would become Catholics, as they did.[3]

How far military and medical jealousy went no one but Miss Nightingale herself can tell. Kinglake says that the military commander Sir George Brown and his successor, Lord William Paulet were warm in her praise and cordially assented when the War Minister wrote: "You will find her most valuable—her counsels are admirable suggestions." Lord Raglan, the Commander-in-chief, spoke of her as an auxiliary general, and gave her, according to Kinglake, frank and cordial support. With him she kept up

[1] *Leaves from the Annals of a Sister of Mercy.* By a Member of the Order. New York, Catholic Pub. Society, 1885.

[2] *Memoirs*, vol. i., pp. 412, 417.

[3] *Leaves from the Annals*, etc. Vol. ii., pp. 157, 161, 163.

a constant interchange of official communications and he visited her in her tent when she had fever. It was naturally the bureaucratic underlings, and those who resented her authority, who disliked her most—the red-tape men, whose dense mediocrity was too rudely shocked by her electric intelligence. The hard-working ward surgeons, and all of those who were trying to do their duty, regarded her as a powerful support. Kinglake says that the overworked and harassed surgeons used her name as a menace when the red-tape men were too intolerable, and were wont to threaten them effectively with the anger of the Lady-in-Chief.

Pincoffs, who has left one of the best accounts of her, and who, as a civilian physician, had small love for his military brothers, tells how the junior medical officers and orderlies of one division had been instructed that "the less they had to do with Miss Nightingale and her people the better it would be for them." [1] (He also records that a splendid dissecting room was built, liberally provided with numerous and excellent instruments, microscopes, chemical apparatus, etc. by the government, at her suggestion.) [2]

It was the red-tape officials who complained that she used to hasten to get her stores out first "for fear" that the supplies would come through the regular channels; that she did not give them

[1] *Op. cit.*, p. 80.
[2] *Ibid.*, p. 55.

"time" ("it was always more time the males wanted," says Kinglake); and these were the men whose feelings were outraged when she commanded the orderlies, on an historic occasion, to break in the door of the storerooms and distribute supplies for which the patients were suffering. (Nolan says that the authorities used to lock up her private stores to make it seem as if they were not needed.) [1] Naturally, too, the incompetent purveyor, Wreford, who was unable to buy anything in Stamboul where there were ample markets, must have disliked her thoroughly.[2]

It is intimated in Sidney Herbert's letters that she must have had serious difficulties with two of the medical officers.   One of these was Dr. Hall, and it is obvious on reading the *Notes on the British Army* that the difficulty here arose from the incompatibility of ineptitude and genius.   The calibre of Dr. Hall is shown in the official correspondence summed up by Miss Nightingale in her *Notes*: on March 12 he wrote to the London office a series of optimistic inaccuracies about the health of the army, and said:

A system of detraction has been commenced against our establishments and has been kept up by interested parties, under the garb of philanthropy.

[1] *The Illustrated History of the War with Russia*, E. H. Nolan Ph.D., LL.D., J. S. Virtue, London, 1857, p. 710.
[2] On this, hypercriticism could scarcely go further than Lord Stanmore's peevish query as to whether she told this purveyor where he could buy. *Memoirs*, vol. i., p. 381.

Some of these detractors, he adds, have become so, "*to regain lost moral reputation, and others to make their mission of importance, and they wish the world to believe that all the ameliorations in our institutions are entirely owing either to their own exertions or those of a few nurses;* and I am sorry to say some of our own department have pandered to this and have been rewarded for it." [1]

Another interesting example of ingenious evasion was the testimony given by Dr. Menzies before the House of Commons committee as to a raw mutton chop having been given to a patient. The explanation given by the purveyor (again Mr. Wreford) was that Miss Nightingale and her nurses took up so much room and time in the general kitchen that the cooks could not do their work. The testimony of the cook himself afterwards proved that "Miss Nightingale and her nurses never set foot in the general kitchen." [2]

Still another misrepresentation, which Miss Nightingale records, is contained in remarks in a letter from Lord Paulet to Lord Panmure in April, 1855, in which he refers to Miss Nightingale's "extensive establishment" as making great extra work, and also remarks that he has "continual applications from the ladies and nurses for extra expenses." [3]

She follows this with exact figures about her sources of private funds and their use which

[1] *Notes on the British Army*, preface to sec. i, pp. xxiv.–xxv. The italics are ours.

[2] *Ibid.*, p. 363.

[3] *Ibid.*, preface to sec. iii, p. xii.

prove the second statement to have been entirely false, and of the former, remarks:

> Miss Nightingale's "extensive establishment," consisting of 40 women, was housed in the Barrack hospital in the same space which, in corresponding quarters, was occupied by three medical officers and their servants, and in about the same space as was occupied by the Commandant. This was done in order to make no pressure for room on an already overcrowded hospital. It could not have been done with justice to the women's health, had not Miss Nightingale later taken a house in Scutari at private expense, to which every nurse attacked with fever was removed.[1]

But, annoying as these incidents may have been at the time, they were swept away in the flood of the devotion of the army, and public gratitude and recognition, which rose to a height rarely known, and remained deep and steadfast with a loyalty seldom equalled. After the labours of the Crimean War were over there were some who felt aggrieved, or perhaps it would be better to say wounded, that where so many had equally striven and borne hardship and unspeakable difficulties, equally braving death and equally risking parting from home and friends, the whole passion of recognition, gratitude, and praise of the English nation should be poured at the feet of one nurse—Miss Nightingale.

Dr. South in a printed pamphlet regretted the

[1] *Notes* on the British Army, pref., sec. iii, xxxii., xxxiii.

absence of any public recognition of the services
of Mrs. Roberts, whom he considered to have been
more experienced and skilled in surgical nursing
than any one in the Crimea. No doubt the friends
and supporters of the other volunteer gentlewomen on the nursing staff may also have felt
that they too should have been more publicly
recognised; especially those who had held super-
visory positions, as Miss Emily Hutton, who was
the lady superintendent of the Koulalee hospital,
or Miss Weare, who had charge of still another,
or Miss Stanley, who showed high devotion and an
exquisite spirit.[1] And the friends of the Sisters
of Mercy, whose endurance and unfailing cheerfulness under hardship had excited the admiration of all who saw them, may have felt the same
thing, for Cardinal Wiseman, in a public sermon,
had said:[2] "It must have been a source of pain
to Roman Catholics that no manifestation of
feeling had ever been witnessed toward them [the
Sisters] while charity that had sprung up suddenly in the world had been honoured by royal
praise and commemorated by lasting monuments."

But the actual significance of the unexampled
homage offered to Miss Nightingale was not
grasped by any one of these critics,—not by Dr.
South, and not by Cardinal Wiseman. From

[1] See her article *Ten Days in the Crimea : A Reminiscence.*
Macmillan's Magazine, Feb., 1862.

[2] Quoted in letter of Emily Hutton, in *Memories of the
Crimea*, by Sister Mary Aloysius, p. 77.

their standpoint they were right; but the truth, vaguely apprehended if not defined by the English people and by thousands of observers in other lands, was that with Miss Nightingale's entrance on the scene there had risen a new ideal and a new estimate of nursing and its possibilities. Gone forever, from the time when she applied her intellect to the problems of the Crimea, was the conception of nursing as a charity, exceedingly meritorious and deserving of the heavenly reward for its self-sacrificing character. The self-sacrifice remained, but under her sway nursing shone forth as a part of the invincible and glorious advance of science; sanitary science, the science of health, first, and of disease only secondarily. Not pity alone, but prevention foremost; not only the amelioration but the reduction of suffering, was now typified in the personality of this woman not only as a possibility, but a positive policy for future generations. As her far-famed little lamp dissipated the gloom of the long corridors at Scutari, so her genius banished old mists of stupidity, misconception, and long-settled customs in the realms of thought.

Sickness, through so many centuries regarded as divine vengeance for "original sin"—fear-inspiring and mysterious—what does she say of it?

Sickness or disease is Nature's way of getting rid of the effects of conditions which have interfered with health. It is Nature's attempt to cure.

And of nursing, long regarded by the devout as the hardest of sacrifices, and by the laity as an occupation inexpressibly low and repugnant?

Nursing is putting us in the best possible condition for Nature to restore or to preserve health, to prevent or to cure disease or injury, . . . to enable Nature to set up her restorative processes; to expel the intruder disturbing her rules of health and life. . . . Partly, perhaps mainly, upon nursing must depend whether Nature succeeds or fails in her attempt to cure by sickness. Nursing is therefore to help the patient to live. Nursing is an art, and an art requiring an organised practical and scientific training. For nursing is the skilled servant of medicine, surgery, and hygiene.[1]

And what says she of the nurse's attitude toward life? For many centuries it had been a favorite dogma of churchmen that an inclination to such work defied the normal human interest and sympathies and could only be based on some transcendental or supernatural motive. But hear her:

I give a quarter of a century's European experience when I say that the happiest people, the fondest of their occupation, the most thankful for their lives, are, in my opinion, those engaged in sick-nursing. It is a mere abuse of words to represent the life, as is done by some, as a sacrifice and a martyrdom. But there have been martyrs in it. The founders and pioneers of almost everything that is best must be martyrs. But these are the last ever to think themselves so.[2]

[1] Article on *Nursing the Sick* from *Quain's Dictionary of Medicine*, Edition of 1894.

[2] Introd. to *Life of Agnes Jones*, pp. xxx-xxxi.

CHAPTER IV

THE NIGHTINGALE SCHOOL FOR NURSES AT ST. THOMAS'S HOSPITAL

THE desire of the British people to offer Miss Nightingale a testimonial had been expressed at a public meeting held at Willis's Rooms, on November 29, 1855. She must long have cherished the wish to found a training school for nurses; for her friends the Sidney Herberts, when consulted as to the form the testimonial might take, were able from their intimate knowledge of her to advise that the one thing she would be willing to accept would be the means of founding such a school. The Duke of Cambridge presided at the meeting and the distinguished company present represented the progressive and freer minds rather than those of any strict or rigid tenets. The bishops of the Church were mostly absent; but Dean Stanley was there; Gladstone sent a letter of apology; Sir James Clark, M.D., Mr. C. Locock, M.D., Mr. H. Bence Jones, M.D., and Mr. W. Bowman of the Royal College of Surgeons were mentioned in the list of those present. The Duke of Cambridge, after stating the object of the meeting, suggested that the offering of the people be raised with a view of establishing a system of nurses under Miss Nightingale's immediate control, and that she should be left unfettered to select her own council. The Marquis of Lansdowne in seconding said:

One of the most useful lessons of the war would be the permanent improvement in the duty of attending the sick and wounded soldiers, as the part taken by the ladies of the country in organising and inspiring that improvement would be among its most glorious reminiscences. . . . [He moved] that the noble exertions of Miss Nightingale and her associates in the hospitals of the East and the valuable services rendered by them to the sick and wounded of the British forces demand the grateful recognition of the British people.

Sir James Pakington proposed a resolution that funds be raised to "enable her to establish an institution for the training, sustenance, and protection of nurses and hospital attendants."

Sir James Clark, for the medical profession, said that he had had the pleasure of being acquainted with Miss Nightingale for many years. Long before the war was thought of he had known her to watch day and night by the bedsides of the sick, and knowing the beauty and goodness of her character it was with no common feelings of admiration he had watched her career in the East. He did not doubt the noble exertions of Miss

Nightingale would prove a permanent blessing to the whole country.

Mr. Sidney Herbert spoke earnestly and to the point. He urged leaving her free to direct her school, for "in her we have a woman of genius." He told of having visited her at Kaiserswerth, of what he had heard from the Fliedners of her great ability; he had no hesitation in saying that during the course of the war Miss Nightingale had exhibited greater powers of organisation, a greater familiarity with details, with a comprehensive view of the general bearings of the subject, than had marked the conduct of any one connected with the hospitals during the war. He told some anecdotes gathered from the soldiers,—how they kissed her shadow as it fell on them:

She would speak to one and another, and nod and smile to as many more, but she could n't do it to all, you know, for we lay there by the hundreds, but we would kiss her shadow as it fell and lay back on our pillows content. [And how one said] before she came there was such cussin' and swearin', but after that it was as holy as a church.

And the meeting ended with great enthusiasm.[1]

In January, 1856, while still in the Crimea, Miss Nightingale had replied to a letter embodying the proposals of the testimonial committee:

Exposed as I am to be misinterpreted and mis-

[1] *The Times*, Nov. 30, 1855.

A number of other public meetings, equally successful, were held in different parts of Great Britain. See *Report of the Committee of the Nightingale Fund*. London, 1856.

understood in a field of action in which the work is new, complicated, and distant from many who sit in judgment on it, it is indeed an abiding support to have such sympathy and such appreciation brought home to me in the midst of labours and difficulties all but overpowering. I must add, however, that my present work is such as I would never desert for any other, as long as I see room to believe that what I may do here is unfinished. May I, then, beg you to express to the committee that I accept their proposal, provided I may do so on their understanding of this great uncertainty as to when it will be possible for me to carry it out.[1]

A pleasing detail, which nurses as a rule do not know, was that the soldiers themselves contributed over £4000 to the Nightingale fund. The military secretary, writing from headquarters in 1856, said:

. . . The subscription has been the result of voluntary individual offerings, and plainly indicates the universal feeling of gratitude which exists among the troops engaged in the Crimea for the care bestowed upon, the relief administered to, themselves and their comrades, at the period of their greatest sufferings, by the skilful arrangements, the unwearying, constant, personal attention of Miss Nightingale and the other ladies associated with her. . . .[2]

When, after Miss Nightingale's return from the Crimea, it was, after a few years of waiting, made evident that her health would not permit her to

[1] Wintle, *op. cit.*, p. 121.
[2] *Ibid.*, p. 122.

direct in person the promised school for nurses, the responsibility was placed in the hands of a committee, and St. Thomas's hospital selected as the place to try the experiment. Dr. Blackwell refers to this period of her life in a letter written to her sister in 1859.

Have just returned from an interview with Miss Nightingale in relation to a school for nurses which she wishes to establish. My old friend's health is failing from the pressure of mental labour. I can't go into the details of her last five years now, but the labour has been and is immense. I think I have never known a woman labour as she has done. It is a most remarkable experience. She indeed deserves the name of a worker. Of course we conversed very earnestly about the numerous plans in which she wished to interest me. She thinks her own health will never permit her to carry out her plan herself and I much fear she is right in this belief.[1]

The new school was not established without much hostile comment and criticism. Flippant society ladies, like Lady Pam, thought the Nightingale fund

great humbug. . . . The nurses are very good now,

[1] *Pioneer Work in Opening the Medical Profession to Women*, Longmans, Green & Co., pp. 217, 218. As, after her return from the Crimea, Miss Nightingale had fought almost single-handed, except for Sidney Herbert's help, the battle to overturn the antiquated but strongly intrenched machinery which had nearly destroyed the British army, those who know the cost at which such work is done may readily conjecture that Dr. Blackwell's remark may have referred to this as the drain on Miss Nightingale's health.

though perhaps they do drink a little, but so do the ladies' monthly nurses, and nothing can be better than them; poor people, it must be so tiresome sitting up all night, and if they do drink a little too much they are turned away and others got!

Strange as it may seem, the majority of the medical men of the day appear to have been, if not distinctly unfriendly, at least far from cordial supporters of the proposed plan, and those who had been directly concerned with the management of the nurses under the old system regarded the new one as a sort of an affront. Such, at least, was the assertion of Dr. South, who wrote a pamphlet adverse to the projected Nightingale school. Dr. South was senior surgeon at St. Thomas's hospital. He was probably quite of the old school, liked to have his nurses on the plane of domestic servants, was patronising and kindly disposed to those who served him, and not too exacting in his own requirements. He was very loyal to Mrs. Roberts, who had been Sister in his wards for over twenty years, and felt some chagrin that she had not received more popular applause for her share of the toils and reforms of the Crimea. His arguments are worth reviewing, because they show so plainly what a different idea was present at that time in the average medical mind of what nursing really might mean, and how little he actually understood of what Miss Nightingale wanted to do. He defended the old-fashioned nursing system as excellent and satisfactory; warmly defended the character and conduct of the Sisters[1] (barely mentioning, however, the servant-nurses, with whom he probably did not come in contact); and gave an account of the work of the nurses and Sisters and the way they were trained.

The training of the Sisters and the general control of the nursing work had been entirely in the hands of the medical staff.   This is an important point to notice, and it was, no doubt, reason enough for the resentment felt by medical men at the proposed change.   The Sisters were not taught by the matron, but by the surgeons and physicians.   They were, however, taken first into the matron's office, and by errands and by substituting in the wards they gradually learned the hospital ways.   They were then put on probation in the wards and were trained into their duties by the physicians.   The terms "nurse" and "wardmaid" were synonymous, and either nurse or Sister might be called upon to remain on duty all night after a day of fourteen hours, during which time, the writer adds incidentally, they "rarely" sat down for five min-

[1] The superior rank of the Sister had been emphasised in 1699, by an ordinance that only the wives of freemen should be appointed Sisters.   In the year 1752 the degradation of hospital work is indicated by an attempt of the governors to change the name "Sister" to "Nurse," and that of nurse to "helper," but custom was too strong and the use of the familiar terms continued. *An Historical Account of St. Thomas's Hospital.*   Benj. Golding, London, 1819, p. 207.

utes." He then considered the proposed meeting
at Willis's Rooms to promote Miss Nightingale's
plan for teaching nurses, and declared that the
proposed school was quite unnecessary and super-
fluous; that statements made as to the nursing
inefficiency and bad conditions in hospitals were
offensive and untrue; that Sidney Herbert's
words, "It was hoped that through Miss Nightingale's proposition nursing would be raised to a
pitch of efficiency never known before," were not
founded on fact—that hospital nursing was not
only efficient but was satisfactory to all the physicians and surgeons.

That this proposed hospital-nurse training-school
scheme has not met with the approbation or support
of the medical profession is beyond all doubt [he
wrote]. Among the signers of subscriptions to the
Nightingale Fund, out of ninety-four physicians and
seventy-nine surgeons from the seventeen hospitals
of London, only three physicians and one surgeon from
one hospital, and one physician from a second, are
found among the supporters of the scheme.

(But the patients were not asked what they
thought of it.) This, to his mind, is proof that
the existing nursing in hospitals was as near as
possible to being what it should be, and sufficient
cause for a natural resentment over attacks made
by persons who had no knowledge of the subject.
He proves, further, that there was no need of more
women for private duty, since St. John's House
and the Institute for Training Nurses (Mrs. Fry's)

were filling the whole field and doing all that was required. He then quoted the following critic- ism on English hospitals, which is taken from the pamphlet on Kaiserswerth written by Miss Nightingale, though he did not appear to know the authorship:

We see [it ran], as every one conversant with hospitals knows, a school, it may almost be said, for immorality and impropriety—inevitable where women of bad character are admitted as nurses, to become worse by their contact with the male patients and young surgeons; inevitable where the nurses have to perform every office in the male wards, which it is undesirable to exact from women of good character —how much more, from those of bad?—inevitable where the examination of females must take place before a school of medical students. We see the nurses drinking, we see the neglect at night owing to their falling asleep.

This pamphlet was printed without Miss Night- ingale's name, and Dr. South's unconsciousness of its source is rather amusing when he says that he does not pretend to know where "he or she" got this information; that it is entirely untrue as regards the nurses and a gross libel on the young surgeons; adding that he "fears the writer has fallen into very bad medical company"! How different was his standard of nursing from Miss Nightingale's can be estimated by com- paring her luminous definition "Nursing is helping the patient to live" with his amiable offhand definition of the duties of the ward nurses:

As regards the nurses or wardmaids, these are in much the same position as housemaids and require little teaching beyond that of poultice-making, which is easily acquired, the enforcement of cleanliness, and attention to the patients' wants.

The nurses need not, he thinks, be of the same class required for Sisters, nor have the same responsibilities, nor do they often stay more than one year or two in the wards. But what became of them then, or if they went out to private duty, he does not ask.[1]

In spite of individual doubts and disapproval, and with the encouragement of the more enlightened members of society,[2] the Nightingale school was opened with fifteen probationers on June 15, 1860, a date for many reasons, and from varied standpoints, the most memorable in the history of nursing. For now was established a set of principles distinctly new or of new ap-

[1] *Facts Relating to Hospital Nurses*, J. F. South. London, 1857.

[2] Mrs. Jameson, who was somewhat in advance of the ideas of her own day, wrote thus: " It is an undertaking wholly new to our English customs, much at variance with the usual education given to women in this country. If it succeeds, it will be the true, the lasting glory of Florence Nightingale, and her band of devoted assistants, that they have broken down a 'Chinese wall' of prejudices, religious, social, professional, and have established a precedent which will indeed multiply the good to all time." Wintle, *op. cit.*, p. 58.

plication to nursing orders. Most significant and
radical was the recognition of science as the supreme authority in the education of the nurse.
No other conflicting authority was henceforth to
separate her path from that of advancing medical
knowledge. With this, as an inevitable corollary,
was the complete secularisation of her calling;
this, combined with a respectable, or it might be
even distinguished, social position, set her free
for enlarged possibilities of usefulness. No less
far-reaching was the tacit rejection of the ancient
corner-stone of poverty, so long held essential for
the nurse, which had, more than anything else,
kept her bound, uneducated, and passive. However partially and experimentally, the new system
started on the direction following which she was
enabled rapidly to gain the basis on which all
other progress rests, that of economic independence. Nursing now ceased to be a penance, a
self-sacrifice, or a merit ensuring a high place
in the next world, and was firmly established as
an honourable, if laborious, means of earning one's
livelihood.

The magnificent plan of the Nightingale school
was that it should above all else prepare women
to go into the hospitals and infirmaries and there
carry on further the work of nursing reformation
and teaching, and this plan has been triumphantly
carried out. The Nightingale probationers, as
they were called, were not trained to be private
duty nurses, as those of the earliest English or-

ganisations had been, but were preëminently encouraged to become pioneers, teachers, and regenerators in hospital management and nursing systems, and St. Thomas's has never had a private nursing department.

As vacancies occurred in the regular staff of the hospital they were filled by Nightingale nurses, so that, eventually, the old style of ward nurse was replaced by the new. It would probably be impossible to record all the hospitals that were regenerated by the Nightingale nurses; the committee preferred, when possible, to send a group under one recognised head to initiate reform in other institutions. This was done in the case of the Royal Infirmary and the great Workhouse Infirmary at Liverpool, the Royal Infirmary at Edinburgh, and a number of other less well known but not less important infirmaries. Important hospitals in Ireland, such as Sir Patrick Dun's, colonial hospitals, such as the infirmary in Sydney and the General hospital at Montreal, obtained their first trained heads from St. Thomas's, as did also St. Bartholomew's; and the Empress Victoria of Germany, then Crown Princess of Prussia, sent Fräulein Fuhrmann, who afterwards developed the Victoria House or training school for nurses in Berlin, to St. Thomas's for her preliminary experience. The War Office recognised Miss Nightingale's work by selecting a superintendent of nurses for the Royal Hospital at Netley in 1869, with a staff of nurses to work under her. Miss Alice Fisher, who regenerated Blockley hospital, was a Nightingale nurse, and Miss Linda Richards, the pioneer nurse of the United States, enjoyed the advantages of post-graduate work in St. Thomas's and of Miss Nightingale's personal, kindly interest and encouragement.

Though later on newer schools, beginning more easily where this had to break the ground, first equalled it and then, for a time, out-distanced it, none can ever forget its debt to this, the mother school, the first one at once secular, non-sectarian, soundly organised, adequate in its hospital facilities, and based on teaching. The head nurses were paid by the Nightingale fund for teaching the probationers, the matron was paid for superintending them, and the medical instructor for his services in lecturing to them. Having been at the outset a most radical and daring innovation, the Nightingale school thereafter went steadily on its way, becoming, in time, conservative through so doing, while the forces it had released to action turned to successive innovations and advanced to fresh revolutions, with which it was not always in sympathy.

The weak point (as it seems now to us, though it must be noted that this is not universally agreed to among superintendents, especially in England, where a superior type of woman is found in domestic service) in the composition of the early English schools was their inheritance and continuation in modified form of the servant-nurse,

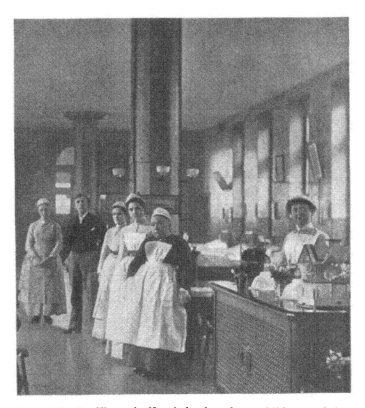

A ward in St. Thomas's Hospital, after the establishment of the training school. One of the old-time nurses in the foreground

though it would have been hard not to accept and
continue to some extent a class distinction which
was ingrained in the social order and had so long
characterised the hospital service under both
lay and religious governing bodies.   Kaiserswerth
had ignored all class distinctions, and so had Mrs.
Fry's Institute, but caste had reappeared in the later
German organisations, and in the nursing orders
of the Anglican Church.   It would perhaps have
been impossible then, at one step, to secure only
probationers who were of the class of gentlewomen
in sufficient numbers to carry on all the work of
the hospitals.   It seems to have been tacitly understood in those early days that private duty
nurses, at least, must be recruited largely from
among those of a lower social grade.   This was
not regarded with disfavour, but rather the contrary, and some English matrons still hold it advisable.   Miss Nightingale's writings in several
places indicate this general view, and she has left
comparisons between the relative advantages of
domestic service and nursing, showing that the
same women might choose to go into either one
or the other.   Though in the school the lower
social class was not prevented from rising to the
superior posts, if fitness was demonstrated, yet
the social difference was not lost sight of, and the
terms "lady nurse," "lady probationer," and "servant class" are found on every page of English
nursing history even late into the present time.
As a result, the nurses of Great Britain have con-

stituted a vertical instead of a transverse section of society. This has been from one standpoint an advantage, for there have always been women of the highest education and social class at the top, to take hospital positions, district nursing work, army nursing work, and to direct and organise; with a plain, mediocre body beneath them to do the routine hard work. But it has been a disadvantage from another point of view, for it has definitely hindered intelligent and loyal organisation among the nurses themselves (this, in effect, has only developed in recent years and since a rising entrance standard has tended to exclude an uneducated class) and so has clogged the feet of the more public-spirited members of the nursing profession, who, early discerning the higher views of intelligent citizenship as obligations of a trained body of workers, have not ceased to aspire to a higher educational and industrial plane.

The greater natural dependence of this class may have been one reason why the earliest English schools after St. Thomas's established their own private duty homes, where their nurses, after completion of their hospital service, were expected and encouraged to remain as were the deaconesses in their motherhouses, or the nurses of the Continental Red Cross societies in their associations, actually a part of the outfit of the institution, to be rented out as one rents utilities. Precarious, then, were their opportunities of receiving calls or hospital positions if they established themselves

independently, for such a thing as the "co-opera-
tive" or alumnæ registry was then unknown.
While they remained in the service of the hospital
they received a salary, while their earnings went
to the institution. This system, an inheritance
bequeathed by the old monastic systems, had the
advantages of the monastery—*i.e.*, security of
home and support, and release from the necessity
of seeking employment. These were strong points,
for, though work is dignified and worthy, it is often
hard and humiliating to look for work. But the
dignity and corporate wealth of the monastery,
with its ample provision for old age, were gone,
and in the average secular institution this system
too often brought in its train a dependent old age,
insufficiently provided for by hospital pensions
and charity. Had it become an enduring system
the condition of nurses would eventually have been
little better in England than on the Continent.
But, it may again be emphasised, in the '60's and
'70's it would hardly have been possible to go
further and emancipate the nurses completely from
the old form, and had they been turned loose into
the world, as is the modern nurse, training schools
would probably have lost the confidence of the
public. We know from Miss Nightingale's writings that she approved keeping the certificated
nurse under the guardianship of her school, chiefly
on the ground that she might always have a home
where she would be under good influence and be
secured from the disintegrating effects of a nomad

existence. For Miss Nightingale herself, it is
without question that only the purest and highest
moral and ethical standards underlay her strong
conviction of the necessity for the nurse's thus living in a home under close permanent tutelage of
her school, but we may think that she has over-
idealised the benefits of private nursing institutions under autocratic control and underestimated
the value of free association on a self-governing
basis.

To the extent to which the Nightingale school
retained the older and more military ideas in this
respect, it has been out of sympathy with the later
development of complete organic separation of the
graduate from her school, and her evolution into
organised self-governing associations.

The reason for the selection of St. Thomas's as a
training field, was to be found in the character and
personality of a very notable woman and self-
trained nurse, little known even to many of her
contemporaries, and whose name to-day would
convey no meaning whatever to the great army
of modern young nurses—so little has the important work which she did for nursing been
remembered,—Mrs. Wardroper, the matron of the
hospital. In the early 50's, Mrs. Wardroper, a
woman of refinement, having been left responsible
for the care of a little family, applied for the post
of Sister or head of a ward in St. Thomas's hospital, and, through the interest of some of the
authorities who knew her, received the post,

though she knew nothing whatever of hospital life. The conditions already often referred to were the rule in the hospital, for the days of Sairey Gamp were in full swing; but in a remarkably short time Mrs. Wardroper instituted a surprising degree of order and cleanliness, as well as sobriety. The committee, seeing and appreciating the improvements she made, gradually gave her more power, until finally she had all the wards under her supervision, and was given the post of matron. Although regular training was not then thought of, yet her selection of candidates for the positions of nurses, her discipline and influence, system and intelligence in the care of patients were such that when the Council of the Nightingale Fund visited the different London hospitals, with a view of making a selection for the new school, St. Thomas's under Mrs. Wardroper's rule was found to be the best managed and most suitable, not including those under the care of Anglican Sisterhoods.[1]

Although no biography of Mrs. Wardroper has been written, there are many nurses who remember her well, some of whom have given little glimpses of her personality. Thus Miss Richards has recalled her dignity, and her habit of always wearing black kid gloves on duty, and the ease with which she wrote with them on. Miss Isla Stewart, the present matron of St. Bartholomew's hospital, has told of the feelings of awe with which she contemplated Mrs. Ward-

[1] From private sources through Miss Diana Kimber.

roper when, one time, visiting the hospital with her father, they had some occasion for conversation, and Miss Stewart wondered how her father could be so self-possessed while talking to a woman in such an exalted position, who seemed little less august than the Queen herself.   Mrs. Strong in 1901 wrote:

For Mrs. Wardroper I would like to say one word. The single-handed combat which she undertook with the general bad condition and the ignorance which prevailed at that time in the nursing world, was being nobly fought when Miss Nightingale, in search of a hospital wherein to establish a school for the training of nurses, came upon and recognised the good work being done by Mrs. Wardroper and chose St. Thomas's hospital as the centre of her operations.[1]

Mrs. Wardroper remained the head of the Nightingale school for many years, and Miss Nightingale herself has left the following memorial, which gives an inimitable picture of her:

One has passed away without noise, without crown or sceptre of martyrdom, who was the pioneer of hospital nursing—the first lay hospital matron, at least of a great public hospital—who was a gentlewoman. Her kingdom was that of the sick.   No public-press heroine was she, yet the countless sick will bless her name though they never heard it; and she opened a new calling for women of all classes, the nursing institutions for the poor.   She did this, a great work, for her country and her sovereign—thrice blessed to

[1] "The Preparatory Instruction of Nurses," *Transactions, Third International Congress of Nurses*, Buffalo, 1901.

those for whom it initiated a divine life of common-
sense in nursing. No Mrs. Gamp could live in her
neighbourhood; Mrs. Gamp was extinct forever. She
was soon gladly acknowledged by the doctors as their
chief in nursing. She led a hard life, but never pro-
claimed it. What she did was done silently. No
herald chanted her praises.

The state of what was by ignorance called nursing when she began hospital work, with the miserable
state, morally and technically, of the nurse, would
scarcely now be credited. Did one who knew it
attempt to describe it, she would be by a universal
jury of her fellows found guilty of exaggeration. . . .

I saw her first in October, 1854, when the expedition
of nurses was sent to the Crimean War. She had been
then nine months matron of the great hospital in
London of which for thirty-three years she remained
head and reformer of the nursing. Training was
then unknown; the only nurse worthy of the name
that could be given to that expedition, though several
were supplied, was a "Sister" who had been pensioned
some time before, and who proved invaluable. I
saw her next after the conclusion of the Crimean
War. She had already made her mark: she had
weeded out the inefficient, morally and technically;
she had obtained better women as nurses; she had
put her finger on some of the most flagrant blots,
such as the night nursing, and where she laid her
finger the blot was diminished as far as possible, but
no training had yet been thought of.

All this led to her being chosen to carry out, in the
hospital of which she was matron, the aim in the training of nurses of the Nightingale Fund which had then
been subscribed. She was named first superinten-

dent of the school, and continued such for 27 years, until her retirement in 1887. That school under her has been more or less the model of all the subsequent nurse training schools, of which now nearly every considerable hospital, and many an inconsiderable, has its own, but they chiefly train for themselves; she, as head of the Nightingale school, trained for many other hospitals and infirmaries.

The principles of this school may be shortly said to be as follows: (1) That nurses should have their technical training in hospitals specially organised for this purpose. (2) That they should live in a "home" fit to form their moral life and discipline. The school under this lady was opened at the old St. Thomas's, near London Bridge, in 1860. St. Thomas's and the Nightingale school were removed to the Surrey Gardens in 1862, and in 1870 to their present abode opposite the houses of Parliament. . . . At the time of her retirement upward of 500 nurses had completed their training and entered into service on the staff of St. Thomas's or other hospitals, and of these over 50 educated gentlewomen were occupying important posts as matrons or superintendents of nurses in hospitals, infirmaries, and nursing institutions for the poor, and not only in the United Kingdom, but also abroad.

It is difficult to describe the character of such a woman—the more so as her praises were never sounded in newspaper or book. . . . Her power of organisation or administration, her courage, and discrimination in character, were alike remarkable. She was straightforward, true, upright. She was decided. Her judgment of character came by intuition, at a flash, not the result of much weighing and consideration; yet she rarely made a mistake, and she would take the greatest pains in her written delineations of character required for record, writing them again and again in order to be perfectly just, not smart or clever, but they were in excellent language. She was free from self-consciousness: nothing artificial about her. "She did nothing because she was being looked at, and abstained from nothing because she was looked at." Her whole heart and mind, her whole life and strength were in the work she had undertaken. She never went a-pleasuring, seldom into society   Yet she was one of the wittiest people one could hear on a summer's day, and had gone a great deal into society in her young unmarried life. She was left a widow at 42 with a young family. She had never had any training in hospital life. There was none to be had. Her force of character was extraordinary. Her word was law. For her thoughts, words, and acts were all the same. She moved in one piece. She talked a great deal, but she never wasted herself in talking: she did what she said. Some people substitute words for acts: *she* never. She knew what she wanted, and she did .it. She was a strict disciplinarian; very kind, often affectionate, rather than loving. She took such an intense interest in everything, even in things matrons do not generally consider their business, that she never tired.

She had great taste and spent her own money (for the hospital). She was a thorough gentlewoman, nothing mean or low about her; magnanimous and generous, rather than courteous.

And all this was done quietly. Of late years the great nursing work has been scarred by fashion on

one side, and by mere money-getting on the other—
two catastrophes sure to happen when noise is substituted for silent work.   Few remember her in
these express-train days, dashing along at 60 years
in a day. "A perfect woman, nobly planned, to warn,
to comfort, and command"; comfort not in the
present meaning of comfortable, easy-chair life, but
comfort in the good old meaning of "be strong with
me."

And so, dear Matron, as thou wast called so many
years, we bid thee farewell, and Godspeed to His
Higher world. . . .[1]

So marked a type of the conscientious dicta-
tor and autocrat as this character-picture shows
would obviously and necessarily be out of touch
with many modern tendencies. Mrs. Wardroper
was the perfect example of the old-fashioned
autocratic, military matron, who, perhaps through
the necessity of ruling severely in most cases, neglected the art of treating those under her as her
equals even when they were so. She was often
severe and hard when it was unnecessary, so that
some of the gentlewomen who worked under her
could not speak of her manner without resentment. She was a convinced individualist; believed in class lines, and aimed at the preservation
of fixed status; wished the Nightingale nurses
to move in a circle by themselves, and regarded
the earliest movements toward a more democratic

[1] "The Reform of Sick Nursing, and the late Mrs.
Wardroper."   By Florence Nightingale.   *British Medical
Journal*,   Dec. 31, 1892.

order with the most intense disapprobation. Miss Nightingale shared these views, to a certain extent at least, though it is always well to remember that we cannot tell how she would have felt toward organisation had she been able to continue her active life. Mrs. Wardroper was undoubtedly, on some lines, conservative even to narrowness; and when, in England, the first steps were taken toward a professional equality and fraternity in the formation of the Royal British Nurses' Association (whose history will be considered in another volume), designed to bring nurses from all schools together for mutual stimulus, protection, and progress, — a thing which was until then unheard-of in the evolution of nursing orders,— Mrs. Wardroper regarded the movement as dangerous and subversive of proper standards, and opposed it with all her power.[1]   Miss Nightingale, too, disapproved, and urged the Nightingale nurses not to enter into this unknown, and, as it seemed then, revolutionary union, which threatened to undermine the authority and restrict the sphere of the matron, and to cut loose the ties which had heretofore kept the nurse closely related to her school.

Anomalous as such views seem to-day, they were very natural then, for the power of ideas made the dependency of the convent seem a hard

[1] St. Thomas's nurses have never formed an association, but have an annual reunion at the school and are encouraged to keep in touch with it.

thing for women to break away from, and the forms of the convent still lay only a very short distance in the past of nursing.

It was, possibly, with some such conservative idea in mind that Miss Nightingale wrote to nurses these words:

Esprit de corps should be encouraged. It is a great help to think, "If I do this I shall be a disgrace to my training school"—"If I do that I shall be an honour to it." Let nurses be proud of their alma mater. Let them think their own training school and their own doctors the first in the world. Let there be a friendly rivalry with other hospitals, and never try to fuse all nurses into one mass—one indistinguishable mass—of all training schools or hospitals. If, however, there has been little or no discipline in the training school, then the *esprit de corps* will tend to harm, and not to good.[1]

The benefit of *esprit de corps* is more keenly realised than ever, but we no longer feel that widespread organisation fuses all nurses in an indistinguishable mass. Solidarity, that word that means so much to-day, had no force for the members of the older training schools.

It is also well known that Miss Nightingale and the matrons of that older school have not supported the modern movement for legal status, though with Miss Nightingale this arose from a belief that it would check progress. She wrote:

[1] Quain's *Dictionary of Medicine*, ed. of 1894. Art., *Training of Nurses.*

Nursing is, above all, a progressive calling. Year by year nurses have to learn new and improved methods, as medicine and surgery and hygiene improve. Year by year nurses are called upon to do more, and better, what they have done. It is felt to be impossible to have a public register that is not a delusion. Further, year by year nursing needs to be more and more of a moral calling.[1]

It is, however, possible that, were Miss Nightingale still out in the world of nurses, she, too, might regard State examination not as a public bureau for certifying the personal character of nurses to employers (which it could never possibly be), but as a bulwark (capable, also, of extension), to protect the fundamentals of a practical training and teaching which she with such rare revolutionary skill, courage, and success built up after having doomed the whole bad system then existing to extinction. We will recur to this later in considering her writings.

While in the principles of nursing, sanitation, hygiene, and enlightened humanitarianism Miss Nightingale may be confidently regarded as, humanly speaking, infallible, there is no lessening of the deep reverence in which she is held to assume that she is not always so when judging of the changing social adjustments under which nurses, following an inexorable compulsion, have been reorganising their living and working conditions.

The time of training of the Nightingale school

[1] Art., *Nursing the Sick.* Quain, 1894, Art., *Training of Nurses.*

was one year. The pupils were called probationers during the entire time. At the end of the
year, if their record was satisfactory, they were
entered in the school register as certified nurses,
to be recommended for employment accordingly.
The training was now usually considered complete, but the nurse did not leave her school and
become independent. On her entrance the probationer had agreed to remain in the service of
the school for three full years after the first year of
training: this was, in effect, a four years' course,
except that class and lecture instruction had
ceased at the end of the first year. The nurses
received certain payments in money and clothing,
and after the four years' service was ended the
Nightingale committee secured hospital positions
for them on salary; but the nurses were not allowed to make engagements except through the
committee, nor to terminate one except after three
months' notice to the committee. By this arrangement the school carried out its design of
training women for hospital work preëminently.

It is interesting to know that the Nightingale
school for many years did not give certificates to
its pupils. Miss Nightingale on this point said:

We do not give the women a printed certificate, but
simply enter the names of all certificated nurses in
the Register as such. This was done to prevent them
in the case of misconduct from using their certificate
improperly.[1]

[1] Art. in *Accounts and Papers*, Metropol. Workhouses," 1867.

This detail was one which later became out of harmony with public sentiment, and certificates are now granted at the end of the three years' course to special probationers, and after four years to the hospital nurses. Long after all the other equally important English hospitals had lengthened to three years the period during which the nurse was in training, and before she received her certificate, St. Thomas's retained its one year, but at the present time its term of training, like the others, is placed on the higher basis. St. Thomas's still recognises two classes of students—

special or paying probationers [who must be gentlewomen, and who come] with the express object of entering the nursing profession permanently by eventually filling superior situations in public hospitals and infirmaries, or by nursing the poor at their own homes under some organised system of district nursing; who pay a fee of £30 [about $150] and agree to remain for two years' service after the first, which is still regarded as the year of training: probationers, or women desirous of working as hospital nurses. Such probationers pay no fee, but continue to receive certain wages and clothing, with instruction, during the first year, and agree to remain for three further years of service, on salary.[1]

As, contrary to the earlier custom, these two classes of pupils now receive certificates, and as these are not given to them until the termination of, respectively, the three and four years' course

[1] Regulations.

to which they bind themselves, this period may
be regarded as a time of pupilage, or training term
of three and four years.[1]

The theoretical teaching was in the form of
lectures, prescribed reading, and examination by
the medical lecturers, but before all else Miss
Nightingale insisted upon the cultivation of the
observation and reflection by written notes of
cases, of work and procedures.   She says:

To train to train needs a system — a systematic
course of reading, laid down by the medical instructor,
hours of study (say two afternoons a week), regular
examinations by him, themselves cultivating their
own powers of expression in answering him.

Those who have to train others are the future
leaders, and this must be borne in mind during their
year's training.

Careful notes of lectures, careful notes of type
cases, and of cases interesting from being not types
but unusual, must be kept by them; their powers of
observation must be improved in every way.

To illustrate the cases they are nursing in the
wards, descriptions of these cases must be pointed
out to them at the time in the books in their library.

They must be encouraged to jot down afterwards,
but while still fresh in the memory, the remarks
made by the physicians and surgeons to their students
in going their rounds.

They must be taught, both by the ward Sisters and

[1] St. Thomas's hospital does not give its nurses a pension,
but provides many permanent positions, with good conditions.   The nurses average ten years' stay there.   *Blue
Book*, " Metropolitan Hospitals," 1890, p. 91.

the medical instructor, to know not only symptoms and what is to be done, but to know the "reason why" of such symptoms, and *why* such and such a thing is done. Else, how can they train others to know the "reason why"?

Time must be given them for this, otherwise they are too likely to degenerate into drudgery in the wards.

They must write out their jottings afterward in the home.[1]

While the attitude of the medical profession towards the new teaching must have been on the whole cordial (or it could not have been carried on), yet the perennial objector did not fail to rise up in the person of Dr. La Garde, who, in an address on "Nursing Sisterhoods and Hospital Schools for Nurses" regarded with alarm this dangerous tendency to communicate professional knowledge of a technical sort to the nurse, whose proper standing he summed up as follows:

A nurse is a confidential servant; but still only a servant. She should be middle-aged when she begins nursing; and if somewhat tamed by marriage and the troubles of a family so much the better.

The medical instruction of the early schools, however, was, in the opinion of Dr. Gill Wylie, who visited St. Thomas's in 1872, not alarmingly complicated. He wrote an account of his visit and impressions which is very lifelike:

[1] From the article on training in *Accounts and Papers*, " Metropolitan Workhouses," 1867.

During the three weeks' stay in London, my lodg-
ings were in St. Thomas's Hospital. Mrs. Wardroper
has been matron of this hospital of 600 beds for eighteen years. She is also lady superintendent of the
Nightingale training school for nurses, and fulfils
the varied duties of these positions in the most
satisfactory manner. Although much occupied, she
was very kind in giving me information, and allowing me every advantage for studying the system of
training.

The arrangements for the nursing staff are as follows: There are in all 16 hospital Sisters or head
nurses, one of whom acts as superintendent of night
nurses and one as matron's assistant. There are
fifty-four nurses and three nursemaids; to five of the
head nurses are assigned two wards each; to seven,
one each, and there is one Sister for the infectious
block; for every large ward there is one day nurse
and one night nurse.

There are 23 wardmaids, and for the cleaning of
the stairs and corridors, and the general work outside the wards, 14 scrubbers. Such nurses as have
charge of a ward sleep in their own rooms adjoining
their respective wards; and the other nurses and wardmaids sleep on the attic floor of the block in which
their respective wards are situated. Each nurse has
a bedroom to herself.

The probationers are employed as assistant nurses
under the immediate direction of the head nurses.
As a general rule two are assigned to each medical and
surgical ward; occasionally, according to the necessities of the case, three to one ward and one to another; they are not employed in the infectious wards.
They pass, during the year's training, successively

through all the different wards, except those of the infectious block. Those who are qualified are employed to take the places of the other nurses during illness or temporary absence.

From this it is seen that to about thirty patients there is one head nurse, one day nurse, one night nurse, two probationer-assistants, and one ward maid.

As to the instructions given outside the wards, a few lectures are delivered each season by Dr. Peacock, on principles of medicine; by Mr. Le Gros Clark, on surgical subjects; and Dr. Bernays, on chemistry and the properties of air and light. All of these are men of reputation, being visiting physicians to the hospital and professors in the medical college. While the lectures are being delivered the probationers take notes, and afterwards write out the lectures. I examined eight or nine of the best written. In most of them the subjects were treated in the simplest style. Mr. Clark himself told me that he merely gave them a talk, telling them what they should not do, rather than anything else. The lectures are too few in number and not at all systematised. It seems to me that to take a woman or man at the age of 30 with only a common education as a basis, and teach them science by lectures, is a doubtful experiment; and that if attempted at all it should be by men who have the time to make the course of instruction a special study.[1]

The general features of hospital life and nursing arrangements at the time that Miss Nightingale's

[1] *Report to the Training School Committee of Bellevue Hospital*, 1872.

reformation was set in motion are very graphically
described in the *British Medical Journal* in a series
of reports by a special commissioner, who compared the conditions of his day (1874) with those
of twenty years earlier.   Then (1854) the average
metropolitan hospital had three classes of nurses:
head nurses, nurses, under nurses.   It was possible, under the system of promotion prevailing,
for the under nurses to become head nurses.   There
was no uniform dress, and (what modern nurse-
pupils would do well to note) besides a salary each
nurse received eight shillings a week in place
of board.   They cooked their food (which they
bought for themselves) and ate their meals in the
ward kitchens or scullery.   The assistant nurses
had the cooking to do for the head nurses and the
patients as well as for themselves.   The night
nurses were on duty from 10 P. M. to 1 P. M., or
fifteen hours.   They occasionally had a leave of
absence for afternoon and evening, but were on
duty at ten as usual; on these occasions being up
for about forty hours at a stretch.   The matron
was someone who perhaps had been nurse or
house-keeper to some influential governor.   She
is described as having been usually a stout lady
with an authoritative voice and wonderful cap.
The head nurses were, in their wards, practically
independent of her, and their loyalty was prin-
cipally shown by imitating her cap.   But that
there were personalities of value among the old-
style nurses is recorded by Sir James Paget, who

has left recollections of some of the old nurses at St. Bartholomew's.

"It is true [he writes] that even fifty years ago there were some excellent nurses, especially among the Sisters in the medical wards, where everything was more gentle and orderly than in the surgical. There was an admirable Sister Hope, who had her leg amputated and then devoted her life to nursing there. . . .

An old Sister Rahere was the chief among them, stout, ruddy, positive, very watchful. She once taught an erring house surgeon where and how to compress a posterior tibial artery. She could always report correctly the progress of a case; and from her wages she saved all she could and left it in legacy to the hospital.[1]

The customs relating to board and wages were of long standing, but had varied a little in different hospitals. St. Bartholomew's had paid its Sisters an average of sixteen shillings a week, and they provided their own food. The nurses received one shilling and twelve ounces of bread daily. St. Thomas's gave its Sisters £37 a year; the nurses had 9 shillings 7 pence a week, and beer. Guy's hospital paid its Sisters and nurses better than any, but at none of the three did they receive any food beyond that mentioned, nor were their wages increased by length of service. At St. George's all the nurses were allowed six pounds of bread a week, one half pint of milk and two pints

[1] *Memoirs and Letters of Sir James Paget*, Longmans, Green & Co., London, 1901, p. 353.

of beer daily, and one shilling a day to buy additional food (board and wages).[1]

The example of the Nightingale school, triumphantly made, was in time followed by every other English hospital of importance. One by one they gave up the old system of nursing for the new, and the English colonies and the United States followed the lead. As time went on it was not always easy to keep the ranks recruited in sufficient numbers to fill all the demands of hospital service, and a feature peculiar to English hospital life appeared in the "lady probationer." The lady probationer came for a term of from three to six months' training, paying a fee for her tuition, and had rather special privileges in that she was allowed to slip over more laborious and routine parts of ward work and to attain superior posts by virtue of her education, intelligence, and social position instead of as the result of the long, hard time of training. She was only a transient figure, and has to-day almost entirely disappeared from English hospitals.[2]

[1] *History of the Middlesex Hospital*, p. 117.
[2] See evidence on "paying probationers" in *Blue Book*, Metropolitan Hospitals, 1890, p. 293.

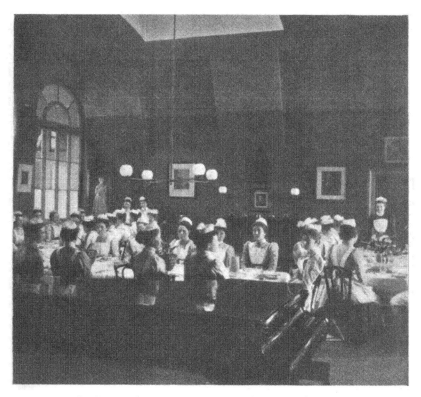

Nightingale Home and Training School for Nurses, St. Thomas's Hospital

CHAPTER V

MISS NIGHTINGALE'S WRITINGS

GREAT as Miss Nightingale was as a nurse, her nursing reflected only a part of her genius. She was, perhaps, even greater as a teacher, and without a doubt greatest as a sanitarian. Though it was by her nursing that she seized and held the hearts and imaginations of men—so that those who know nothing further of her know that she was the heroine of the Crimea and the reformer of nursing,—it is the intellectual quality of her deep insight into problems of health that keeps her work and will always keep it fresh and vivid. It is not possible to study her writings without being strongly stirred by her ardent realisation of all that makes for health. She was an enthusiast for health and happiness. Said Dr. Blackwell, " *To her* chiefly I owe the awakening to the fact that *sanitation* is the supreme goal of medicine, its foundation and its crown." In considering her practical and technical knowledge, so extensive, so minute, so exact, and above all so intelligent is it found to be that it is perhaps not too much to call her the foremost sanitarian of her age, as uniting in a rare measure technical knowledge with organising capacity. Practical hygiene underlay all her teachings throughout her long life, beginning with her individual visits in the cottages near her country home.

A very remarkable example of the originality of this teaching is her *Notes on Nursing; What It Is, and What It Is Not*. In this unrivalled monograph she does not concern herself with so much as a glance at the carrying out of "orders" in the application of treatment, nor describe a single method of technical procedure, nor hint at the relation of the nurse to the patient, the physician, the family, nor describe the symptoms of a single disease, nor outline the special nursing care of any special case. That which makes this book an immortal classic is its teaching of sanitary truths and principles as applied in the care of sickness, and of a boundless and exquisite humaneness towards the patient; principles which will never change, while procedures, professional etiquette, and methods will. In its presentation of these truths and the practical application made of them, it stands unique, unapproached, and complete. In selecting quotations from the *Notes* we are impressed afresh with its rare characteristics, and are impelled to urge upon every woman— not only every nurse, but every woman who reads these words—to possess herself of it and make its teaching a part of her mental equipment.

In watching disease, both in private houses and in

public hospitals, the thing which strikes the experienced observer most forcibly is this, that the symptoms or the sufferings generally considered to be inevitable. and incident to the disease, are very often not symptoms of the disease at all, but of something quite different—of the want of fresh air, or of light, or of warmth, or of quiet, or of cleanliness, or of punctuality and care in the administration of diet, of each or of all of these.   And this quite as much in private as in hospital nursing.

The reparative process which Nature has instituted and which we call disease, has been hindered by some want of knowledge or attention, in one or in all of these things, and pain, suffering, or interruption of the whole process sets in.

If a patient is cold, if a patient is feverish, if a patient is faint, if he is sick after taking food, if he has a bed-sore, it is generally the fault, not of the disease, but of the nursing.

I use the word nursing for want of a better.   It has been limited to signify little more than the administration of medicines and the application of poultices. It ought to signify the proper use of fresh air, light, warmth, cleanliness, quiet, and the proper selection and administration of diet—all at the least expense of vital power to the patient.

It has been said and written scores of times that every woman makes a good nurse.   I believe, on the contrary, that the very elements of nursing are all but unknown. . . .

The art of nursing, as now practised, seems to be expressly constituted to unmake what God had made disease to be, viz., a reparative process. . . . If we were asked, Is such or such a disease a reparative

process?   Can such an illness be unaccompanied with
suffering?   Will any care prevent such a patient from
suffering this or that?—I humbly say, I do not know.
But when you have done away with all that pain and
suffering, which in patients are the symptoms, not of
their disease, but of the absence of one or all of the
above-mentioned essentials to the success of Nature's
reparative process, we shall then know what are the
symptoms of and the sufferings inseparable from the
disease. . . .

    . . . The very elements of what constitutes good
nursing are as little understood for the well as for the
sick.   The same laws of health, or of nursing, for they
are in reality the same, obtain among the well as among
the sick.   The breaking of them produces only a less
violent consequence among the former than among the
latter,—and this sometimes, not always. . . . O mothers
of families, do you know that one of every seven infants
in this civilised land of England perishes before it is one
year old?   That in London two in every five die before
they are five years old?   And in the other great cities
of England, nearly one out of two?   "The life duration
of tender babies" (as some Saturn, turned analyt-
ical chemist, says) "is the most delicate test" of sanitary conditions.   Is all this premature suffering and
death necessary?   Or did Nature intend mothers to
be always accompanied by doctors?   Or is it better
to learn the pianoforte than to learn the laws which
subserve the preservation of offspring? . . .

    The very first canon of nursing, the first and the
last thing, upon which a nurse's attention must be
fixed, the first essential to a patient, without which
all the rest you can do for him is as nothing, with
which, I had almost said, you may leave all the rest

alone, is this: *to keep the air he breathes as pure as the external air, without chilling him.* Yet, what is so little attended to? Even where it is thought of at all, the most extraordinary misconceptions reign about it. Even in admitting air into the patient's room or ward few people ever think where that air comes from. It may come from a corridor into which other wards are ventilated, from a hall always un-aired, always full of the fumes of gas, dinner, of various kinds of mustiness; from an underground kitchen sink, washhouse, water-closet, or even, as I myself have had sorrowful experience, from open sewers loaded with filth; and with this the patient's room or ward is aired, as it is called—poisoned, it should rather be said. . . . Never be afraid of open windows, then. People don't catch cold in bed. This is a popular fallacy. . . . Dr. ———'s air test, if it could be made of simple application, would be invaluable to use in every sleeping- and sick-room. . . .

And O, the crowded national school, where so many children's epidemics have their origin, what a tale an air-test would tell! We should have parents saying, and saying rightly, "I will not send my child to that school, the air-test stands at 'Horrid.'" And the dormitories of our great boarding-schools! Scarlet fever would be no more ascribed to contagion, but to its right cause, the air-test standing at "Foul." . . .

The extraordinary confusion between cold air and ventilation even in the minds of well-educated people illustrates this. To make a room cold is by no means necessary to ventilate it. Nor is it at all necessary, to ventilate a room, to chill it. . . . Another extraordinary fallacy is the dread of the night air. What air can we breathe at night but night air? The choice

is between pure night air from without and foul night
air from within.   Most people prefer the latter.   An
unaccountable choice.   What will they say if it is
proved to be true that fully one half of all the disease
we suffer from is occasioned by people sleeping with
their windows shut?

.   .   .   .

If a nurse declines to do these things for her patient,
"because it is not her business," I should say that
nursing was not her calling.   I have seen surgical
"Sisters," women whose hands were worth to them
two or three guineas a week, down upon their knees
scouring a room or hut, because they thought it otherwise not fit for their patients to go into.   I am far
from wishing nurses to scour.   It is a waste of power.
But I do say that these women had the true nursing
calling—the good of their sick first, and second only
the consideration what it was their "place" to do;—
and that women who wait for the housemaid to do
this, or for the charwoman to do that, when their patients are suffering, have not yet the *making* of a nurse
in them.

.   .   .   .

Is it not living in a continual mistake to look upon
diseases, as we do now, as separate entities, which
must exist, like cats and dogs, instead of looking
upon them as conditions, like a dirty and a clean condition, and just as much under our own control, or
rather as the reactions of a kindly nature against the
conditions in which we have placed ourselves?
I was brought up, both by scientific men and igno-

rant women, distinctly to believe that small-pox, for instance, was a thing of which there was once a first specimen in the world, which went on propagating itself, in a perpetual chain of descent, just as much as that there was a first dog (or pair of dogs), and that small-pox would not begin of itself any more than a new dog would begin without there having been a parent dog.

Since then I have seen with my own eyes and smelt with my nose small-pox growing up in first specimens, either in close rooms or in overcrowded wards, where it could not by any possibility have been "caught," but must have begun.

Nay, more, I have seen diseases begin, grow up, and pass into one another. Now, dogs do not pass into cats.

I have seen, for instance, with a little overcrowding, continued fever grow up: and with a little more, typhoid fever: and with a little more, typhus, and all in the same ward or hut.

Would it not be far better, truer, and more practical, if we looked upon diseases in this light? For diseases, as all experience shows, are adjectives, not noun substantives.

. . . .

There are five essential points in securing the health of houses: 1. Pure air. 2. Pure water. 3 Efficient drainage. 4. Cleanliness. 5. Light. God lays down certain physical laws. Upon His carrying out such laws depends our responsibility (that much abused word); for how could we have any responsibility for actions the results of which we could not foresee?—which would be the case if the carrying out of His laws were not certain.   Yet we seem to be continually expecting that He will work a miracle, *i. e.*, break His own laws expressly to relieve us of responsibility.

. . . .

5.   A dark house is always an unhealthy house, always an unaired house, always a dirty house.   Want of light stops growth, and promotes scrofula, rickets, etc., among the children.

People lose their health in a dark house, and if they get ill, they cannot get well again in it.

. . . .

Don't imagine that if you, who are in charge, don't look to all these things yourself, those under you will be more careful than you are.   It appears as if the part of a mistress now is to complain of her servants, and to accept their excuses—not to show them how there need be neither complaints made nor excuses.

But again, to look to all these things yourself does not mean to *do* them yourself.   "I always open the windows," the head in charge often says.   If you do it, it is by so much the better, certainly, than if it were not done at all.   But can you not insure that it is done when not done by yourself?   Can you insure that it is not undone when your back is turned?   This is what "being in charge" means.   And a very important meaning it is, too.   The former only implies that just what you can do with your own hands is done.   The latter, that what ought to be done is always done.

. . . .

Wise and humane management of the patient is the best safeguard against infection.

There are not a few popular opinions in regard to which it is useful at times to ask a question or two.   For example, it is commonly thought that children must have what are commonly called "children's epidemics," "current contagions," etc. — in other words, that they are born to have measles, whooping-cough, perhaps even scarlet fever, just as they are born to cut their teeth, if they live.

Now, do tell us, why must a child have measles?

Oh, because, you say, we cannot keep it from infection: other children have measles, and it must take them, and it is safer that it should.

But why must other children have measles?   And if they have, why must yours have them too?

If you believed in and observed the laws for preserving the health of houses, which inculcate cleanliness, ventilation, whitewashing, and other means, and which, by the way, *are laws*, as implicitly as you believe in the popular opinion—for it is nothing more than an opinion—that your child must have children's epidemics, don't you think that upon the whole your child would be more likely to escape altogether?

All the results of good nursing, as detailed in these notes, may be spoiled or utterly negatived by one defect, viz., in petty management, or in other words, by not knowing how to manage that what you do when you are there shall be done when you are not there.   The most devoted friend or nurse cannot be always *there*.   Nor is it desirable that she should. . . . It is as impossible in a book to teach a person in charge of sick how to *manage* as it is to teach her how to nurse.   Circumstances must vary with each different case.   But it *is* possible to press upon her to think for herself. . . . To be "in charge" is certainly not

only to carry out the proper measures yourself but
to see that every one else does so too: to see that no
one, either wilfully or ignorantly, thwarts or prevents
such measures.   It is neither to do everything yourself nor to appoint a number of people to each duty,
but to ensure that each does that duty to which he is
appointed.   This is the meaning which must be attached to the word by (above all) those "in charge"
of sick, whether of numbers or of individuals. . . .

.   .   .   .

Never to allow a patient to be waked, intentionally
or accidentally, is a *sine quâ non* of all good nursing.
If he is roused out of his first sleep, he is almost certain
to have no more sleep.   It is a curious but quite intelligible fact that, if a patient is waked after a few hours'
instead of a few minutes' sleeep, he is much more
likely to sleep again.

.   .   .   .

Unnecessary noise, then, is the most cruel absence
of care which can be inflicted either on sick or well.
For, in all these remarks, the sick are mentioned as
suffering in a greater proportion than the well from
precisely the same causes.

All hurry or bustle is peculiarly painful to the sick.
And when a patient has compulsory occupations to
engage him, instead of having simply to amuse himself, it becomes doubly injurious.   The friend who
remains standing and fidgeting about while a patient
is talking business to him, or the one who sits and
poses, the one from an idea of not letting the patient
talk, the other from an idea of amusing him, each is
equally inconsiderate.   Always sit down when a sick
person is talking business to you, show no signs of

hurry, give complete attention, and full consideration, if your advice is wanted, and go away the moment the subject is ended.

Always sit within the patient's view, so that when you speak to him he has not painfully to turn his head round in order to look at you.   Everybody involuntarily looks at the person speaking.   If you make this act a wearisome one on the part of the patient you are doing him harm.   So also if by continuing to stand you make him continuously raise his eyes to see you.   Be as motionless as possible, and never gesticulate in speaking to the sick. . . .

These things are not fancy.   If we consider that, with sick as with well, every thought decomposes some nervous matter, that decomposition as well as re-composition of nervous matter is always going on, and more quickly with the sick than with the well;— that to obtrude abruptly another thought upon the brain while it is in the act of destroying nervous matter by thinking is calling upon it to make a new exertion,—if we consider these things, which are facts, not fancies, we shall remember that we are doing positive injury by interrupting, by "startling a fanciful" person, as it is called.   Alas!   It is no fancy. . . .

One hint I would give to all who attend or visit the sick, to all who have to pronounce an opinion upon sickness, or its progress.   Come back and look at your patient *after* he has had an hour's animated conversation with you.   It is the best test of his real state we know.   But never pronounce upon him from merely seeing what he does, or how he looks during such a conversation. . . .

Irresolution is what all patients most dread.   Rather than meet this in others, they will collect all their data,

and make up their minds for themselves. A change
of mind in others, whether it is regarding an operation,
or rewriting a letter, always injures the patient more
than the being called upon to make up his mind to the
most dreaded or difficult decision.

With regard to the reading aloud in the sick-room
my experience is that when the sick are too ill to read
themselves they can seldom bear to be read to. . . .

The extraordinary habit of reading to oneself in a
sick-room and reading aloud to the patient any bits
which will amuse him, or more often the reader, is
unaccountably thoughtless. What *do* you think the
patient is thinking of during your gaps of non-reading?
Do you think that he amuses himself upon what you
have read for precisely the time it pleases you to go
on reading to yourself, and that his attention is ready
for something else at precisely the time it pleases you
to begin reading again? . . .

. . . Volumes are now written and spoken upon
the effect of the mind on the body. Much of it is
true. But I wish a little more was thought of the
effect of the body on the mind. . . .

. . . I think it is a very common error among the
well to think that "with a little more self-control" the sick might, if they chose, "dismiss painful
thoughts," which "aggravate their disease," etc. Believe me, almost *any* sick person, who behaves decently well, exercises more self-control every moment
of his day than you will ever know till you are sick
yourself. Almost every step that crosses his room
is painful to him; almost every thought that passes
his brain is painful to him; and if he can speak without being savage, and look without being unpleasant,
he is exercising self-control. . . .

How little the real sufferings of illness are known or understood! How little does any one in good health fancy him- or even *her*-self into the life of a sick person!

Do, you who are about the sick, or visit the sick, try and give them pleasure, remember to tell them what will do so. How often in such visits the sick person has to do the whole conversation, exerting his own imagination and memory, while you would take the visitor, absorbed in his own anxieties, making no effort of memory or imagination, for the sick person!

. . . "What can't be cured must be endured" is the very worst and most dangerous maxim for a nurse which ever was made. Patience and resignation in her are but other words for carelessness or indifference—contemptible if in regard to herself, culpable if in regard to her sick.

The most important practical lesson that can be given to nurses is to teach them what to observe, how to observe, what symptoms indicate improvement, what the reverse, which are of importance, which are the evidence of neglect, and of what kind of neglect.

All this is what ought to make part, and an essential part, of the training of every nurse. At present how few there are, either professional or unprofessional, who really know at all whether any sick person they may be with is better or worse. . . . It is a much more difficult thing to speak the truth than people commonly imagine. There is the want of observation *simple*, and the want of observation *compound*, compounded, that is, with the imaginative faculty. The information of the first is simply defective. That of the second is much more dangerous. The first gives, in answer to a question asked about a thing that has been before his eyes perhaps for years, information exceedingly imperfect, or says he does not know. He has never observed. And people simply think him stupid.

The second has observed just a little, but imagination immediately steps in, and he describes the whole thing from imagination merely, being perfectly convinced all the while that he has seen or heard it; or he will repeat a whole conversation as if it were information which had been addressed to him: whereas it is merely what he has himself said to somebody else. This is the commonest of all. These people do not even observe that they have *not* observed, nor remember that they have forgotten.

Courts of justice seem to think that anybody can speak "the whole truth, and nothing but the truth," if he does but intend it. It requires many faculties combined of observation and memory to speak "the whole truth," and to say "nothing but the truth."

In dwelling upon the vital importance of *sound* observation, it must never be lost sight of what observation is for. It is not for the sake of piling up miscellaneous information or curious facts, but for the sake of saving life and increasing health and comfort. The caution may seem useless, but it is quite surprising how many men (some women do it too) practically behave as if the scientific end were the only one in view, or as if the sick body were but a reservoir for stowing medicines into, and the surgical disease only a curious case the sufferer has made for the attendant's special information. . . .

For it may safely be said, not that the habit of ready and correct observation will by itself make us useful nurses, but that without it we shall be useless with all our devotion.

It seems a commonly conceived idea among men and even among women themselves that it requires nothing but a disappointment in love, the want of an object, a general disgust or incapacity for other things, to turn a woman into a good nurse.

This reminds one of the parish where a stupid old man was set to be a schoolmaster because he was "past keeping the pigs."

Apply the above receipt for making a good nurse to making a good servant; and the receipt will be found to fail.

. . . The everyday management of a large ward, let alone of a hospital, the knowing what are the laws of life and death for men, and what the laws of health for wards (and wards are healthy or unhealthy mainly according to the knowledge or ignorance of the nurse), are not these matters of sufficient importance and difficulty to require learning by experience and careful inquiry, just as much as any other art? [1]

Notes on Nursing for the Labouring Classes is, in some respects, the most noteworthy of the revisions of *Notes on Nursing*. It incorporates the most vital portions of the latter work and contains an inspiring and most practical chapter on "The Health of the House," with special reference to and detail for rural cottages.[2]   It sounds, more-

[1] Extracts from *Notes on Nursing*, 1860. By permission of D. Appleton & Co., New York.

[2] The Rural Housing and Sanitation Association, with offices at 9 Southampton St., Holborn, W. C., London, is carrying on this work to-day, but even yet conditions are painfully the same as when the *Notes* was written.

over, an ardent plea for the better housing of
workers, and expresses her deep pity and distress
over bad factory conditions and the disasters of
sweated home industries:

How much sickness, misery, and death are produced by the present state of many factories, ware-
houses, workshops, and workrooms! The places
where poor dressmakers, tailors, letter-press printers,
and other similar trades have to work for their living
are generally in a worse condition than any other portions of our worst towns. Many of these places of
work were never constructed for such an object. They
are badly adapted garrets, sitting-rooms, or bedrooms, generally of an inferior class of houses. No
attention is paid to the cubic space or ventilation.
The poor workers are crowded on the floor to a greater
extent than occurs with any other kind of overcrowding. . . . In such places, and under such circumstances of constrained posture, want of exercise,
hurried and insufficient meals, long and exhaustive labour, and foul air. . . . is it wonderful that a great
majority of them die easily of chest disease? . . .
Employers seldom consider these things. Healthful
working rooms are no part of the bond into which
they enter with their working people. They pay
their money . . . and for this wage the worker has to
give up work, health, and life. . . . Working people
should remember that health is their only capital, and
should come to an understanding among themselves
to secure pure air in their places of work, which is one
of the principal agents of health. This *would* be
worth a "trades-union," almost worth a "strike."
. . . If tenants would be so wise as to refuse to

occupy unhealthily built homes, builders would soon
be brought to their senses. . . .

Presently, with her own inimitable irony, she
throws this remark in a footnote:

This very year, 1868, a health report has appeared
in Manchester which is virtually to this effect: Let
the town breed as much infectious disease as it likes;
put the cases into big infirmaries: this is the way to
cure Manchester—to build hospitals to cure people
after they have been killed.

This edition also contains a chapter on "Minding Baby," the sweetest, brightest, intimate and
simple talk to girls imaginable.

And now, girls, I have a word for you. You and
I have all had a great deal to do in minding baby,
though "baby" was not our own "baby."

Thus she begins, and goes on to a talk on the
health and care of infants that is a perfect model
of important truths and simple style. Few are
the words over one syllable, and yet the most
thorough scientist might willingly own its authorship. The entire book is sanitary teaching in its
most convincing and persuasive form.

Of her *Notes on Hospitals*, it has been said
that it has "probably done more than any other
treatise to promote sound views of hospital
economy."[1]

This, as well as two notable papers on India,

[1] *Tent Hospitals*, by J. Foster Jenkins. *Amer. Soc. Sci.
Journ.*, May, 21, 1874.

were first read at the meetings of the English National Association for the Promotion of Social Science, afterwards being reprinted in book form, and it has been said that they are the most able papers ever presented to that association.

Miss Nightingale's genius was early recognised by Sidney Herbert, and utilised by him in the work of army reorganisation. Though now the least known of her writings, her various monographs on the army had in their day an immense influence, and show most strikingly her remarkable mental grasp and generalship. This is particularly true of her *Notes on Matters affecting the Health, Efficiency, and Hospital Administration of the British Army*, presented by request to the Secretary of State for War, and published in 1858. This (a work of considerable size) takes up the entire field of army organisation from every aspect except that which is purely military, and discusses, first, the entire official correspondence and the records of the whole Crimean campaign, pointing out in minutest detail every defect in organisation of the commissariat, the purveying, the medical departments, dieting and cooking, transport, statistics, regimental and general hospitals, sanitary (or unsanitary) conditions, laundry, canteens, and conditions of the soldier's social and family relations.

Every criticism is accompanied by a constructtive recommendation. Every riddling of clumsy inadequacy is followed by a picture of a practical and efficient working method. Every exposure of stupidity is linked with a corresponding plan for attaining clear sanitary benefits.

Miss Nightingale's brilliant perception even re-constructed the whole medical hierarchy; she dis-cusses the pay and promotion of medical officers, medical education, sanitary officers for hospitals and encampments; gives actual and proposed forms for medical statistics in the army, and shows the importance of a scientific study of the diseases incident to army life.

All that the Japanese have recently so brilliantly demonstrated could be done, to reduce the death rate from preventible causes to a minimum, she here and elsewhere besought the English govern-ment to do.

It is not denied that a large part of the British force perished from causes not the unavoidable or necessary results of war. . . . (10,053 men, or sixty per cent. per annum, perished in seven months, *from disease alone*, upon an average strength of 28,939. This mor-tality exceeds that of the Great Plague) . . . . The question arises, must what has here occurred occur again?

No tribunal has ever yet tried this question. It hardly seems to have occurred to the national mind.

. . . Immediately after the troops went to the East, the practical inefficiency of the Army Medical Department began to shew itself.

Abstracts of correspondence follow, showing failures to adopt recommendations made in advance by a commission in charge of the health of the army.

It would, indeed, be difficult to frame a system of administration more likely to lose an army at any time than this. Here is the first downward step of our noble army to destruction.

Abstracts of records follow showing the failure to supply proper rations to the army in the field, absence of vegetables, and appearance of scurvy.

The great calamity is now drawing to its height. . . . Had half the ingenuity exercised in sending out lime juice been expended in making that article unnecessary, the army might have returned to England alive and well. From this point, the correspondence seems to read as if the medical office was to register *post-mortem* appearances, instead of keeping the patient in health—as if the business of the police was to record murders instead of preventing them.

In order to make this intelligible, it is necessary to give a short summary of what the army did receive in vegetables and blankets. . . .

The summaries follow, all calamitous facts.

. . . For three months this army had not had the means of cleanliness (no soap) either as to their persons or clothing: and what the state of the men was, on arriving at Scutari, let those who saw it testify. . . .

Abstracts of letters between Drs. Smith and Hall follow, saying "symptoms of scurvy" are appearing among the men.

The expression "symptoms of scurvy" seems quite inexplicable, as well as that of its "not having made much progress." The army was dying, and of scurvy. More than half the infantry was sick in hospital during this month (January, 1855). . . . Yet there is nothing in these letters to indicate that either Principal Medical Officer or Director-General know that an army is dying, or that, if it is, it is any business of theirs. January 24, Dr. Smith objects to the issue of unground coffee (the troops had, for four months, had only *green* coffee beans issued to them). . . .

Now, also, arrived the lime juice so painstakingly sent, Dr. Hall having received all the notifications, but six weeks after its arrival it had not been given out. The winter having passed, commissions were appointed.

One would think that the fact, well known by this time, of an army having all but perished would have been of itself a sufficient reason for the severest animadversion from the head of the army medical department. But no. The Sebastopol Committee is to have the doings of that department before it, and Dr. Smith writes to his principal medical officer:

"I beg you to supply me, and that immediately "— with what?—"with every kind of information which you may deem likely to enable me to establish a character for it " (the department), "which the public appears desirous to prove that it does not possess." What hope for the army after this? He might as well have said, Never mind anything if you only enable me to free the department from blame. . . .

Analyses of lists of medical supplies, and light

diets, etc., called "medical comforts," are then made and compared with the numbers of the sick, showing glaring insufficiency.

On Jan. 1, 1855, the number of patients who had arrived in the hospitals of the Bosphorus during the last fortnight amounting to 2532, followed by 1044 more in the next six days, the superintendent of nurses, according to her invariable custom of ascertaining first whether the articles for which requisition was made upon her by medical officers were or were not in the purveyor's stores, in order that no ostentatious display or unnecessary issue might be made by her, received the following return—

in brief, of plates, candlesticks, tin drinking cups, pails for tea, bolsters, slippers, knives, forks, spoons, flannel shirts, socks, and drawers, there were *none*; of bedpans, *some*; and of night-caps, *a few*.

Let it not be said, "It is all past, let bygones be bygones." A future war is not past. We are speaking for the future. Otherwise it may be prophesied . . . that, exactly in the proportion in which similar circumstances recur, will similar destruction recur. We shall do as before and lose again half an army from disease. . . .

Methods of sanitary administration are then discussed fully.

If you treat your Director-General like a schoolboy you will have a schoolboy for your Director-General.

The mischief to the public service is produced in this way: Scientific men are placed in a position re-

quiring them to give advice whether they be asked for
it or not. *Other considerations not known to their department* are then acted upon.   This is a certain way
of destroying the sense of responsibility. . . .   The
consequence will be that there will be *no* scientific
men in the department.

Recommendations for an ideal sanitary service
then follow, practically covering every detail
which the Japanese have since then put into
practice.

As to laundry matters, Miss Nightingale states
that in the Barrack hospital the number of towels
washed by the purveyor during November, December, and January, with from 2000 to 2400
patients in the wards, was 132 towels.   The amiable Mr. Wreford wrote in February, "The necessity for a subsidiary washing establishment has
never been made apparent to me." . . .

As to the lack of hospital comforts, Miss Nightingale says, "This has been denied, will be denied
again; a few official records are therefore annexed."

Of the nursing service Miss Nightingale says
here:

If, with a party of female volunteers so suddenly
formed, . . . the labours of female nurses could be
carried on for nearly two years advantageously (as it
is presumed) to the soldier, and without injurious dis-
turbance to the medical and military departments of
hospital government, it must necessarily be admitted
that the female nursing element may be introduced
into military hospitals in future, concurrently with a

better system of orderlies: the number of nurses being restricted and the duties better defined. It must be added that it is absolutely necessary that the high character and respectability of the female must be maintained, both as to her personal and official conduct; and no motives of supposed utility should be allowed to require or lead her to do that which would lower her morally or officially. . . .

Miss Nightingale notes the fact, observed by other nurses later, that discipline in military hospitals does not approach that of civil institutions. Of special interest also, of her writings on the army, is her "Army Sanitary Administration and its Reform under the late Lord Herbert," [1] for in this she sets forth in order all the different branches of reform which we know (though she does not say so) were in reality the outcome of her practical and suggestive reports made to him privately. She says:

. . . In times past, war has been conducted in more or less forgetfulness, sometimes in total oblivion, of the fact that the soldier is a mortal man, subject to all the ills following on wet and cold, want of shelter, bad food, excessive fatigue, bad water, intemperate habits, and foul air. . . . And who can tell how much systematic attempts made by all nations to diminish the horrors of that great curse, war, may not lead the way to its total disappearance from the earth? The faithful records of all wars are records of preventible suffering, disease and death. It is needless to

[1] Read at the London meeting of the *Congrès de Bienfaisance*, June, 1862.

illustrate this truth, for we all know it.   But it is only from our latest sorrow, the Crimean catastrophe, that dates the rise of army sanitary administration in this country. . . . No provision was made for the systematic care of the soldier's health, but only for his sickness. . . . In all our wars, our general hospitals have been signal failures, fatal examples of how to kill, not to cure.

She calls Herbert "highest among the savers of men," and says of him:

Sidney Herbert, although his passion, his hereditary occupation to which he was born and bred was politics, yet made his administrative labours greater, set his administrative objects higher, recoiled from none of its dry fatigue, and attained its highest usefulness.

. . . .

He did not sink in politics the powers which were meant for mankind. . . .   The first war minister who seriously set himself to the task of saving life. . . . Let us hope that the great lesson which has been taught will have its weight with those charged with the duty of protecting the public health.

The *Sanitary State of the Army in India*[1] is likewise written in her most masterly, lucid, and trenchant style. Her comments on the details of the report, her summary of the whole, and her indictment of the conditions and systems allowed to exist are scathing and unsparing.

[1] Being observations on the evidence contained in the statistical report submitted to her by the Royal Commission.

Native caste prejudice [she observes] appears to have been made the excuse for European laziness as far as regards our sanitary and hospital neglects of the native."

With an unswerving hand she dissects the feeble and futile attempts of governments to regulate vice and drink. "Common-sense is the same as moral sense in these things," she concludes.

In her article on Village Sanitation in India[1] her inexhaustible human sympathies are shown again in her reference to the ancient customs of the vanished Hindoo civilisation. This catholic sympathy was the mainspring of her energy.

Under the old village organisation [she said] the villagers, working under their head man, managed, in their humble way, every department of business required for their local wants, and it was the duty of certain low caste village servants to remove dead animals and perform other sanitary work. But, unfortunately, in a large part of India the village system has been allowed to fall into decay. The ancient patriarchal methods have ceased to be effectual, while as yet little has been done to find any modern substitute. The results are very deplorable.

She then quotes from the report of a sanitary commission, and says she had had the advantage of corresponding with these commissions and with educated Indian gentlemen who were interested

[1] Read before the Tropical Section of the 18th International Congress of Hygiene and Demography, Buda-Pesth, September, 1894.

in this subject, adding that it was clear the chief
improvements needed were a diminution of overcrowding, the carrying away of sewage, and a
better water supply, and continues:

As regards removal of sewage and care of water-
supply, much may be done by the villagers themselves
if they can be made to understand the terrible result
of neglect and the benefits of the most simple remedies.
I have therefore appealed to my educated Indian
friends to instruct their poorer brethren in these vital
truths.   And I have ventured to suggest to them that
health missioners might be sent among the villagers,
men (and women also, to convert the rural mothers,
whose influence in this matter is great and whose dearest interests are at stake) well versed in the principles
of sanitation and at the same time sympathetic and
conciliatory.   Lectures and practical demonstrations
might be given out in the village school-rooms.   But
the lectures would only be the first beginning of the
teaching: a lecturer who had made himself acceptable
to the people, would go around the village and show
the people how to dispose of their refuse: he would
explain to them the dangers of depositing it in
their little close courtyards. . . .

Then he would go with them and examine their
water-supply, and show them certain simple precautions to be observed. . . .   The Hindoo religion
enjoins so much purity and cleanliness that the influence of religious teachers and of all caste Panchayats
(or councils) might be usefully appealed to.   With a
gentle and affectionate people like the Hindoos much
may be accomplished by personal influence. . . .   The
government is powerful . . . but in such delicate

matters, affecting the homes and customs of a very conservative people, almost more may be done by personal influence, exercised with kindly sympathy and respect for the prejudices of others. . . .

On the same lines, and overflowing with care for, and eager interest in, the homes of the people, was her paper on "Rural Hygiene."[1] She refers therein to the woman health missioners who were hoped for in India, and exclaims:

Let not England lag behind, especially in the conviction that nothing can be done without personal friendship with the women to be taught. It is a truism to say that the women who teach in India must know the language, the religious superstitions and customs of the women to be taught in India. It ought to be a truism to say the same for England. We must not talk to them, or at them, but with them. . . .

. . . What is the existing machinery of public health in what are called, with a grim sarcasm, our rural sanitary districts? Is health or sickness, life or death, the greatest miracle in the present condition of things? To some of us the greatest miracle, repeated every day, is that we can live at all in the surroundings which our ignorance and neglect create.

After reviewing the conditions, legislation, and its difficulties, she says:

These are the facts as they are. Now let us consider what they ought to be.

We want independent medical officers of health,

[1] Presented at the Conference of Women Workers, Leeds, November, 1893.

appointed by the county council, and removable only
by them—men trained for this as a profession; we
want sanitary inspectors with a proper qualification,
appointed with the medical officer's approval; we
want that each medical officer should be informed as
to all approaches of dangerous disease, and bound in
his term to supply the information for other neighbouring districts: we want sanitary inspectors who are
duly qualified by examination acting under the directions of medical officers, in order that they may feel
themselves responsible for their appointment, and
co-operators in their work, sanitary inspectors who
are not removable unless for neglect of duty, and certain to be removed if they do persistently neglect it
We want a fully trained nurse for every district, and
a health missioner: we want a water-supply to each
village, rain-water properly stored; earth closets;
scavenging—as necessary a public duty as paving and
lighting: gardens near houses, and allotments where
refuse and privy contents are used; . . . cottage
owners made amenable to sanitary laws, compelling
the landlord to give his cottages the essentials for
health so far as construction is concerned; school
teaching of health rules made interesting and clear by
diagrams showing dangers of foul drains, etc. (But
we must not expect too much practical result from
this. It has failed, except as a book or lesson, where
it has been tried in India. The schoolmaster himself
should be a health apostle.)

After describing in detail the absence of a good
sanitary condition in villages she scorches and
flays public apathy:

In these days of investigations and statistics,

where results are described with microscopic exactness and tabulated with mathematical accuracy, we seem to think figures will do instead of facts, and calculation instead of action.   We remember the policeman who watched his burglar enter the house, and waited to make quite sure whether he was going to commit robbery with violence or not, before interfering with his operations.   So as we read such an account as this we seem to be watching, not robbery, but murder going on, and to be waiting for the rates of mortality to go up before we interfere.   We wait to see how many children playing around the houses shall be stricken down.   We wait to see whether the filth will really trickle into the well, and whether the foul water will really poison the family and how many will die of it. And then, when enough have died, we think it time to spend some money and some trouble to stop the murders going further, and we enter the results of our "masterly inactivity" neatly in tables, but we do not analyse and tabulate the saddened lives of those who remain, and the desolate homes of our "sanitary districts."

.   .   .   .

Now let us come to what the women have to do with it, *i. e.*, how much the cottage mothers, if instructed by instructed women, can remedy or prevent these and other frightful evils? . . . .

Then follows the best syllabus of instruction in domestic sanitation that has ever been put together, and through it all throbs the spiritualised maternal instinct which is hers in rare fullness.

Sympathy with interest in the poor so as to help

them can only be got by long and close intercourse
with each in her own house—not patronising—"talking down" to them, not "prying about." Sympathy
which will grow in insight and love with every visit:
which will enable you to show the cottage mother on
the spot how to give air to the bedroom, etc. You
could not get through the daily work of the cottage
mother, the cooking, washing, cleaning, mending,
making. . . . And don't think the gain is all on
their side. How much we learn from the poor, how
much from our patients in the hospital, when heart
meets heart. . . . The criticism on all this will be:
' What an enormous time it will take. You are describing a process that will not take weeks, but months
and years. Life is not long enough for this." Our
reply is that for centuries there have been superstitions, for centuries the habits of dirt and neglect
have been steadily and perseveringly learnt, and that,
if we can transform by a few years' quiet, persistent
work the habits of centuries, the process will not have
been slow, but amazingly rapid. What is "slow"
in more senses than one is the eternal lecturing that is
vox et præterea nihil—words that go in one ear and out
the other. The only word that sticks is the word that
follows work. The work that "pays" is the work of
the skilful hand directed by the cool head and inspired by the loving heart. Join heart with heart,
and hand with hand, and pray for the perfect gift of
love to be the spirit and the life of all your work.

Can there be any higher work than this? Can any
woman wish for a more womanly work? Can any
man think it unworthy for the best of women?

We are inclined to class with her teachings on

hygiene and sanitation her work on *Lying-In Hospitals*, a book of some size, characteristically dedicated to the "Shade of Socrates' Mother."

The introduction tells how, in the year 1862, the Nightingale committee, with a view of extending the advantages of the Nightingale school, made arrangements with the authorities of St. John's House by which wards were fitted up in the new part of the King's College hospital, opening out of the great staircase but closed in behind their own doors, for the reception of midwifery patients. The wards and nursing were under the charge of the lady superintendent, and every precaution (as it was thought) was taken to secure the well-being of the patients. But the record of puerperal sepsis was so grave, even though not as bad as in other institutions, that the Nightingale committee decided to close up the wards.

Miss Nightingale then, though in ill-health, gave her attention to making a thorough study of the subject and the conditions under which maternity hospitals were conducted. She found striking vagueness and inexactness in the statistics of many institutions, as well as in the prevalent medical theories on puerperal sepsis. True, medical writers had not been lacking to declare its communicable character,[1] yet others, of whom

[1] In 1843 Oliver Wendell Holmes had read his article "The Contagiousness of Puerperal Fever" to the Medical Society and declared that it could be carried from patient to patient by physician and nurse. In this essay Holmes quoted a long

Miss Nightingale quotes Le Fort, held that it could
originate *de novo*.   In her investigations Miss
Nightingale found that the restrictions laid down
as to the admission of students to the lying-in
wards at King's College hospital had been disre-
garded; also that a post-mortem theatre had been
erected almost under the ward windows.   While
she made no criticism on persons, she emphasised
principles strongly, and declared that those
hospital authorities incurred grave responsibility
who did not assure themselves that students admitted to maternity practice gave up, for the time
being, all connection with general wards or with
anatomical schools.

She characterised existing hospital records and
death-rate statistics as grotesque (except that the
subject was so serious), pointing out that child-
birth was not a disease and should not be entered
as such, and that it was especially unjust to class
it as a "miasmatic disease."   She concluded by
summing up the evidence and showing that no
lying-in ward should be connected with a general
hospital service, and then presented plans and
schedules for separate buildings and a properly
organised separate service with midwifery teaching for women.

In coming to the subject of training and organ-

list of distinguished physicians who had pointed out its con-
tagious character, going back to Dr. Gordon of Aberdeen in
1795.   See the writings of Oliver Wendell Holmes.   Houghton
& Mifflin, Boston, 1891, vol. ix., p. 131 *et seq.*

ising a nursing staff, in which Miss Nightingale's genius shines so brilliantly, no better introduction could be planned than her own exposition of her studies and observations of nursing systems as they existed in 1862. This set of data stands as an appendix to the *Notes on Hospitals*, where, it is much to be feared, few persons ever see it, though the rare pithiness, acumen, and judgment shown in its balancing and weighing of the different systems give it an interest and a value far too great to be reconciled with oblivion. In its acute observation and its crisp, fresh comments it is delightfully characteristic of its author and contains some of her most pertinent aphorisms.

At the time it was written, it gave the names of certain hospitals as examples of each system described. As, however, to-day, many of these have altered their schemes of nursing, all names have been omitted, as well as some personal allusions.

[It may, however, be noted that, at the present day, there may still be found, in Italy, many examples of class No. 1; that examples of Class 2 may be found in this country and Canada; that Class 3 is illustrated, in this country, by the Cook County hospital, Chicago, with the Illinois training school, and by Bellevue hospital with the school attached to it; that the General hospital in Vienna, Austria, which was mentioned by Miss Nightingale as belonging in Class 4, still belongs there, with unchanged system, and that Class 5 includes certain military hospitals, and departments in some hospitals for the insane.]

ON DIFFERENT SYSTEMS OF HOSPITAL NURSING AS EXISTING IN THE YEAR 1862

In the important question of accommodation for nurses, so much depends upon the method of nursing chosen that an appendix is devoted to this.

The methods of nursing the sick [then] adopted in the public hospitals of Europe may be distinguished under five classes:

1. Where the nurses belong to a religious order, and are under their own spiritual head: the hospital being administered by a separate and secular governing body.

2. Where the nurses are of a religious order, the head of which administers both order and hospital.

3. Where the nurses are secular under their own head: the hospital having its own separate and secular gove nment.

4. Where the nurses are secular, and under the same secular authority as that by which the hospital where they nu se is governed.

5. Where the nurses are all men and seculars and under the same secular male authority as the hospital.

Of these systems of nursing—

No. 1, where the nu ses belong to a religious order, and are under their own spiritual head—the hospital being administered by a separate and secular governing body—is, on the whole, best calcu ated to secure good nursing for the sick, and the general well-being of both patients and nurses. . . . But in giving this unqualified opinion in favour of nursing by sister-hoods, *provided* the administration be secular, I must add a caution against two mistakes, whether committed in France or in England, in Roman Catholic or in Protestant institutions, *viz.*, (1) the female head of the Sisters *must* reside in the institution nursed by them and neither in a "nurses' home," or "*Maison Mère*," [which is] *not* the hospital, nor in a "home" where other works of charity, not hospital ones, are carried on. If she has other works of charity which appear to her more important, then she had better not undertake hospital ones. Hospital nursing is jealous, and demands her whole heart. It will not have a divided allegiance. It will not be too much of her whole life to gather experience and learn to govern such institutions. If she has several hospitals, as the Augustinians of Paris, the female head must live where the novices, or probationers, or whatever they are called, are trained. She must be at once matron of the hospital, which means of the nursing of it, and superintendent of the nurses. It will not do for her to head the nurses or probationers in their "home" and to leave the heading of them in the hospital to a matron, or other superior.

No. 2. The Sisters must not be the heads of wards merely in order to use "moral influence," as the inexperienced sometimes fancy will be sufficient. If a lady has, in addition, the same knowledge and experience as an old-fashioned hospital head nurse, which indeed many nuns, but only in secularly governed hospitals, have, good: she is fit to be Sister or head nurse; if not, not.

No. 3, where the nurses are secular under their own secular female head—the hospital having its own sep-

arate and secular government—is unquestionably the
system which secures the best nursing, after No. 1.

Out of the other systems of nursing, Nos. 2, 4, and 5,
in each of which there is but one sole authority, although in No. 2 a religious one, in Nos. 4 and 5 a secular one, over both nurses and administration, are
equally to be deprecated—

Nos. 4 and 5 because the nurses, whether male or
female, are under the sole command of the male hospital authorities: in this case the arrangements as
to hours, proprieties, and sanitary rules generally,
would strike any one as all but crazy.   Such
are the rules which give nurses twenty-four hours
"on duty" in a ward, or which put them to
sleep with the sick, of which the extreme case is where
a female nurse is made to sleep in a man's ward, etc.

In No. 2, on the contrary, the nursing staff, whether
Protestant or Roman Catholic, whether its heads be
male or female, or both, is in entire and sole command
of the hospital: in this case the arrangements are
generally nearly as crazy as in the former, although
the objects and results are widely different.   Such
are the letting a patient die of a bed-sore because
the nurse may spread the dressing for it but must not
look at it; the leaving the wards at night, or at times
when the "community" assembles, in sole charge of
subordinates.

In Case No. 4 the nurses are destroyed bodily and
morally, but the patients are generally, not always,
better nursed.

In Case No. 2 the patients are not always, but generally worse nursed; the sick are less cared for, while
the spiritual good of the nurses is consulted.   But the
care of the sick is the object of hospitals.

The collision, often disagreeable, but generally salutary for the care of the sick, between the secular
administration and the nursing staff (whether this consist of nuns, brothers, deaconesses, or nurses), as is the
case in the hospitals of London and Paris, keeps each
belligerent party to his duty, and reacts beneficially
on the interests of the sick.　Even the mutual impertinence, just as often to be heard between nuns and
doctors as between doctors and nurses, is far better
for the management of a hospital, and any neglect of
the sick is far less likely to pass unnoticed, than where
the authority is solely invested in one of the two ways
above mentioned: *i. e.*, either vested in the secular
male authorities of the hospital, or in the spiritual
head of the nursing establishment by either Protestant
or Roman Catholic orders.　Take the nuns, brothers,
deaconesses out of the parent institution, and set them
to work in a great secular hospital, in daily contact
with the (often vexatious) exigencies of doctors and
governors, and they will work admirably.

Take Case 2.　Theory differs widely from practice in these things.　If we were perfect, no doubt an
absolute hierarchy would be the best kind of government for all institutions.　But, in our imperfect state
of conscience and enlightenment, publicity, and the
collision resulting from publicity, are the best guardians of the interests of the sick.　A patient is much
better cared for in an institution where there is the
perpetual rub between doctors and nurses or nuns,
between students, matrons, governors, treasurers,
and casual visitors, between secular and spiritual
authorities (for this applies quite as much to Roman
Catholic as to Protestant institutions) than in a hospital under the best governed order in existence where

the chief of that order, be it male or female, is also sole chief of the hospital.

Taking the imperfect general run of human things —for we are considering men, and not angels—public opinion is a higher average standard than individual opinion. For many years I have been trying to find how this could be, since public opinion is made up of individual opinions. I think it is because A will be much more rigid in making B mind B's business than in minding his own. Public opinion is good for this. The remark is not a high-minded one, but it is true.

Orders, whether Roman Catholic or Protestant, unless held in check by the rude curb of public opinion, or by the perpetual rub and collision with the secular authority of the hospital, are inclined to make into a special object the spiritual (often fancied) good of their members, and not the general and real good of the inmates of the hospital (for whom, nevertheless, the hospital was intended, and not for working out the salvation of the order).

It is bad for the activity of any one to have always his own way. And if it were only for this, *viz.*, that no great sanitary or administrative improvements have ever come out of orders, or out of seculars whose authority is undivided, it would be enough to condemn them.

Nos. 2 and 4. Where the nurses, religious or secular, are governed by the same authority, religious or secular, which governs the hospital, the destruction of health of the members both of orders and secular institutions often takes place in a period of about five years. This consumption of human beings is the worst policy in every sense. Its operative causes are under-feeding, want of proper sleep, want of the most ordinary sanitary precaution—the result of austerity in orders, of an ignorant economy in secular institutions. In the latter, want of the most ordinary means for propriety and morality is often a fourth cause.

No. 2. In some institutions nursed by brotherhoods, abroad, a good Augustinian nun, or good hospital nurse from London, would turn everything out of window (though the former could not do all she wou'd wish), and be as disgusted as we are with their pestilential filth. But, al:s! this has been seen even in those nursing *sisterhoods* where the salutary check of the secular administ ation was not.

No. 2. Where institution and sisterhood alike are under the same authority. The following remark applies exclusively to orders, and to orders where no secular authority is in play, but much more to Protestant than to Roman Catholic orders, which latter have better sense:

There is a constant change of occupation of each member of the o der, for the sake of detaching said member from earthly things. To-day he or she is in the kitchen, to morrow in a surgical ward, next week in a medical ward, the week af er in he laundry. The perplexed medical attendant, when giving his directions about the patients, sees a new face, at least every fortnight, to give his directions to.

In the best Roman Catholic orders, especially where, as in 1, the secular authority comes into action, there is far more lat ude given to individual character, and scope to individual capacity, than we are at all aware of. Each member is much more independent in his or her own occupation than is the case under arrangement No. 2.

Nos. 2, 4, and 5. Where there is but one authority

over both hospital and nurses, whether that authority
be religious or secular. The following remark implies
alike to some institutions, both religious and secular,
to all military, and to some civil, to Protestant and
Roman Catholic establishments:

The want of one defini e head in permanent charge
of each ward, or set of wards, invariably acts disas-
trously for the patients. There should always be
some one person in acknowledged responsibility for
the nursing, wi h servants—call them lay Sisters or
Brothers, or assistant nurses, or what you will—under the head.

Religious motives in some orders, a want of any
practical ystem of nursing in many military and some
civil hospitals, reproduce the above defect, in the most
varied forms, in institutions of the most opposite
character.

No. 4. Where nurses and institutions are under
the same secular authority. The following remark
applies solely o institutions secu'arly nursed:

The practice of having man and wife in oin charge
of a ward or wards has in it more evil than good for the
patien s. It is rue that a woman had better flirt
with her husband than with a studen or patient: it
is true that the common ph ase "settling" (which
means marrying in some classes) has its significance
here, for some women never are "settled" till they
are married. But it is no less true that the interest
of the husband henceforth come before that of the
patients, in hones as in dishonest ways. The woman
is no longer attached to her ward, but o her husband,
and the patients are, more or less, neglected. This
is still more eminently the case in regimental hospitals, where it is a common practice to choose married

hospital sergeants, as being more "respectable," and to have the wife to live in the hospital. As well might the hospital head nurse have her husband to live with her in the room off her ward.

Nos. 1 (where the sisters are of a religious order, but the nurses are secular), 3 and 4 (where all the nurses are secular, whether governed by a separate head from that which governs the hospital, or by the same head). The cardinal sin of paid nu ses, of all classes, of all nations, is taking petty bribes and making petty advantages (of many different sorts and sizes) out of the patients. From this sin all orders, whether Roman Catholic or Protestant, are exempt, but from it their servants are by no means exempt.

The rules of hospital head nurses in London, were they really religious women, who would neither take any present themselves, nor be guilty of any kind of impropriety, would enable them to exercise a far more efficient surveillance over assistant nurses, as to both these things, than can be exercised by Roman Catholic or Protestant orders living in community. All kinds of things between nurses and patients may and do go on in the Sisters' wards, when the Sisters are out of the way. A hospital head nurse is (or ought to be) always in command of her ward.

To sum up: Case 1. There is a higher average of care of the sick and a higher universal sense of morality among hospital Sisters, Protestant and Roman Catholic, provided the hospital authority be a secular one. Case 2. There is a lower average care of the sick, although an equally high morality, among hospital nuns, Protestant and Roman Catholic, if the hospital authority be not a secular one. Case 3. There is a far greater average care of the sick, although a lower morality, among nurses under a secular female head, the authority of the hospital being a secular and separate one, than in Case 2: and there is a somewhat higher average care of the sick in Case 4 than in Case 2, and no morality at all, but an awful destruction of both life and soul, among nurses, where both nurses and hospital are under the same secular (male) authority.   Case 5.   There is no care of the sick and no morality, not even discipline, in hospitals where the nurses are men, and where both nurses and hospital are under the same secular (male) authority. This is the worst state of things of all.   Case 2 is perhaps the second worse.   For, take it which way you will, the idea of the "religious order" is always, more or less, to prepare the sick for death: of the secular, to restore them to life.   And their nursing will be accordingly.   There will be instances of physical neglect (though generally unintentional) on the part of the former: of moral neglect on that of the latter.   Unite the two, and there will be fewer of either.

Of course to all this there are exceptions.   This appendix is dealing only with systems of nursing *as systems*.[1]

The proper position of the matron or head of the nurses has been defined by Miss Nightingale with insistent reiteration.   It is a point she never fails to dwell on, and often recurs to in her writings.   In one of her first papers on hospital organisation she says:

[1] From *Notes on Hospitals*, by permission of the publishers, Longmans, Green & Co., London.

"Equal in importance to the provision of trained nurses is the nature of the hospital authority under which these nurses are to perform their duties. For, unless an understanding is come to on this point the very existence of good nursing is an impossibility. In dealing with this question I may state at once that to turn any number of trained nurses into any workhouse infirmary to act under the superintendent or the instructions of any workhouse master or matron or medical officer would be sheer waste of good money. This is not matter of opinion but of fact and experience. . . . Experienced administrators will scarcely suppose that I mean to imply an independence or to ask for uncontrolled hospital authority for the nursing staff. . . . The matron or nursing superintendent must be held responsible for her own efficiency and the efficiency of all her nurses and servants. . . . All that the medical department or the governing body has a right to require is that the regulation duties shall be faithfully performed. . . . Neither the medical officer nor any other male head should ever have the power to punish . . . his duty should end with reporting the case to the female head. . . .[1]

Again, on this point, she wrote:

I may perhaps again point out that the superintendent should herself be responsible to the constituted hospital authorities and that all her nurses and servants should, in the performance of these duties, be responsible to the superintendent only.

[1] From a paper on training and organising nurses for the sick poor in workhouse infirmaries in *Accounts and Papers*, vol. lx. " Metropolitan Workhouses." 1867.

No good ever comes of the constituted authorities placing themselves in the office which they have sanctioned her occupying.

No good ever comes of any one interfering between the head of the nursing establishment and her nurses. It is fatal to discipline.

All complaints on any subject should be made directly to the superintendent, and not to any nurse or servant.

She should be made responsible, too, for her results, and not for her methods.

Of course, if she does not exercise the authority entrusted to her with judgment and discretion, it is then the legitimate province of the governing body to interfere, and to remove her.

It is necessary to dwell strongly on this point, because there has been not unfrequently a disposition shown to make the nursing establishment responsible on the side of di cipline to the medical officer, or the governor of a hospital.

Any attempt to introduce such a system would be merely to try anew and fail anew in an attempt which has frequently been made. I n disciplinary matters a woman only can understand a woman.

It is the duty of a medical officer to give what orders, in regard to the sick, he thinks fit, to the nurses. And it is unquestionably the duty of the nurses to obey or see his orders carried out.

Simplicity of rules, placing the nurses in all matters regarding management of sick absolutely under the orders of the medical men, and all disciplinary matters absolutely under the female superintendent (matron), to whom the medical officers should report all cases of neglect, is very important. At the outset there must be a clear and recorded definition of the limits of these two classes of jurisdiction.

.   .   .   .

The matron must be one whose desire is that the probationers shall learn; a rarer thing than is usually supposed.

But beside this there is a constant, motherly, intangible supervision and observation to be exercised, for there are qualities which no written tests and no examination can reach. The probationers must really be the matron's children: the "home" Sister must really be their elder sister.

A training school without a mother is worse than children without parents. And in disciplinary matters none but a woman can understand a woman.

.   .   .   .

In view of some modern tendencies these words of Miss Nightingale are also of interest:

With regard to an oft-disputed question whether it is desirable to train probationers entirely in a public hospital I should say, without hesitation, it is *there only* that they *can* be trained; and every well-judging superintendent will tell you that the students, governors, stewards, etc. (disagreeable as the collisions with them sometimes are), are the most valuable assets in the training of her nurses. Whether in opposition or in kindness she hears of all their shortcomings through the secular bystanders which she would hear of in no other way. I have rarely known a nurse worth the bread she ate—Catholic, Lutheran, or Anglican Sister or paid—who had not been trained under a hospital discipline consisting partly of the secular man authority of the hospital and partly of her own female superintendent. I don't know which is the worst managed—the hospital which is entirely under the secular men heads, or the hospital which is entirely under the superintendent of the nurses, whether religious or secular, whether male or female." [1]

So, too, in principles of training hers are the most clear-cut definitions, penetrating, complete, and unanswerable. In small domestic or local details time and varied conditions may easily prove some of her directions to be out of date, as when she insists that the nurse should always live in the hospital (it is to be remembered, though, here, that what she was contending against was a system which allowed the nurse to be a married woman living at home with her family and coming by day or by night only to the ward), or when she says that the Sister should command her ward day and night, meaning that the head nurse must have her living and sleeping room adjacent to or even opening out of the ward,—but her ethics and principles are for all time.

Training is to teach not only what is to be done, but how to do it. The physician or surgeon orders what is to be done. Training is to teach the nurse how to do it to his order, and to teach not only how to do it, but *why* such and such a thing is done, and not such and such another ; as also to teach symptoms, and

[1] Quoted in article: "Training Schools for Nurses," *Journal of Social Science* (*Transactions* of the American Association), by F. B. S., p. 294, September, 1874.

what symptoms indicate what of disease or change,
and the "reason why" of such symptoms.

Nearly all physicians' orders are conditional. Telling the nurse what to do is not enough and cannot be
enough to perfect her, whatever her surroundings.
The trained power of attending to one's own impressions made by one's own senses, so that these should
tell the nurse how the patient is, is the *sine quâ non*
of being a nurse at all. The nurse's eye and ear must
be trained; smell and touch are her two right hands—
and her taste is sometimes as necessary to the nurse
as her head. Observation may always be improved
by training, will indeed seldom be found without
training: for otherwise the nurse does not know what
to look for. Merely looking at the sick is not observing. To look is not always to see. It needs a high
degree of training to look so that looking shall tell
the nurse aright, so that she may tell the medical officer aright what has happened in his absence—a higher
degree in medical than in surgical cases, because the
wound may tell its own tale in some respects; but
highest of all, of course, in children's cases, because
the child cannot tell its own tale: it cannot always
answer questions. A conscientious nurse is not necessarily an observing nurse, and life or death may lie
with the good observer. Without a trained power
of observation, the nurse cannot be of any use in reporting to the medical attendant. The best one can
hope for is that he will be clever enough not to mind
her, as is so often the case. Without a trained power
of observation, neither can the nurse obey intelligently
his directions. It is most important to observe the
symptoms of illness; it is, if possible, more important
still to observe the symptoms of nursing: of what is

the fault not of the illness, but of the nursing. Observation tells *how* the patient is; reflection tells *what* is to be done. Training and experience are, of course, necessary to teach us, too, *how* to observe, *what* to observe, *how* to think, *what* to think. Observation tells us the fact, reflection the meaning of the fact. Reflection needs training as much as observation. To obey *is* to understand orders, and to understand orders is really to obey. A nurse does not know how to do what she is told without such "training" as enables her to understand what she is told, or without such moral disciplinary "training" as enables her to give her whole self to obey. A woman cannot be a good and intelligent nurse without being a good and intelligent woman. Therefore, what "training" signifies in the wide sense, what makes *a good training school*, what moral and disciplinary "training" means, and how it is to be obtained, is to be clearly understood.

The essentials of a training school (or, indeed, for a nurse-establishment of any kind) may be shortly given thus:

(*a*) That nurses should be technically trained in hospitals *organised for the purpose*.

(*b*) That they should live in "homes" fit to form their moral lives and discipline.

The untrained nurse, like other people called quacks, easily falls into the confusion of *on account of*, *because after*—the blunder of the "three crows." The nurse is told by the medical attendant, "If such and such a change occur, or if such or such symptoms appear, you are to do so and so, or to vary my treatment in such and such a manner." In no case is the physician or surgeon always there. The woman must have trained powers of observation and reflection, or she cannot obey. The patient's life is lost by her blunders, or "sequelæ" of incurable infirmity make after-life a long disease, and people say, "The doctor is to blame;" or, worse still, they talk of it as if God were to blame— as if it were God's will. God's will is *not* that we should leave our nurses, in whose hands we must leave issues of life or death, without training to fulfil the responsibilities of such momentous issues.

A nurse without training is like a man who has never learnt his alphabet, who has learnt experience only from his own blunders. Blunders in executing physicians' or surgeons' orders upon the living body are hazardous things, and may kill the patient. Training is to enable the nurse to see what she sees—facts; and to do what she is told, to obey orders not only from the rule of thumb, but by having the rule of thought, of observation, to guide her. Otherwise she finds out her own mistakes by experience, acquired out of death rather than life, or does not find them at all.

. . . Training is to teach a nurse to know all her business, that is, to observe exactly, to understand, to know exactly, to do, to tell exactly, in such stupendous issues as life and death, health and disease. Training is to enable the nurse to act for the best in carrying out her orders, not as a machine, but as a nurse; not like Cornelius Agrippa's broomstick which went on carrying water, but like an intelligent and responsible being. Training has to make her, not servile, but loyal to medical orders and authorities. True loyalty to orders cannot be without the independent sense or energy of responsibility, which alone secures real trustworthiness. Training makes the

difference in a nurse that is made in a student by making him prepare specimens for himself instead of
merely looking at the prepared specimens.   Training
is to teach the nurse how to handle the agencies within
our control which restore health and life, in strict
obedience to the physician's or surgeon's power and
knowledge, how to keep the health mechanism prescribed to her in gear.   Training must show her how
the effects of life on nursing may be calculated with
nice precision—such care or carelessness, such a sick
rate; such a duration of case, such a death-rate.

And *discipline* is the essence of training.

. . . Discipline embraces order, method, and, as
we gain some knowledge of the laws of nature (God's
laws) we not only see order, method, a place for everything, each its own work, but we find no waste of material or force or space; we find, too, no hurry, and we
learn to have patience with our circumstances and
ourselves, and so, as we go on learning, we become
more content to work where we are placed, more anxious to fill our appointed work than to see the result
thereof; and so God, no doubt, gives us the required
patience and steadfastness to continue in our "blessed
drudgery,"which is the discipline he sees best for most
of us."[1]

. . . .

What a Nurse is to Be.—A really good nurse must
needs be of the highest class of character.   It needs
hardly be said that she must be (1) chaste, in the sense
of the Sermon on the Mount—a good nurse should

[1]From " The Training of Nurses," Quain's *Dictionary of
Medicine*, ed. of 1894.   By permission of the publishers,
Longmans. Green & Co., London.
    VOL. II.—17.

be the Sermon on the Mount herself. It should naturally seem impossible to the most unchaste to utter
even an immodest jest in her presence. Remember
this great and dangerous peculiarity of nursing, and
especially of hospital nursing, namely, that it is the
only case, queens not excepted, where a woman is
really in charge of men. And a really good, trained
ward "Sister" can keep order in a men's ward better
than a military ward-master or sergeant. (2) Sober,
in spirit as well as in drink, and temperate in all
things. (3) Honest, not accepting the trifling fee or
bribe from the patients or friends. (4) Truthful, and
to be able to tell the truth includes attention and observation, to observe truly; memory, to remember
truly; power of expression, to tell truly what one has
observed truly; as well as intention to speak the truth;
the whole truth, and nothing but the truth. (5)
Trustworthy, to carry out directions intelligently and
perfectly, unseen as well as seen, "to the Lord" *as well
as* unto men—no mere eye-service. (6) Punctual
to a second, and orderly to a hair—having everything
ready in order before she begins her dressings or her
work about the patients: nothing forgotten. (7)
Quiet, yet quick: quick without hurry, gentle without
slowness; discreet without self-importance, no gossip.
(8) Cheerful, hopeful, not allowing herself to be discouraged by unfavourable symptoms; not given to
distress the patient by anticipations of an unfavourable result. (9) Cleanly to the point of exquisiteness
both for the patient's sake and for her own; neat and
ready. (10) Thinking of her patient and not of herself, "tender over his occasions" or wants, cheerful
and kindly, patient, ingenious and *feat*. The
best definition can be found, as always, in Shakes-

peare, where he says that to be "nurse-like" is to be—

"So kind, so duteous, diligent,
So tender over his occasions, true,
So feat." [1]

The most remarkable summing-up of all her previous dicta on training and ideals is found in the paper which Miss Nightingale contributed to the Nursing Section of the Congress on Hospitals, Dispensaries, and Nursing at the time of the World's Fair in Chicago.   In reading this paper, masterly in its scope and grasp, it seems as if Miss Nightingale must have foreseen, in prophetic vision, the mushroom growth of the quackery which had not then developed, but which has since grown to menacing proportions.   Had she then read the flowery circulars issued by commercial enterprises, belittling the practical and the disciplinary training, and lauding to the skies all that is superficial and flimsy, she could not better have answered their sophistries.   But by one of the ironies of fate, and a lamentable one, she foresees the wave of pinchbeck nursing education as something linked with regulation and examination by the state or an authorised central body, instead of, as it actually is, the irreconcilable enemy of state protective legislation, which demands practical service as the *sine quâ non* for obtaining its shield and ægis.

[1] "Nursing the Sick." Quain's *Dictionary of Medicine*, ed. of 1894. By permission of the publishers, Longmans, Green & Co., London.

And so throughout this impressive address runs an appeal to the nurses of America *not* to do this thing which they have done and have had to do in order to strengthen the basis of sound hospital training against the sapping of teaching by correspondence and by the elimination of all real work. When this paper was read before the American nurses none of them could have foreseen that ten years after they had heard it they would be steadfastly and unitedly banded together against sham in nursing education. That, in so doing they have done what Miss Nightingale herself would have done, and have kept before them her own standard, cannot be doubted; that in so doing they have taken a road which she believes to be astray, the road of state protection for a fixed basis of requirement, has been inevitable, and in this necessary divergence lies much that is to be deplored, for it has meant an apparent disregard of the advice of one whose advancing years and honour call for all respect and consideration.

I. A new art and a new science has been created since and within the last forty years. And with it a new profession—so they say: we say, *calling*. One would think this had been created or discovered for some new want or local want. Not so. The want is nearly as old as the world, nearly as large as the world, as pressing as life or death. It is that of sickness. And the art is that of *nursing the sick*. Please mark— nursing the *sick*, *not* nursing sickness. We will call the art nursing proper. This is generally practised by

women under scientific heads—physicians and surgeons.   This is one of the distinctions between nursing
proper and medicine. though a very famous and successful physician did say, when asked how he treated
pneumonia, "I do not treat pneumonia.   I treat the
person who has pneumonia."   This is the reason why
nursing proper can only be taught by the patient's
bedside, and in the sick-room or ward.   Neither can
it be taught by lectures or by books, though these are
valuable accessories, if used as such; otherwise, what
is in the book stays in the book.

· · · · · ·

II.   But, since God did not mean mothers to be
always accompanied by doctors, there is a want older
still and larger still.   And a new science has also been
created to meet it, but *not* the accompanying art, as
far as the households are concerned, families. schools.
workshops, though it is an art which concerns every
family in the world, which can only be taught from
the home, in the home.

This is the art of health, which every mother, girl,
mistress, teacher, child's nurse, every woman ought
practically to learn.   But she is supposed to know it
all by instinct, like a bird.   Call it *health nursing* or
general nursing—what you please.   Upon womankind
the national health, as far as the household goes, depends.   *She* must recognise the laws of life, the laws of
health, as the nurse proper must recognise the laws
of sickness, the causes of sickness, the symptoms of
the disease, or the symptoms, it may be, not of the
disease. but of the nursing, bad or good.

It is the want of the art of health, then, of the
cultivation of health, which has only lately been

discovered, and great organisations have been made to meet it, and a whole literature created.   We have medical officers of health, immense sanitary works. We have not nurses, "missioners" of health-at-home.

How to bring these great medical officers to bear on the families, the homes and households, and habits of the people, rich as well as poor, has not been discovered, although family comes before Acts of Parliament. One would think "family" had no health to look after.   And woman, the great mistress of family life, by whom everybody is born, has not been practically instructed at all.   Everything has come before health. We are not to look after health, but after sickness. Well, we are to be convinced of *error* before we are convinced of right: the discovery of sin comes before the discovery of righteousness, we are told on the highest authority.

Though everybody *must* be born, there is probably no knowledge more neglected than this, nor more important for the great mass of women, *viz.*, how to feed, wash, and clothe the baby, and how to secure the utmost cleanliness for mother and infant.   Midwives certainly neither practise nor teach it.   And I have even been informed that many lady doctors consider that they have "nothing to do with the baby," and that they should "lose caste with the men doctors" if they attempted it.   One would have thought that the ladies "lost caste" with themselves for *not* doing it, and that it was the very reason why we wished for the "lady doctors," for them to assume these cares which touch the very health of everybody from the beginning.   But I have known the most admirable exceptions to this most cruel rule.

I know of no systematic teaching, for the ordinary

midwife or the ordinary mother, how to keep the baby in health, certainly the most important function to make a healthy nation. The human baby is not an invalid, but it is the most tender form of animal life. This is only one, but a supremely important instance of the want of health-nursing.

.   .   .   .

III. As the discovery of error comes before that of right, both in order and in fact, we will take first (*a*) sickness, nursing the sick: training needful; (*b*) health, nursing the well at home: practical teaching needful. We will then refer (IV) to some dangers to which nurses are subject, (V) benefit of combination, and (VI) our hopes for the future.

What is sickness? Sickness or disease is nature's way of getting rid of the effects of conditions which have interfered with health. It is nature's attempt to cure. We have to help her. Diseases are, practically speaking, adjectives, not noun substantives. What is health? Health is not only to be well, but to be able to use well every power we have. What is nursing? Both kinds of nursing are to put us in the best possible conditions for nature to restore or to preserve health, to prevent or to cure disease or injury. Upon nursing proper, under scientific heads, physicians or surgeons must depend partly, perhaps mainly, whether nature succeeds or fails in her attempts to cure by sickness. Nursing proper is therefore to help the patient suffering from disease to live, just as health nursing is to keep or put the constitution of the healthy child or human being in such a state as to have no disease.

What is training?   Training is to teach the nurse
to help the patient to live.   Nursing the sick is an art,
and an art requiring an organised, practical and scientific training, for nursing is the skilled servant of medicine, surgery, and hygiene.   A good nurse of twenty
years ago had not to do the twentieth part of what
she is required by her physician or surgeon to do now;
and so, after the year's training, she must be still
training under instruction in her first and even second
year's hospital service.   The physician prescribes for
supplying the vital force, but the nurse supplies it.
Training is to teach the nurse how God makes health,
and how He makes disease.   Training is to teach a
nurse to know her business, that is, to observe exactly
in such stupendous issues as life and death, health and
disease.   Training has to make her, not servile, but
loyal to medical orders and authorities.   True loyalty to orders cannot be without the independent
sense or energy of responsibility, which alone secures
real trustworthiness.   Training is to teach the nurse
how to handle the agencies within our control which
restore health and life, in strict, intelligent obedience
to the physician's or surgeon's power and knowledge:
how to keep the health mechanism prescribed to her
in gear.   Training must show her how the effects on
life of nursing may be calculated with nice precision
—such care or carelessness, such a sick-rate; such a
duration of case, such a death-rate.

What is discipline?   Discipline is the essence of
moral training.   The best lady trainer of probationer nurses I know says: "It is education, instruction, training—all that, in fact, goes to the full
development of our faculties, moral, physical and
spiritual, not only for this life, but looking on this

life as the training ground for the future and higher
life.   .   ."

What makes a good training school for nurses?
The most favourable conditions for the administration
of the hospital are;

First. A good lay administration with a chief executive officer, a civilian (be he called treasurer or
permanent chairman of committee), with power
delegated to him by the committee, who gives his
time. This is the main thing. With a consulting
committee, meeting regularly, of business men, taking
the opinions of the medical officers. The medical
officers on the committee must be only consulting
medical officers, not executive. If the latter, they
have often to judge in their own case, which is fatal.
Doctors are not necessarily administrators (the executive), any more than the executive are necessarily
doctors. Vest the charge of financial matters and
general supervision, and the whole administration
of the hospital or infirmary, in the board or committee
acting through the permanent chairman or other officer who is responsible to that board or committee.

Second. A strong body of medical officers, visiting and resident, and a medical school.

Third. The government of hospitals, in the
point of view of the real responsibility for the conduct
and discipline of the nurses, being thrown upon the
matron (superintendent of nurses), who is herself a
trained nurse, and the real head of all the female
staff of the hospital. Vest the whole responsibility
for nursing, internal management, for discipline and
training of nurses in this one female head of the
nursing staff, whatever called. She should be herself
responsible directly to the constituted hospital

authorities, and all her nurses and servants should, in the performance of their duties, be responsible in matters of conduct and discipline to her only. No good ever comes of the constituted authorities placing themselves in the office which they have sanctioned her occupying. No good ever comes of any one interfering between the head of the nursing establishment and her nurses. It is fatal to discipline. Without such discipline, the main object of the whole hospital organisation, viz. to carry out effectively the orders of the physicians and surgeons with regard to the treatment of the patients, will not be attained.

Having then, as a basis, a well organised hospital, we require as further conditions:

(1) A special organisation for the purpose of training, that is, where systematic technical training is given in the wards to the probationers; where it is the business of the ward "Sisters" to train them, to keep records of their progress, to take "stock" of them; where the probationers are not set down in the wards to "pick up" as they can.

(2) A good "home" for the probationers in the hospital, where they learn moral discipline—for technical training is only half the battle, perhaps less than half; where the probationers are steadily "mothered" by a "home" Sister (class mistress).

(3) Staff of training school. (a) A trained matron over all, who is not only a housekeeper, but distinctly the head and superintendent of the nursing. (b) A "home" Sister (assistant superintendent)—making the "home" a real home to the probationers, giving them classes, disciplining their life. (c) Ward Sisters (head nurses of wards) who have been trained in the school—to a certain degree permanent, that is, not

constantly changing. For they are the key to the
whole situation, the matron influencing through them
nurses (day and night), probationers, wardmaids,
patients. For, after all, the hospital is for the good
of the patients, not for the good of the nurses. And
the patients are not there to teach probationers upon.
Rather, probationers had better not be there at all
unless they understand that they are there for the
patients, and not for themselves.

There should be an *entente cordiale* between matron,
assistant matrons, "home" Sister, and whatever
other female head there is, with frequent informal
meetings, exchanging information, or there can be
no unity in training.

Nursing proper means, besides giving the medicines
and stimulants prescribed, or the surgical appliances,
the proper use of fresh air (ventilation), light, warmth,
cleanliness, quiet, and the proper chousing and giving
of diet, all at the least expense of vital power to the
sick. And so health-at-home nursing means exactly
the same proper use of the same natural elements
with as much life-giving power as possible to the
healthy.

We have awakened, though still far from the mark,
to the need of training or teaching for nursing proper.
But, while a large part of so-called civilisation has
been advancing in direct opposition to the laws of
health, we uncivilised persons, the women, in whose
hands rests the health of babies, household health,
still persevere in thinking health something that
grows of itself (as Topsy said, "God made me so long,
and I grow'd the rest myself"), while we don't take
the same care of human health as we do of that of
our plants, which, we know very well, perish in the

rooms, dark and close, to which we too often confine human beings, especially in their sleeping rooms and workshops.

The life duration of babies is the most "delicate test" of health conditions. What is the proportion of the whole population of cities or country which dies before it is five years old? We have tons of printed knowledge on the subject of hygiene and sanitation. The causes of enormous child mortality are perfectly well known: they are chiefly want of cleanliness, want of fresh air, careless dieting and clothing, want of whitewashing, dirty feather-beds and bedding—in one word, want of household care of health. The remedies are just as well known, but how much of this knowledge has been brought into the homes and households and habits of the people, poor or even rich? Infection, germs, and the like are now held responsible as carriers of disease. "Mystic rites," such as disinfection and antiseptics, take the place of sanitary measures and hygiene.

The true criterion of ventilation, for instance, is to step out of the bedroom or sick-room in the morning into the open air. If on returning to it you feel the least sensation of closeness, the ventilation has not been enough, and that room has been unfit for either sick or well to sleep in. Here is the natural test provided for the evil.

The laws of God—the laws of life—are always conditional, always inexorable. But neither mothers nor school-mistresses, nor nurses of children are practically taught how to work within those laws which God has assigned to the relations of our bodies with the world in which He has put them. In other words, we do not study, we do not practise the laws which make these bodies, into which He has put our minds, healthy or unhealthy organs of those minds: we do not practise how to give our children healthy existences.

It would be utterly unfair to lay all the fault upon us women, none upon the buildings, drains, water-supply. There are millions of cottages, more of town dwellings, even of the rich, where it is utterly impossible to have fresh air.

As for the workshops, work-people should remember health is their only capital, and they should come to an understanding among themselves not only to have the means, but to use the means to secure pure air in their places of work, which is one of the prime agents of health. This would be worth a "trades union," almost worth a strike.

And the crowded national or board school—in it how many children's epidemics have their origin! And the great school dormitories! Scarlet fever and measles would be no more ascribed to "current contagion," or to "something being much about this year," but to its right cause: nor would "plague and pestilence" be said to be "in God's hands," when, so far as we know, He has put them into our own.

The chief "epidemic" that reigns this year is "folly." You must form public opinion. The generality of officials will only do what you make them. *You*, the public, must make them do what you want. But while public opinion, or the voice of the people, is somewhat awake to the building and drainage question, it is not at all awake to teaching mothers and girls practical hygiene. Where, then, is the remedy for this ignorance?

Health in the home can only be learnt from the

home and in the home. Some eminent medical officers, referring to ambulance lectures, nursing lectures, the fashionable hygienic lectures of the day, have expressed the opinion that we do no more than play with our subject when we "sprinkle" lectures over the community, as that kind of teaching is not instruction, and can never be education: that as medicine and surgery can, like nursing, only be properly taught and properly learnt in the sick-room and by the patient's side, so sanitation can only be taught properly and learned properly in the home and house. Some attempts have been made practically to realise this, to which subsequent reference will be made.

Wise men tell us that it is expecting too much to suppose that we shall do any real good by giving a course of lectures on selected subjects in medicine, anatomy, physiology, and other such cognate subjects, all "watered down" to suit the public palate, which is really the sort of thing one tries to do in that kind of lectures.

It is surely not enough to say, "The people are much interested in the lecture." The point is, Did they practise the lecture in their own homes afterwards? did they really apply themselves to the household health and the means of improving it? Is anything better worth practising for mothers than the health of their families?

The work we are speaking of has nothing to do with nursing disease, but with maintaining health by removing the things which disturb it, which have been summed up in the population in general as "dirt, drink, diet, damp, draughts, drains."

But, in fact, the people do not believe in sanitation

as affecting health, as preventing disease. They think it is a "fad" of the doctors and rich people. They believe in catching cold and in infection, catching complaints from each other, but not from foul earth, bad air, or impure water. May not some remedy be found for these evils by directing the attention of the public to the training of health-nurses, as has already been done with regard to the training of sick-nurses?

The scheme before referred to for health-at-home nursing has arisen in connection with the newly-constituted administration of counties in England, by which the local authority of the county (County Council) has been invested by Act of Parliament with extended sources of income applicable to the teaching of nursing and sanitary knowledge, in addition to the powers which they already possessed for sanitary inspection and the prevention of infectious diseases. This scheme is framed for rural districts, but the general principles are also applicable to urban populations, though, where great numbers are massed together, a fresh set of difficulties must be met, and different treatment be necessary.

The scheme contemplates the training of ladies, so-called health missioners, so as to qualify them to give instruction to village mothers in: (1) The sanitary condition of the person, clothes and bedding, and house. (2) The management of health of adults, women before and after confinement, infants and children. The teaching by the health missioners would be given by lectures in the villages, followed by personal instruction by way of conversation with the mothers in their own homes, and would be directed to: (1) The condition of the homes themselves in a sanitary point of view; (2) the essential principles of keeping the body in health, with reference to the skin, the circulation, and the digestion; and (3) instruction as to what to do in cases of emergency or accident before the doctor comes, and with reference to the management of infants and children. In the addendum to this paper will be found a scheme for training health-at-home missioners, a syllabus of lectures given by the medical officer to the health missioners, and a syllabus of health lectures given by the health missioners to village mothers.

IV. Dangers. After only a generation of nursing arise the dangers: (1) Fashion on the one side, and its consequent want of earnestness. (2) Mere money-getting on the other. Woman does not live by wages alone. (3) Making nursing a profession, and not a calling.

What is it to feel a *calling* for anything? Is it not to do our work in it to satisfy the high idea of what is the right, the best, and not because we shall be found out if we don't do it? This is the "enthusiasm" which every one, from a shoemaker to a sculptor, must have in order to follow his "calling" properly. Now, the nurse has to do not with shoes or with marble, but with living human beings.

How, then, to keep up the high tone of a calling, to "make your calling and election sure"? By fostering that bond of sympathy (*esprit de corps*) which community of aims and of action in good work induces: a common nursing home in the hospital for hospital nurses and for probationer nurses; a common home for private nurses during intervals of engagements, whether attached to a hospital, or separate; a home for district nurses (wherever possible). where four or five can live together; all homes under loving, trained, moral, and religious, as well as technical superintendence, such as to keep up the tone of the inmates with constant supply of all material wants and constant sympathy. Man cannot live by bread alone, still less woman. Wages is not the only question, but high home-helps.

The want of these is more especially felt among private nurses. The development in recent years of trained private nursing, *i. e.*, of nursing one sick or injured person at a time at home, is astonishing. But not less astonishing the want of knowledge of what training is, and, indeed, of what woman is. The danger is that the private nurse may become an irresponsible nomad. She has no home. There can be no *esprit de corps* if the "corps" is an indistinguishable mass of hundreds, perhaps thousands, of women unknown to her, except, perhaps, by a name in a register. All community of feeling and higher tone absents itself. And too often the only aim left is to force up wages. Absence of the nursing home is almost fatal to keeping up to the mark. Night nurses even in hospitals, and even district nurses (another branch of trained nursing of the sick poor without almsgiving which has developed recently), and above all private nurses, deteriorate if they have no *esprit de corps*, no common home under wise and loving supervision for intervals between engagements. What they can get in holidays, in comforts, in money, these good women say themselves, is an increasing danger to many. In private nursing the nurse is sometimes spoilt, sometimes "put upon," sometimes both.

In the last few years, private trained nursing, district trained nursing, have, as has been said, gained immeasurably in importance, and with it how to train, how to govern (in the sense of keeping up to the highest attainable in tone and character, as well as in technical training), must gain also immeasurably in importance, must constitute almost a new starting-point. Nursing may cease to be a calling in any better sense than millinery is. To have a life of freedom, with an interesting employment, for a few years—to do as little as you can and amuse yourself as much as you can—is possibly a danger pressing on.

(4) There is another danger, perhaps the greatest of all. It is also a danger which grows day by day. It is this; as literary education and colleges for women to teach literary work start and multiply and improve, some, even of the very best women, believe that everything can be taught by book and lecture,[1] and tested by examination—that memory is the great step to excellence.

Can you teach horticulture or agriculture by books, *e. g.*, describing the different manures, artificial and natural, and their purposes? The being able to know every clod, and adapt the appropriate manure to it, is the real thing. Could you teach painting by giving, *e. g.* Fuseli's lectures? Fuseli himself said, when asked how he mixed his colours, "With brains, sir"—that is, practice guided by brains. But you have another, a quite other sort of a thing to do with nursing: for you have to do with living bodies and living minds, and feelings of both body and mind.

It is said that you give examinations and certificates to plumbers, engineers, etc. But it is impossible to compare nurses with plumbers, or carpenters, or en-

[1] Miss Nightingale is greatly mistaken in this statement. Instead of "women" she should have said "men," though they are not the best.

gineers, or even with gardeners.   The main, the tremendous difference is that nurses have to do with these living bodies and no less living minds: for the life is not vegetable life, nor mere animal life, but it is human life—with living, that is, conscious forces, not electric or gravitation forces, but human forces. If you examine at all, you must examine all day long, current examination, current supervision, as to what the nurse is doing with this double, this damaged life entrusted to her.

The physician or surgeon gives his orders, generally his conditional orders, perhaps once or twice a day, perhaps not even that.   The nurse has to carry them out, with intelligence of conditions, every minute of the twenty-four hours.

The nurse must have method, self-sacrifice, watchful activity, love of the work, devotion to duty (that is, the service of the good), the courage, the coolness of the soldier, the tenderness of the mother, the absence of the prig (that is, never thinking that she has attained perfection or that there is nothing better). She must have a threefold interest in her work—an intellectual interest in the case, a (much higher) hearty interest in the patient, a technical (practical) interest in the patient's care and cure.   She must not look upon patients as made for nurses, but upon nurses as made for patients.

There may also now—I only say *may*—with all this dependence on literary lore in nurse training, be a real danger of being satisfied with diagnosis, or with looking too much at the pathology of the case, without cultivating the resource or intelligence for the thousand and one means of mitigation, even where there is no cure.

And never, never let the nurse forget that she must look for the fault of the nursing, as much as for the fault of the disease, in the symptoms of the patient.

(5) Forty or fifty years ago a hospital was looked upon as a box to hold patients in. The first question never was, Will the hospital do them no harm? Enormous strides have had to be made to build and arrange hospitals so as to do the patients no sanitary or insanitary harm. Now there is danger of a hospital being looked upon as a box to train nurses in. Enormous strides must be made not to do them harm, to give them something that can really be called an "all-around" training.

Can it be possible that a testimonial or certificate of three years' so-called training or service from a hospital—*any* hospital with a certain number of beds—can be accepted as sufficient to certify a nurse for a place in a public register? As well might we not take a certificate from any garden of a certain number of acres, that plants are certified valuable if they have been three years in the garden?

(6) Another danger—that is, stereotyping, not progressing. "No system can endure that does not march." Are we walking to the future or to the past? Are we progressing or are we stereotyping? We remember that we have scarcely crossed the threshold of uncivilised civilisation in nursing: there is still so much to do. Don't let us stereotype mediocrity.

To sum up the dangers;

I. On one side, fashion, and want of earnestness, not making it a life, but a mere interest consequent on this.

II. On the other side, mere money-getting: yet man does not live by bread alone, still less woman.

III. Making it a profession, and not a calling. Not making your "calling and election sure"; wanting, especially with private nurses, the community of feeling of a common nursing home,[1] pressing towards the "mark of your calling," keeping up the moral tone.

IV. Above all, danger of making it book-learning and lectures—not an apprenticeship, a workshop practice.

V. Thinking that any hospital with a certain number of beds may be a box to train nurses in, regardless of the conditions essential to a sound hospital organisation, especially the responsibility of the female head for the conduct and discipline of the nurses.

VI. Imminent danger of stereotyping instead of progressing. "No system can endure that does not march." Objects of registration not capable of being gained by a public register. Who is to guarantee our guarantors? Who is to make the inquiries? You might as well register mothers as nurses. A good nurse must be a good woman.

V. The health of the unity is the health of the community. Unless you have the health of the unity there is no community health.

Competition, or each man for himself, and the devil against us all, may be necessary, we are told, but it is the enemy of health. Combination is the antidote—combined interests, recreation, combination to secure the best air, the best food, and all that makes life useful, healthy, and happy. There is no such thing as

---

[1] In the United States it is probable that private nurses are of higher education than in England. On the other hand, they have the doubtful dignity of graduates.

independence.   As far as we are successful, our success
lies in combination.   .

The Chicago Exhibition is a great combination
from all parts of the world to prove the dependence
of man on man.

What a lesson in combination the United States
have taught to the whole world, and are teaching!

In all departments of life there is no apprenticeship
except in the workshop.   No theories, no book-learning can ever dispense with this or be useful for anything, except as a stepping-stone.   And rather more
than for anything else is this true for health.   Book-
learning is useful only to render the practical health
of the health-workshop intelligent, so that every
stroke of work done there should be felt to be an illustration of what has been learned elsewhere—a driving
home, by an experience not to be forgotten, what has
been gained by knowledge too easily forgotten.

Look for the ideal, but put it into the actual—"not
by vague exhortations, but by striving to turn beliefs
into energies that would work in all the details" of
health.   The superstitions of centuries, the bad habits of generations, cannot be cured by lecture, book, or
examination.

VI.   May our hopes be that, as every year the technical qualifications constituting a skilful and observing nurse meet with more demands on her from the
physicians and surgeons, progress may be made year
by year, and that not only in technical things, but in
the qualifications which constitute a good and trustworthy woman, without which she cannot be a good
nurse.   Examination papers, examinations, public registration, graduation, form little or no test of these

qualifications. The least educated governess, who
may not be a good nurse at all, may, and probably
will, come off best in examination papers, while the
best nurse may come off worst. May we hope that
the nurse may understand more and more of the moral
and material government of the world by the Supreme
Moral Governor, higher, better, holier than her "own
acts," that government which enwraps her round,
and by which her own acts must be led, with which
her own acts must agree in their due proportion in
order that this, the highest hope of all, may be hers;
raising her above, *i. e.*, putting beneath her, dangers,
fashions, mere money-getting, solitary money-getting,
but availing herself of the high helps that may be
given her by the sympathy and support of good
"homes"; raising her above intrusive personal morti-
fications, pride in her own proficiency (she may have
a just pride in her own doctors and training school),
sham, and clap-trap; raising her to the highest
"grade" of all, to be a fellow-worker with the Supreme
Good, with God! That she may be a "graduate" in
this, how high! that she may be a "graduate" in
words, not realities, how low!

We are only on the threshold of nursing.

In the future, which I shall not see, for I am old,
may a better way be opened! May the methods by
which every infant, every human being, will have the
best chance of health, the me hods by which every
sick person will have the best chance of recovery, be
learned and practised! Hospitals are only an inter-
mediate stage of civilisation, never intended, at all
events, to take in the whole sick population.

May we hope that the day will come when every
mother will become a health-nurse, when every poor

sick person will have the opportunity of a share in a district sick-nurse at home! But it will not be out of a register: the nurse w.ll not be a stereotyped one. We find a trace of nursing here, another there; we find nothing like a nation, or race, or class who know how to provide the elementary conditions demanded for the recovery of their sick, whose mothers know how to bring up their infants for health.

May we hope that when we are all dead and gone leaders will arise who have been personally experienced in the hard, practical work, the difficulties and the joys of organising nursing reforms, and who will lead far beyond anything we have done! May we hope that every nurse will be an atom in the hierarchy of the ministers of the Highest! But then she must be in her place in the hierarchy, not alone, not an atom in the indistinguishab e mass of the thousands of nurses. High hopes, which will not be deceived!

Aside from nursing proper Miss Nightingale's sympathetic interest and the magic power of her name have been given to innumerable causes and campaigns of right against wrong. Among such we may instance especially the long struggle made by a few heroic women (finally successful) for the repeal of odious laws regarding the regulation of vice in England. Miss Nightingale's name was placed on a petition for repeal. She has also always held broad impersonal views on the subject of public service. An illustration of this attitude is given by some of her words in *Notes on Nursing*.

I would earnestly ask my sisters to keep clear of

both the jargons now current everywhere (for they *are* equally jargons): of the jargon, namely, about the "rights" of women, which urges women to do all that men do, including the medical and other professions, merely because men do it, and without regard to whether this *is* the best that women can do; and of the jargon which urges women to do nothing that men do, merely because they are women, and should be "recalled to a sense of their duty as women," and because "this is women's work," and "that is men's," and "these are things which women should not do," which is all assertion, and nothing more. Surely woman should bring the best she has, *whatever* that is, to the work of God's world, without attending to either of these cries. . . . But you want to do the thing that is good, whether it is "suitable for a woman" or not.

It does not make a thing good that it is remarkable that a woman should have been able to do it. Neither does it make a thing bad, which would have been good had a man done it, that it has been done by a woman.

Oh, leave these jargons, and go your way straight to God's work, in simplicity and singleness of heart.[1]

She has been a life-long advocate of suffrage for women, says the *Woman's Journal*, and when asked one time for her reasons, said:

I have no reasons. It seems to me almost self-evident, an axiom, that every householder and tax-payer should have a voice in the expenditure of the money we pay, including, as this does, interests the most vital to a human being.

[1] *Notes*, p. 135.

An interesting testimony to her constant interest in and attention to progressive social steps was a letter written by her in 1892, to a public official, in which she said:

We must create a public opinion which will drive the Government, instead of the Government having to drive us—an enlightened public opinion, wise in principles, wise in details. We hail the County Council as being or becoming one of the strongest engines in our favour, at once fathering and obeying the great impulse for national health against national and local disease. For we have learned that we have national health in our own hand—local sanitation, national health. But we have to contend against centuries of superstition and generations of indifference."

One of the most interesting published expressions of her views on social questions, showing, as it does, that from her sick-room she constantly with eager hope followed the tendencies of political and voluntary social action, is an article written in 1873:

What will this world be in August, 1999 . . . what shall we wish then to have been doing, and what shall we wish not to have been doing? . . . Will the views of family life, of social life, of the duties of social life, be the same then as now? Will the distribution of riches, of poverty, of the land . . . be the same then as now? Will religion consist then, as now, not in whether a man is "just, true and merciful" . . . but whether the man "had believed what he was told to believe" . . . What shall we then wish to have

been doing now?   Is it reading or writing mere articles? . . . or is it working, solving by real personal
work the great questions, or rather problems, which,
as they are solved or unsolved, will make 1999 what
it will be?—such as depauperisation, colonisation,
education, reformation, legislation, making religion
and God a real personal presence among us, not a
belief in a creed, a going to a room or church, "for
what we call our prayers."

In this article all of her life-long elemental, fervent hatred of sham and conventional lies breaks
forth again : it is an expression of revolt—of rejection of current smugness of thought.

Religion, sermons, consist now either in telling us
to believe what we are " told to believe," and to attend
the "means of grace"—never enquiring whether
there be not other "means of grace," or else, in
telling us to practise certain so-called religious or
social virtues in that " state of life" (or state of mind)
"to which it has been pleased to call us," leaving life
just as it is, taking for granted that that " state of life "
is the one *we are born into*.

But, in 1999, shall we not wish to have worked out
what life, family life, social life, political life, *should*
be, and not to have taken for granted that family
life, social life, political life, are to be as they are, and
we to get as much enjoyment out of them as we can?

. . . It never seems to be thought that it is more
difficult to discover the ways of creating the kingdom
of heaven upon earth than to discover the ways of
the solar system—yet no one would ever think of
recommending the study of astronomy to be pursued

in the weak, pretentious, sententious manner that we are preached to about pursuing Life. Yet life is a harder study than astronomy, if we are really to succeed in it, really to succeed in bringing about a little corner of the kingdom of heaven.

We are never lectured about the study of anything else in the wild, wishy-washy, womanish terms that we are preached to about life. And this is thought Christian—as if Christ had not been the boldest preacher that ever went about reforming life. . . .

In a new and striking form she re-embodies her life-long insistence on thorough preparation as necessary for efficiency:

Freedom is indeed not doing as we like, not everybody following his or her own way, even if that were possible, but self-control. Self-control, plus a control or command of our subject, gives "freedom"; but a person who has no control over any subject, or right use of any faculties, cannot have freedom. It all comes to the same thing, viz., the necessity of doing what we do well, of what we do being what is well to do, if we are to attain what is commonly called "humility" (disregard of self, useful care for others, efficient service of God and of our brethren).

The work of Arnold Toynbee had evidently aroused her keenest sympathy. She alludes to his work, without mentioning him by name, and urges the need of social workers:

The kingdom of heaven is within, but no one laboured like Christ to make it *without*. He actually recommended people to *leave* their own lives to do this, so much was he penetrated by the conviction, filled by the enthusiasm, that we *must alter* the "state of life" (*not* conform to it, no, oh thrice, ten times, no! a hundred times, no!) into which we are born, in order *to bring about* a "kingdom of heaven." Never was anything less like remaining within good intentions than Christ's teaching, than Christ's example. . . . We must go forth into the world to bring about the kingdom of heaven. . . . If we *did* the things people now *prate* about, write about, speechify, debate, report about, that *would* be—Administration.

She closes with some of her own inimitable aphorisms—keen-edged as a surgeon's knife. She comments on the widespread epidemic of fruitless talk and compares the common tendency to overlook the most real and necessary for the less important to the words of a famous surgeon, who said of a patient on whom a notable operation had been performed, "*He died cured.*"

Discussion nowadays almost precludes consideration—it leaves no time for thought. . . . The only discussion that can be of any use is that between persons who have thought out something about the subject, who bring some contribution of individual thought or of personal knowledge to the common stock. What a valuable rule it would be, for every half hour spent in discussion spend two previous half hours in thought!

Discussion will not govern the world, nor even a single home in it.

Language, says Talleyrand, was given us to conceal our thoughts. Even that is better than what we see now, when language seems to be given us to conceal our want of thoughts.[1]

To sum up such a character as Miss Nightingale's, as displayed in her writings, in scattered personal testimony, and in the multiplied proofs of her energising influence on others, is a task worthy of more able minds than any that have yet attempted it. So rich a combination as hers has rarely been found of dominant, masterful intellectual genius, of creative thought, of individual executive ability to transform thought into effective action, while health lasted, and, when health vanished, still to effect this transformation through a rare force of influence on others; of maternal tenderness for all helpless and suffering life, of cosmopolitan sympathies and diverse interests, of a glorious capacity for righteous anger, with kindliness, and forgetfulness of self; of free, fearless opinions. These characteristics suggest a personality of rare proportions, for whose heroic lines her keen satirical wit, her severity of judgment of incapacity and futility, her intolerance of mediocrity and commonplaceness form only the needed shade and colouring.[2]

[1] A Sub-'Note of Interrogation,' by Florence Nightingale, *Fraser's Magazine*, July, 1873.

[2] Dr. Abraham Jacobi has characterised her as one "who has proved how to become immortal without enjoying high office, or playing on a cannon, or tyrannising nations, or being born on a throne."

CHAPTER VI.

MISS NIGHTINGALE'S CO-WORKERS.

THE most piteous of the caravansaries for the sick, and the very last to be cared for, were the infirmary wards of the great workhouses or almshouses. These, the last refuge of the incurable and chronic poor, beyond which no further transfer was possible save into the grave, appear to have been left quite without the pale of human pity or even interest until as late as the middle of the nineteenth century, when a small group of women, chief and most untiring among whom was Miss Louisa Twining, began a veritable siege to break down the walls of official callousness and ignorance behind which the dependent poor were virtually imprisoned. This siege has lasted throughout the half-century, for Miss Twining still lives, with the happiness of knowing that the battle has been won, though final outposts of stupidity still remain to be taken.

The whole story of these women's persistent and undiscouraged efforts—of the obstacles placed in their way; of the rebuffs which a jealous officialdom, fearing the light of public inquiry and resenting criticism, offered them; of their long, slow, patiently-striven-for gains and advances, resulting in the gradual separation of the sick from the other dependents and in the introduction of enlightened methods of caring for all classes of dependents—is a most impressive one, and it is safe to say that, had it been a campaign of war between nations, it would have been found worthy of volumes upon volumes of description.

Miss Twining's work has gone side by side and hand in hand with the reform of nursing, and to-day, though there is still much to be done, a marvellous change has taken place in the workhouses, many of which now have hospitals and trained nursing of distinguished excellence.

Miss Twining began visiting the workhouses in 1853. She first went to see an old woman whom she had known at home, and from this circumstance may be said to date the beginning of all systematic effort for the organised visiting of workhouses both in London and in the country.[1]

A few years later, Miss Elliott and Miss Frances Power Cobbe also becoming deeply interested in the problem of the incurably ill poor, independently, at first, of Miss Twining's work, did much to stir popular sympathy by issuing (in 1861) the first published articles advocating the separation of incurable and chronic patients from the ordi-

[1] *Recollections of Workhouse Visiting and Managing during Twenty-five Years*, by Louisa Twining. Kegan Paul & Co., London, 1880, p. 6.

nary workhouse population, and urging, further, that official permission should be given for private philanthropy to introduce little comforts and pleasures for the sick; for, incredible as it may seem, this simple effort of good-will, when tried by individuals, met with suspicion and peremptory refusals from the officials in charge of workhouses. Miss Elliott and Miss Cobbe together wrote a circular letter embodying these propositions, and sent it to some six hundred and sixty Unions (guardians of the poor), and through their efforts the Association for the Promotion of Social Science which had been founded in 1856 was enlisted in the cause of workhouse reform.[1]

That was a time when the most ordinary promptings of common-sense and humanity were regarded in some quarters as visionary, for Miss Cobbe (who tells many ludicrous and humorous tales) recalls a dictum of the *Morning Post*, whose editor regarded one of the ablest men in England as unquestionably "cracked" because he believed that it was possible to reform juvenile criminals.[2]

The wretched system of nursing by drunken and degraded paupers, then prevalent, was steadily assailed by all these women. Miss Cobbe speaks of the "monster evil of the unqualified nurse," and concentrated her interest upon this special department.

[1] *Life of Frances Power Cobbe, as told by Herself.* Swan Sonnenschein, London, 1904, p. 315.

[2] " Social Science Congresses and Women's Part in Them," by Frances Power Cobbe, *Macmillan's Magazine*, 1861.

She and Miss Elliott wrote the pamphlets *The Workhouse as a Hospital, Destitute Incurables, The Sick in Workhouses*, etc. As time went on Miss Cobbe became absorbed in other interests, while Miss Twining, who from the first had applied herself to no less a purpose than that of revolutionising the entire workhouse system, made the nursing side one of her reforms, but not the only one. In following out her entire programme she did much to induce a better class of women to take up nursing. Her pamphlet *Nursing for the Sick, with a Letter to Young Women*, London, 1861, is a stirring appeal to the latent tenderness of human nature and gives a pitiful picture of the dreadful conditions in the workhouses.

What some of these conditions were may be gathered from official reports. In 1865 a report of the Poor Law Board printed for the House of Commons showed 6400 sick in forty-one London workhouses, of whom one third were patients suffering from acute, curable diseases. To this mass of patients there were seventy-one paid nurses (and it must be remembered that even these were of the Gamp class), some workhouses having only one nurse apiece. Thirteen of these institutions had no paid nurses at all, but only pauper helpers, many of whom were over seventy and even eighty years of age, while a full one fourth were over sixty. Nor did the term "paid nurse" mean anything very desirable from the labour standpoint.

Some of these nurses were paid the lavish sum of one penny per week, while others received extra diet, or clothing, as payment. The medical officers, who sometimes had as many as three hundred sick under their care, were compelled to buy the medicines for the patients out of their salaries. It is probable that in those wards treatment by the excessive use of drugs was regarded with disapproval.

The instructive thing about all of this tragedy is that the male officials who were in charge quite generally felt that these methods were satisfactory and that improvement was unnecessary. No wonder, with such standards, that the visits of women from outside, who dared to criticise and question, were regarded as unendurable and prying impertinences.

After visiting the south-western counties, with fifty-eight workhouses, the report of the Poor Law Inspector said: "Nursing generally satisfactory; almost every infirmary having one paid nurse, and one or more helpers." And yet this district had one infirmary where there were two hundred and fifty-one sick, including the insane, and only six nurses with nineteen pauper helpers, while there was no night nursing existent in any of the workhouses. Another Poor Law Inspector must be commended as having a little more intelligence than the first mentioned. After visiting one workhouse where no division was made between medical and surgical patients, where the itch was classed as "vagrancy," where one wash-basin and one roller-towel were allowed weekly in wards of from eight to fourteen patients, where one woman nurse with a male helper had charge of seventy insane patients of both sexes, and where one other nurse had under her sole care one hundred and fifty sick persons, this man of rare perception and firmness said, "Although the medical officer is contented with the existing conditions of the infirmary, I do not consider it in a satisfactory state." [1]

In 1855 a proposal was made by a society of physicians, of whom Dr. Sieveking was foremost, to train the numerous able-bodied women in the workhouses as nurses. Miss Twining in speaking of this could not approve the plan, as these women were usually of bad character, and although it was sanctioned, and the Board of Guardians had instructions to carry it out, it never actually took form. [2]

In 1857 an association was formed through Miss Twining's efforts called the Central Society for the Promotion of Workhouse Visiting, and two years later it started its own journal. This society, affiliated with the Social Science Association, carried on the work of workhouse reform. The greatest circumspection was necessary, for Miss Twining relates the incident of a body of visitors

[1] *A Century of Nursing.* Reports of the State Charities Aid Association of New York State, 1876. Quoting from Parliamentary Papers, vols. lx.–lxi., 1866–68.

[2] *Recollections*, p. 17.

being dismissed from a London workhouse in consequence of complaints of well-nigh unendurable grievances endured by the inmates and noticed by a lady—a person of influence and position, as well as humanity.[1]

In 1866 the *Lancet* made an exhaustive investigation into the sick wards of the London workhouses, and brought many abuses to light.

Not until 1872 was the great gain made of having a woman appointed as official inspector of the metropolitan workhouses.[2] Not easily could men be brought to see the necessity of this, for, as Miss Carpenter had once said, "There never yet lived a man so clever but the matron of an institution could bamboozle him about every department of her business."[3]

A lovely outcome of Miss Twining's work was the establishment of the Flower Mission, which has brought solace to so many bedridden patients. She soon found that flowers were the one gift that excited no animosity, and began in 1858 taking them systematically to her sick people. From this grew up in time the organised society which has since then done so much to bring joy into hospital wards.

The education of the public carried on by Miss Twining through all these years has been of simply enormous extent. Her most irresistible weapon has been the absolute accuracy of her every state-

[1] *Recollections*, p. 60.   [2] *Ibid.*, p. 66.
[3] Frances Power Cobbe, *Life*, p. 306.

ment. Moderate and exact in the use of words, steadfast, merciful, and convincing, she has been to the workhouses what Mrs. Fry was to the prisons and Miss Nightingale to the hospitals.

The introduction of trained nursing into workhouse infirmaries was accomplished by Agnes Elizabeth Jones, one of the most beloved of the pioneers in nursing, and one who was a martyr to the cause, but it was the well-planned undertaking of Mr. Wm. Rathbone, a Quaker of Liverpool, who has had a very important part in the progress of English nursing.

The illness and death of his wife in 1859 first turned Mr. Rathbone's attention to nursing. The thought of how the poor must suffer in illness prompted him to try an experiment, and he engaged the woman who had been his wife's nurse, and who was capable and kindly, to work among the poor of the city. He paid her a salary, and provided nourishment and appliances for the sick. The results encouraged him and he wished to extend the service, but there were no more nurses to be had. He went to Miss Nightingale for advice, and she counselled him to try to train nurses in Liverpool, at the Royal Infirmary. The committee of this hospital was anxious to improve the nursing, and offered Mr. Rathbone a seat on their board. His response was to offer to build a training school and home for nurses and give it to the infirmary. He wrote to Agnes Jones to offer her the position of superintendent, but, as we shall see, this was not to be, and finally Miss Merry-weather went to St. Thomas's for training, then took the post, and gave admirable service there. She trained nurses for the wards and for district nursing, and the city was divided into eighteen districts with a nurse and a group of lady visitors for each. So practical was Mr. Rathbone that for a whole year he made rounds regularly with some one of the nurses, to see conditions for himself.

The next thing that impressed him was to learn that the poor abhorred the thought of going to the parish infirmary, and he studied its conditions. There were twelve hundred sick there, in every stage of misery, and none but pauper untrained help. Mr. Rathbone urged bringing in a trained superintendent with a group of nurses, and, as the authorities were very unwilling to incur any expense, he offered to defray the whole cost of the experiment for three years' time. They agreed to this, and he now offered this second and infinitely more difficult piece of work to Agnes Jones, secured twelve Nightingale nurses to assist her, and on the 16th of May, 1865, this little group of women began their renovation of the infirmary with eighteen probationers and fifty-four of the old pauper nurses.[1]

Agnes was born in Cambridge in 1832, and from her early girlhood she was restless with the eager

[1] *William Rathbone*: *A Memoir*, by Eleanor F. Rathbone. Macmillan & Co., London, 1905, pp. 156–173.

desire to be of real usefulness. Beside a natural gift for bringing help and cheer to those around her she was also of excellent executive ability and mental acumen. She was deeply imbued with the excessive evangelical, sentimental piety prevalent at that time (the continuous outpourings of which in speech and writings seem now so self-conscious and unctuous), but had the true missionary spirit. In her travels on the continent she visited Kaiserswerth and other deaconess establishments, and was at first greatly drawn to that life, though later, as she recorded in her diary, she concluded that one could do as well out of as in the deaconess order. For seven years after her visit she longed to go to Kaiserswerth for training, and at last her family, who were of the leisured and cultured class, rather unwilling to have her take this then unusual step, consented, and she spent a year there, from 1860 to 1861. Her letters from Kaiserswerth, and her descriptions of the life are very interesting and give realistic and graphic pictures of the daily round. While in training a number of opportunities of work offered themselves to her—one to go to Syria, another to help Mrs. Ranyard in the Bible Mission and district work, and Mr. Rathbone's first offer to come to Liverpool.

She felt drawn to each, as an ardent explorer does to new countries, but her chief purpose then was to proselytise. It cannot but strike one oddly that she should write to Mr. Rathbone, himself

one of the salt of the earth, a very pillar of goodness, in this pedantic tone: "You send me the
ground plan of the building, but I would ask, Is
its foundation and corner-stone to be Christ and
Him crucified, the only Saviour? Is the Christian
training of nurses to be the primary and hospital
skill the secondary object? . . . I shall not em-
bark in any work whose great aim is not obedience to the command 'Preach the Gospel to every
creature.' . . . "

As the results of this attitude might have been
doubtful in hospital work, the plan went no further
then, and Agnes completed her term at Kaiserswerth and returned to London. She became
more and more attracted to the definite work of
nursing, and consulted Miss Nightingale about the
advisability of entering St. Thomas's for the training. Her family was unwilling to have her take
this step, and even she herself hesitated, partly because of the social inferiority of most of the older
type of nurses; but at last, after some work with
Mrs. Ranyard in the Mission, and more travels to
centres of work and training abroad, her mother
finally consented and, having first had a personal
interview with Mr. Rathbone, she went to St.
Thomas's as a Nightingale nurse, and afterwards,
with twelve other Nightingale nurses revolutionised the great workhouse infirmary at Liverpool,
established order, training, a moral atmosphere, cheerfulness, cleanliness, and good nursing,
giving a wonderful demonstration of what can be

accomplished by skill and devotion. Her achieve-
ment was accented by her death. After three
years of labour so untiring and exacting that she
scarcely had time to write letters to her family,
she died of typhus fever in the hospital.

From her splendid demonstration in the Liverpool workhouse extended all the reforms in the
nursing methods of similar institutions. During
her brief illness Miss Nightingale wrote to her family, "I look upon hers as one of the most valuable
lives in England, in the present state of the poor
law and of workhouse nursing." And after her
death she wrote the exquisite tribute to her memory which forms the preface to her biography.[1]

Another figure stands out prominently among
the pioneers of that day and followers of Miss
Nightingale — Miss Florence Lees, now Mrs. Dacre Craven, whose chief distinction was in improving the district nursing service. Although
she did much more than this, it is with this that
her name is especially associated, as Agnes Jones's
with the workhouses and Mrs. Wardroper's with
the training of nurses. Florence Lees was one of the
first four pupils who entered the Nightingale
school.   She has been called the most highly
trained nurse of her day, and probably was
so.   After training at St. Thomas's she had
post-graduate courses in Berlin, Dresden, and

---

[1] See *Una and her Paupers*: *Memorials of Agnes Elizabeth
Jones*, by her Sister.   First American from the second English ed.   London, James Nisbet Co., 1885; New York, 1872.

Kaiserswerth; was surgical Sister in Kings College hospital; then made a tour of inspection through the hospitals of Holland and Denmark. She was then able to gain entrance for training in the Hôtel-Dieu, Lariboisière, and Enfant Jésus hospitals of Paris, and later served under the Sisters of Charity of St. Vincent de Paul in two military hospitals, where she was allowed to pass through every department, from the kitchens and linen-rooms to the operating theatre. In the Franco-Prussian war she had charge of a military hospital before Metz, and of the ambulance service supported by the Crown Princess of Germany.[1]

After Mr. Rathbone's experiment with his first district nurse his example was quite widely imitated, and in London the East London Society, organised for the sole benefit of the poor, was formed in 1868.

In 1874[2] the order of St. John of Jerusalem inaugurated the National Nursing Association to provide more fully trained nurses for the poor, and under the auspices of this association a very important investigation was carried on under the direction of Miss Lees, who was chairman of the Committee of Inquiry. It was found that the whole system of district nursing then existing was very amateur, slovenly, and haphazard. The nurses

[1] See pp. xvi–xvii *Handbook for Hospital Sisters*, by Florence S. Lees. Preface by Henry Acland, M.D., F.R.S. W. Isbister Co., London, 1874.

[2] See *Times*, June 23, June 26, 1874.

were often almoners rather than nurses, and the connection with the physician was very lax. The nurses often prescribed, and boasted of "curing wounds which no doctor had ever seen."[1]

With this report Miss Lees made the recommendation and carried the point which has proved to be of such conspicuous benefit to the service and with which her name must always be associated, *viz.*, that, district nurses should be entirely recruited from the class known as gentlewomen. It was at first regarded as an impossibility. Even Miss Nightingale doubted, and said to Miss Lees, "I don't believe you will find it answer; but try it—try it for a year." Miss Lees's arguments for her side were those which are to-day regarded as axiomatic, and need not be repeated. She was able to carry them into practice, and the results amply justified her. The association was extended as indicated by the title Metropolitan and National Nursing Association, and Miss Lees became the first superintendent of the Central Home.

To the English system of permanency of Sisters or head nurses and of staff nurses or seniors, which was retained and not discarded when the reform of nursing took place, is chiefly due the homelike, serene, and cheerful atmosphere so characteristic of English hospitals, which are, in a final compari-

[1] See Mrs. Dacre Craven's paper on "District Nursing," read at the Congress of Charities and Correction, World's Fair, Chicago, 1893. *Transactions* of Section on Hospitals, Dispensaries, and Nursing. p. 547.

son, the pleasantest and most comfortable for the
patients in the world.   The Sister remains at the
head of her ward for years; only leaving, often, to
retire from service: the staff nurses or seniors also
remain for long periods, five, eight, ten years; the
probationers come and go, during their three or
four years' course, and the entire current is more
steady, more settled, less strenuous, less kaleido-
scopic than is possible when an entire hospital
nursing force changes throughout in two or even
three years' time.[1]   The English matrons, also,
have a more permanent tenure of office than ours;
their duties, privileges, boundaries, and authority
are more clearly recognised, and less frequently
disputed or encroached upon.   They, too, often
remain for a working lifetime at the head of their
households as contentedly as a mother at the head
of her family.   It is true that this security of tenure may conduce to a narrow outlook or excessive
conservatism, but these errors are avoided by contact with the world, and exist as well in our more
unstable environment.   Though changes, under
the English system, are more slowly made, even
when desirable, they are more definitely settled
and more generally acquiesced in when once made.

[1] It is common to see in the English nursing press such notes
as these:

"Miss Eliza Whitmore, known to medical men and nurses
at St. George's hospital as 'Sister Nannie,' has retired from
active work after twenty-five years of devoted service to the
hospital."

"A presentation was recently made at the Norfolk and

The report already mentioned, written for the *British Medical Journal* in 1874, may now be turned to again for a graphic and well touched-up picture of the general conditions of the hospitals at that date, fourteen years after the opening of the Nightingale school. The earlier conditions have been described; now, in 1874, there were the St. John's House Sisters at King's College and at Charing Cross; the Sisters of All Saints at University College hospital, and the Nightingale Sisters at St. Thomas's. At St. George's and the Middlesex the Sisters, though not ladies, were of rather a better social class than the nurses. The old plan of having a permanent and rather inferior class of night nurses was still in force at St. Mary's, St. George's and the London.

St. Bartholomew's had had until recently the German system of each nurse taking in turn one night duty every third night, making nearly thirty hours of continuous duty. Then (1874) each nurse had one week of night duty alternating with two weeks' day duty.

The old plan of giving board money was nearly extinct. It still lingered in a modified form at St. Bartholomew's, where the Sisters had to provide a great part of their own food, whilst the nurses received uncooked rations of meat, flour, and vegetables.

Norwich hospital of a purse of fifty-five sovereigns to Sister Bessey, who is about to retire after thirty-eight years' service. She entered the hospital for training in 1868 and was appointed Sister in 1875."

The special commissioner speaks of the question of the "lady nurse" as a "burning" one. It really meant an entire reorganisation of hospital work, and some hospital directors were much opposed to "lady nurses," because of the necessity it involved of a separate staff for rough housework. It was hard for some men to hear that the nurse must cease being a scrubber; but others pointed out the difficult and unpleasant nature of many purely nursing duties and insisted on the absurdity of taking up the time of trained persons to do unskilled labour, making it clear that the division of labour proposed did not mean that scrubbing was degrading or menial, but that the nurse should be free to *nurse*, and not be taken away from the patient to scrub. A great improvement was recorded in the general average of education among nurses. Thus in 1867 in a large provincial hospital seven out of twenty nurses could not read or write, and three of these were head nurses. But in 1874 no hospital would accept nurses unless they could read and write. There was a distinct improvement in the quality of woman applying, and in the majority of London hospitals the Sisters were ladies.

The improvement advanced but slowly, writes Mrs. Strong:

In the Glasgow infirmary at the beginning of the last quarter century (about 1870) a nurse had to begin as a semi-wardmaid under the name of assistant nurse and work her way without any direct instruction.

She was called at 3 A.M., and began work at 4, cleaning grates, scullery, and bath-room, sweeping and dusting the ward, etc. She also carried the food for the
ward supply, washed the dishes, and did much heavy
carrying which is now done by men. Her duties
ended at 8.30 P.M., without any definite time off duty.
Most of the women slept in small rooms adjoining the
wards and took their meals, with the exception of
dinner, in the ward kitchens. Nurses and servants
shared the same dining-room and had to carry a knife,
fork, and glass with them.[1]

The deliberation with which the English hospitals adopted the new order is shown in a delightfully gossipy reminiscence of one of the Sisters of
the first class of probationers at St. Bartholomew's hospital (which later rapidly moved to the
very front of progress on practical, social, and
educational lines) when the change was instituted
there:

A Reformation.— . . . I came in on May 1, 1877,
just five and twenty years ago. I was one of a batch
of twelve probationers, the first to be trained at St.
Bartholomew's hospital. Before we came there was
no sort of training for the nurses, and of nursing as
one understands it now there was simply none. The
matron, Mrs. Drake, greatly disapproved of such an
innovation as "lady nurses," and tried hard to dissuade
me from entering when I came up to be interviewed.
There was no entrance examination. We all arrived
one morning and proceeded to put on our uniform.

[1] "Preliminary Work," by Mrs. Strong. International
Congress of Nurses, Buffalo, 1901. *Transactions.*

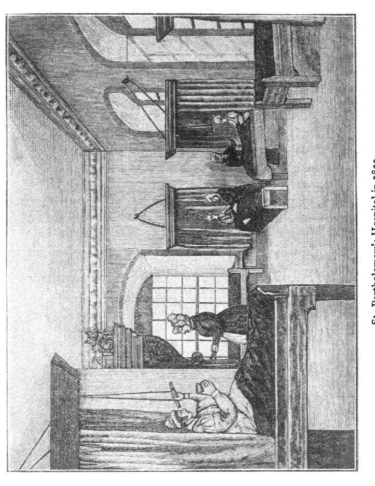

St. Bartholomew's Hospital in 1833

From an old water colour in the hospital

Handbuch der Krankenversorgung u. der Krankenpflege. Liebe, Jacobsohn u. Meyer, Berlin, 1899

What was it? The present probationer's uniform, with the exception of the caps, which were small caps without strings. This was quite different from the uniform of the so-called "staff-nurses," who wore brown merino dresses, aprons without bibs, collars, no cuffs, caps or no caps as they liked, and, when worn, of any description. I remember hearing some weeks after we arrived that the head dispenser had pronounced us "an ornament to the square."

In the afternoon we attended a lecture by Sir Dyce (then Dr.) Duckworth in the lecture-theatre. Though especially for our benefit, it was an open lecture. A few of the Sisters and staff nurses were there, and many students. . . . Curiosity brought them, I suppose. We were something quite new and caused a considerable stir in the place.

That night I was sent to "Harley," where I shared a room opening into the ward (the "dressing-room") with the staff nurses. I did not get much rest. To begin with, my roommate was very drunk and very sick. Being ignorant of the symptoms I wasted much pity on her. When I did fall off to sleep, I was awakened by frightful screams and shouts of "Murder! Fire!" I proceeded to wake my companion, who growled, "Be quiet: it's only 18." Drunkenness was very common among the staff nurses, who were chiefly women of the charwoman type, frequently of bad character, with little or no education, and few of them with even an elementary knowledge of nursing. Some of them might have worked previously at some other hospital, but as often as not they had had no experience whatever when engaged as staff nurses. One woman, I remember, who came some little time after I did and under whom I worked, had been a lady's-maid, and had never done a day's nursing. She was, however, of a decidedly superior class to any of the others, and was, moreover, quite respectable. It was very usual for the friends to bring in presents of gin to bribe the nurses to be kind to the patients. The worst women we had were those who used to come in to look after bad cases, more particularly at night. They were called "night extras." They were most dreadful persons, possessing neither character nor ability, who used to apply here for work much as women now apply for charing. I remember being so horrified soon after I came at the idea of a very bad case (a man whose leg was amputated at the thigh) being left to the tender mercies of one of these creatures, that I summoned up courage to ask Sister Harley to put me on as "special" instead. She consented, and I looked after him in the daytime; at night, of course, he had the "lydy" from outside.

Among the Sisters there was already some improvement. Some there still were of whose virtues the less said the better, and some were wholly untrained, a knowledge of nursing not being in those days a necessary qualification for a Sister. Sister Pitcairn, however, had been for a year or two in Pitcairn, and was undoubtedly much the most highly trained nurse then in the hospital, and Sister Eyes was the ophthalmic Sister, the first to be appointed for that special work. A few, also, had been trained in the Nightingale Home. We should not think much now of the training they had had, but it was a good deal for that time. They also had had considerable experience, and were, moreover, clever and capable women of superior character.

How were we taught? Well, by the Sisters very

little. (The staff nurses were not capable of teaching anything.) Few of the Sisters both could and would teach us. I do not think any Sister taught me anything except Sister Matthew (as she was then) and Sister Pitcairn. Sir Dyce Duckworth or Mr. Willett lectured to us or gave a practical demonstration once a week. Mr. Willett used to have in his out-patient children and teach us to bandage, put on splints, to make and apply plasters, bandages, and so on. Sir Dyce would take us into the wards and give us a lesson on bed-making, poultice-making, or on the contents of the doctor's cupboard, or down to the bath-rooms, where he and old Williams, the bathman, used to show us the best way to get patients in and out of the bath, and how to prepare special baths of various kinds. We were known as "Ducky's lambs." . . . The present bath-rooms off the wards were only just being built. Before we had them all patients who were in fit condition were bathed in the baths under the out-patient department. The only baths in the wards were in the kitchens, and were covered over with wooden covers, which often served as a table on which to carve the dinners.

Then, we picked up what we could, and the resident staff and students taught us a good deal. . . . We were quite a novelty, and every one took a great interest in us. Dr. Griffith, I think, taught me to take temperatures. He was a dresser. The thermometers in use then were very much longer than those we use now, and had to be read while in position, as they ran down at once when removed from the mouth or armpit. They cost twelve shillings sixpence each. The Sisters and nurses never used a thermometer, the dressers and clerks took the temperatures when required.   We probationers were expected to learn the use of the clinical thermometer, but there was generally a row if a Sister caught us with one.

To show you how little we were shown our work, I must tell you two things I remember having to do within my first month.   One day a sweep was brought into Harley straight from his work with six fractured ribs.   "Pro," said Sister, "go and wash that patient." I had never been shown how to set about such a task, and his hair alone, which was full of soot, nearly drove me to despair. Another day I was ordered to give soap-and-water injections to the same man, and also to a man with a very bad compound fracture of the femur.   I had never given one before, and had no instructions whatever given to me.   I know I was in tears before I had finished, and so, I fear, were the patients.   We had always to find out things for ourselves.

"How did we get on with the staff nurses?   On the whole, very well.   You see, our coming brought about several improvements.   To begin with, before then all the three nurses (night and day) shared the one small bedroom, sleeping "Box and Cox."   When we came the "night home" was arranged to accommodate the night nurses, which left only the two day nurses to sleep in the ward bedroom.   Then a dining-room was also made (part of our present library), where breakfast and dinner were provided.   Tea we had in the ward (not in the kitchen), and for supper we had only what we chose to get for ourselves before going to bed.   Before we came all the nurses' food was cooked and eaten in the wards, as also the Sisters'. The Sisters had no dinner provided.   They were given a chop (uncooked) on Sundays only. They lived entirely in their rooms, which were half the size most of them are now.

What hours? We were on duty from 7 A.M., until 10 P.M. Twice a week we were supposed to go off duty for two hours, 6 to 8 P.M., and to have a half-day (3 to 9) once a fortnight. I say "supposed," as we never got off punctually: the work could not be finished in time. When we came in we went on duty again until ten o'clock.

. . . .

Of course, nursing as you understand it now was utterly unknown. Patients were not "nursed" then; they were "attended to," more or less, but there was only one nurse on each side of the ward, and the work was very hard—lockers, locker-boards, and tables, of course, to scrub every day. We did not, as a rule, scrub the floors, though I have scrubbed the whole of the front ward of Matthew (Faith) on a special occasion before 6 A.M. Luke was the only ward where the floor was scrubbed daily, each nurse doing her half, and Sister herself lending a hand if they were very busy. (Luke was considered a particularly smart ward in those days, and Sister always wore a black silk dress when she went round with the visiting physician.) The patients had their beds made once a day, the bad cases had their sheets drawn at night. In Matthew all of the patients got out of bed every day, even the typhoids—it was considered rather smart. Then one thought nothing of having fourteen or fifteen poultices to change. All wounds, of course, suppurated, and required dressing or poulticing twice or three times a day. I well remember Mr. Willett saying, when lecturing to us on wounds, "There are three modes of healing: the first, most to be desired but never seen, by first intention; the second by granulation; and the third, which is always seen, by suppuration."

What was our life in the home like?   There was nothing of the sort.   We had breakfast and dinner in the home; otherwise, when off duty, if we did not go out, we sat in the ward kitchens or in our bedrooms. The food was fairly good.   There was no one to over-look our behaviour or to see that we went to bed at the right time, or anything of that sort.   Indeed, I often sat up very late, and when in Faith went round frequently with Sister and the house physician when they made the night round.   I learned a good deal then.   I generally had to write my lectures out before I got up in the morning, between five and six.   It was the only quiet time and the only time of the day when my head was clear enough: at night I was too tired.

At the end of the year we passed an examination held much on the same lines as now, but I believe that marks were not awarded by the matron until after Miss Manson came (Mrs. Bedford-Fenwick).   We were awarded certificates and offered posts as staff nurses, which few were bold enough to accept on account of the existing condition of things.

We objected to associating constantly and sharing rooms with the staff nurses, to changing our clean cotton uniforms for their brown stuff dresses, and to carrying the soiled linen from the wards to the laundry (which the staff nurses had then to do), and various other things.   The treasurer promised to try and alter these things, and did by degrees.

Things improved little by little.   One or two out

of every batch of probationers (they came in every three months) stayed on after passing the examination. Then Miss Machin, who became matron in 1879, increased the period of training to two years, so that we had a certain number of second-year nurses on whom we could depend. It was not, however, until after Mrs. Bedford-Fenwick, then Miss Manson, came in 1881 that the old ,untrained Sisters and nurses were gradually weeded out and the training lengthened to three years.

A tremendous change? Yes, greater than you can imagine. I have really no words in which to describe the state the hospital was in when I came as probationer, and if I had, you would say the account was not fit for publication. When first I became Sister I often stayed up all night because there was no one to look after my patients but an old woman probably both drunk and disreputable, and unable either to read or write.

It was many years before the nursing staff in general was treated with anything approaching respect.[1]

[1] Sister "Casualty," in "League News," *Journal of St. Bartholomew's Nurses' League*, No. 5, May, 1902. p. 134 *et seq.*

CHAPTER VII.

THE TREATY OF GENEVA AND THE RED CROSS.

IN reading of war nursing and the relief of the wounded to-day, the activity of the Red Cross would loom large on every page, mitigating and repairing the horrors and-brutalities of battle between man and his fellows; but no such beneficent agency existed at the time of the Crimean War. This was one of the last great wars to be carried on before a general humanity organised its counter-army of relief. Miss Nightingale and her aides had to cover as best they might the whole ground now cared for by a highly systematised network of medical, surgical, nursing, and general relief service.

In whose mind had the thought of neutrality for the wounded first arisen? Who shall say how far back it had been germinating? There was Haldora, of Iceland, who lived about the year 1000—"a fair woman, and she had a good temper"; she was also a woman of great intellectual faculty, and she had "a lovely mind." After a deadly battle, Haldora had said to the women of her house, "Let us go and dress the wounds of the warriors, be they friends or foes." She herself sought the wounded in every direction, and came upon the chieftain of the enemy, prostrate with a ghastly wound of the chest through which his lungs could be seen. Haldora dressed the wound, stayed by him all day, nursed him assiduously, and he lived, owing his life to her. "This happened," says Mrs. Norrie, "some years before the people of the North adopted Christianity, and it was not until 1863 that the treaty of Geneva saw the light."[1] Again, in the war of 1813, three women of Frankfort had issued a call which brought together all the women of the city in a union to provide care for the wounded without distinction between friends and enemies. This "Frauenverein" anticipated the spirit of the Red Cross.

M. Moynier instances the work of the Knights Hospitallers as a sort of Red Cross work, and mentions the creation of a medical service attached to armies as having been regarded, through the past three centuries, as all that could be required for the emergencies of war.[2]

The origin of modern army medical service is ascribed to Isabella, Queen of Spain, who in the wars of her time founded tent hospitals for the soldiers and supplied them with medicines, appliances, and attendants to assist the physicians.

[1] "Nursing in Denmark," by Charlotte Gordon Norrie, *American Journal of Nursing* Dec., 1900, pp. 183–184.

[2] *The Red Cross: Its Past and its Future*, by Gustav Moynier, President of the International Red Cross Committee. London, Paris, New York, 1883, p. 12.

Until the time of Miss Nightingale's overthrow of army traditions society had rested satisfied in the belief that no more could be done for the soldier in time of war.[1]

The modern organisation known as the Red Cross owes its inception to Henri Dunant, a Swiss gentleman who, while travelling in Italy in 1859, visited the battle-field after the bloody day of Solferino. Nearly forty thousand men had been lost in this battle, and the wounded were widely distributed over an extensive region. So inadequate was the relief, although the inhabitants of neighbouring towns did all in their power, that the wounded and dead alike lay on the ground for days untended, and many who might have been saved died of neglect. The scenes of needless suffering made so deep an impression on Dunant, who joined as a volunteer in the melancholy task of attempting to succour a few at least of the wounded, that a little later he wrote a description of all that he had seen, under the title *A Souvenir of Solferino.* in a pamphlet that created a profound and general impression. In it he strongly advocated the organisation of some sufficient way of caring for the wounded after battle, and he followed up the impression his publication had made by lecturing, and bringing the subject in every way before the public conscience. In Geneva he secured the sup-

[1] At a meeting of the Red Cross societies of the world held in London in June, 1907, unanimous resolutions were passed honouring Miss Nightingale and declaring that her work was the beginning of the Red Cross activities.

port of M. Gustav Moynier, the president of the
Society of Public Utility and a citizen of rare
qualities, who called the society together to consider "a proposition relative to the formation of
permanent societies for the relief of wounded soldiers." On the 9th of February, 1863, Dunant
appeared before the Society of Public Utility,
and set forth his plan, which was, in brief, to have
organised in each country central associations
which should be responsible for the administration of relief in war, and which, while independent
of each other, should each be formed under the
protection of its own country's laws, all being
affiliated together in an international voluntary
bond.   The plan met with the warmest support
of the hearers, who were men representing the
highest and finest types of civilisation, and the
Society of Public Utility took action by appoint-
ing a committee to take the proper steps toward
organisation.   As the outcome of the doings of
this committee, an international congress was
called to meet in Geneva in October, 1863, to consider how the horrors of war might be lessened
for the wounded and the sick.   The official representatives of fourteen nations attended the congress, which was in session for four days.   There
were also present the representatives of benevolent associations, notably the order of St. John of
Jerusalem.   All the chief nations of Europe, except Russia, sent delegates, but the United States,
then distracted with its own civil war, made no

response to the call. It was agreed by the delegates that a second conference should take place in Geneva in the next year, 1864, and that a formal agreement or treaty should then be presented, providing for the neutrality of hospitals on the fields of battle. At this second meeting the famous articles known as the Geneva convention or treaty were adopted; they are nine in all, but a section of the last, referring only to the details of procedure, is sometimes printed as a tenth.[1] They provided for the neutrality of all ambulances and hospitals and their supplies, equipment, and personnel, and adopted a flag, badge, and uniform to distinguish and protect them. The insignia agreed upon for the new society was a modification of the Swiss colours, which show a white cross on a red field. It was decided to reverse the colours, and thus the red cross on a white ground, to be placed conspicuously on ambulances, equipments, and accoutrements of hospital service, and to be worn upon the arm of aides,—the *brassard*,—was adopted as the badge of the society, which was henceforth to be known in every country as the "Red Cross." It is interesting to recall here that many centuries ago the Knights of St. John of Jerusalem in carrying on a work of similar purpose adopted the same in-

[1] Their full text is given in the *History of the Red Cross, the Treaty of Geneva, and its Adoption by the United States* (published by the American Association of the Red Cross; printed by the Government Printing Office, 1883), pp.51–53, and in Moynier, *op. cit.*,pp. 177–179.

signia and were known as " Knights of the Red Cross."

Free and liberal Switzerland is the only country internationally organised, and is the head and centre of international Red Cross relations. Its standing committee, of which M. Moynier became president, is a clearing-house for Red Cross work all over the world. The committee stimulated organisation in countries not yet in the bond, disseminated information, promoted research for the improvement of methods and equipment, and in general guided the whole network of affiliation. Switzerland and France were the first nations to sign the treaty; others held back a little at first, but soon ten others signed, and a little later all of those present. So great was the popular approval that, at the time when only ten signatures had been affixed to the treaty, there were already twenty-five central committees organised in as many countries.[1]

The four leading principles on which the founders of the Geneva treaty based their plans were, as has been well explained by Miss Clara Barton (for many years the president of the American society)—1. Centralisation: Efficiency of relief in time of war depends on unity of direction; therefore each country must have its central commission or body. 2. Preparation: To be ready

[1] The countries that first signed were Italy, Baden, Belgium, Denmark, Holland, Spain, Portugal, France, Prussia, Saxony, Würtemburg, and Switzerland.

for service in war or other calamity incessant preparation must be carried on in times of peace.   3.
Impartiality: National societies are not always
in a position to reach their own soldiers; therefore
all societies must equally be ready to rescue friends
or foes.   4.   Solidarity: Neutral nations must be
enabled, through the central committee, to furnish aid to belligerents without infraction of the
non-interference to which their governments may
be pledged.

From the outset it was recognised as being of
the first importance that the national societies
should have the definite recognition of their home
governments, as without this all volunteer efforts
in time of war must be crippled and inadequate.
As a consequence the conference of 1863 recommended all central committees to put themselves
in relation with their various governments.   Nor
were the rulers of Europe slow to see the importance of official recognition and co-ordination between the executive and military departments
and this powerful volunteer army.

Thus were brought into existence the now world-
wide ramifications which have made it possible
for organised mercy, pity, and common-sense to
bring a counter-influence to bear on all the various
and conflicting problems of war.   Rescue, repair,
even prevention and constructive force have risen
in opposition to destructive elements, and possibly
at some time in the future the ultimate extinction
of war from the earth will be dated from the day

when Henry Dunant wrote his appeal to the people. The natural, even if unconscious, influence of such an organisation as the Red Cross is first to mitigate and then to abolish international cruelty and murder. But that, even from the outset, the abolition of war as an ultimate possibility was present in the minds of the noble group of men who called the international conference is clear from the words that were spoken in that first convention—"The Red Cross shall teach war to make war upon itself." Nursing was recognised in the resolution passed: "On the demand, or with the concurrence, of the military authority the committee shall send volunteer nurses to the field of battle, where they will be under the direction of military chiefs."

The plans and principles of the Red Cross were energetically propagated by the International Committee, and met with a warm response. A deep and abiding enthusiasm spread from country to country and from city to town. Local committees were formed with extraordinary rapidity, and the work of preparation for succour and relief went on all over Europe without remission. Germany especially excelled in organisation, and advanced rapidly to an astonishing perfection of service. To stimulate and inform the public, exhibitions were held in different countries, at which the latest and best in equipment and outfitting was shown, and, developing from these exhibits, permanent Red Cross museums have been established in several cities, such as Stockholm, St. Petersburg, Carlsruhe, Moscow, and Paris.

The Red Cross societies of the continent of Europe have taken a prominent and energetic part in the development of nursing on a secular and systematic basis.   As they undertook to be responsible for service in war, it became necessary for them to train nurses, for the existing mother-houses of religious orders and the ill-taught personnel of the public hospitals offered no reserve of sufficient proportions or adaptability.   In order to train nurses, it was necessary to command hospitals; hence, one of the first and most arduous tasks of the local societies was to collect funds and build hospitals which should be under their own management and be capable of being utilised as training centres.   These institutions, therefore, performed a double duty—to the community in which the hospital was located, and to the country at large.   This initiated a woman's movement of vast proportions, for, while men and women, in a large measure, worked side by side on terms of harmony and equality under the Red Cross, it nevertheless followed from the very nature of the details that women often took a foremost and major share in the responsibility.   They not only raised money, gathered the supplies, built, often administered and helped to support the hospitals, but also went into them as nurses.   Women's relief societies developed numerously as auxiliaries, and became thoroughly organised, especially

in Germany.   The general line on which the nursing personnel of the Red Cross societies was developed among the nations of the continent was then
as follows: A central or local hospital, managed
by the local society, and at least partly supported
by revenue from pay patients, became the nucleus
or motherhouse for a nursing staff.   Women were
received to be trained as nurses, with the understanding that they would contract themselves for
at least a certain given period, mutually renewable, and possibly lasting for the nurse's lifetime.
While this mutual contract lasted, the nurse
was practically a part and parcel of the general
equipment of the Red Cross society.   In time of
war she was ready for military service, her place
in the hospital being, very possibly, filled for the
time being by a lay volunteer.   In time of peace
she was employed to the best advantage of the
society with which she was united; thus she might
be sent to private duty, her earnings coming into
the society treasury, or to work in other hospitals,
which often found it easier and cheaper to contract with a nursing association for a given staff
of nurses than to train and be responsible for their
own.   If she remained permanently with the society, she was promised support and care in her old
age but, if she finally left it for an independent
life she gave up all claim on its employment of
or responsibility for her.   Her conditions, in
short, were closely modelled after those of military
service.   Her life was one of the strictest

discipline; she was a soldier of a great relief army.

As a social movement and as an emancipatory factor the Red Cross nursing movement of the continent was of an importance that is hardly to be over-estimated. It was distinctly a long step forward toward social and economic equality, though by a hard road. Caste lines received a severe blow from the extension of Red Cross work, and "confessional" exclusiveness was even more seriously damaged, for the necessity of keeping their quota of nurses filled compelled the Red Cross to disregard sectarian religious prejudices. An intellectal freedom never enjoyed by the deaconesses was thus possible for the nurses of the Red Cross (as they were always called, so long as they remained in the employ of a Red Cross society), and a freer social element gave a more normal atmosphere to their communities. Most important of all, for evolutionary purposes, was the fact that it was far easier to terminate the contract and honourably leave the Red Cross service to take up self-support on independent lines than it was to leave the deaconesses' Motherhouse, for a certain sense of public decorum (or narrowness) was shocked in the latter case but not in the former. Indeed, the very conditions of Red Cross service almost compelled a steady exodus of nurses from its control; for, while on the one hand it was important and necessary to train as large a number as possible, on the other hand it rapidly became a financial impossibility to support all their nurses decently in old age and sickness, because of the continued obligation to hold funds and resources of all kinds in readiness for the possible demands of war time.   Important as the phase represented by the deaconesses' movement had been as a step toward democracy and education, that of the Red Cross went far beyond it in secularisation of the nurse's calling and as a preparation for still further advances in the definition of her status and in her training.

On the technical side of nursing the Red Cross has been a factor both for good and for poor standards.   Its nurses in Continental countries have often been well and carefully trained.   In some countries the Red Cross nurses, as they are called, stand in the very front rank for ability and thorough preparation.   On the other hand, the very nature of the Red Cross societies encourages volunteer service, and while this arm of the service can and does do magnificent work in general relief, the same cannot be said of it in nursing, which a superficial training must always render incompetent.   Lay workers of all social grades, from attendants to princesses, have had a passion for so-called army nursing, which has promoted short courses in bandaging and in first aid, often hastily . given in the presence of some emergency.   This has been especially true of those countries where the Red Cross has been least thoroughly organised and has most retained a volunteer character;

but this criticism is far less, or even not at all, applicable in those countries where the Red Cross system has been most seriously looked upon as an important arm of the public service.

In countries where the ancient nursing orders had thrown out modern offshoots, as in Austria, where the Teutonic Knights already had quite an active rôle in the relief of the wounded in war time, the Red Cross, not without the exercise of considerable diplomacy, framed harmonious working agreements with them. The order of St. John of Jerusalem, whose modern branches in Germany, Italy, and elsewhere had grown aristocratic, and practised a somewhat academic philanthropy, was stimulated to some modification of its old-time ways by the vigorous, democratic, enthusiastic young society of the Red Cross, and in some countries co-operation between the two developed to a satisfactory degree, while in others, where church lines and hereditary titles are too exclusive, they have not united, but recognise each other amicably.[1]

The first great test of the Red Cross organisation came with the war of 1871, and was triumphantly met. Miss Clara Barton, who afterwards established the work in the United States, was privileged to accompany the Swiss committee through the war of 1871, and wrote as follows of her experience there, comparing it with her recollections of the Civil War in America, when she had

[1] *The Red Cross*, Gustav Moynier, pp. 39-40.

also given active volunteer service on the battle-field, and had seen untold horrors:

As I journeyed on, and saw the work of the Red Cross societies in the field, accomplishing in four months under their systematic organisation what we failed to accomplish in four years without it,—no mistakes, no needless suffering, no starving, no lack of care, no waste, no confusion, but order, plenty, cleanliness, and comfort wherever that little flag made its way—as I saw all this, and joined and worked in it, I said to myself, "If I live to return to my country I will try to make our people understand the Red Cross and that treaty." [1]

[1] *History of the Red Cross*, p. 59.

CHAPTER VIII.

THE DEVELOPMENT OF NURSING IN AMERICA.

WHEN the pilgrim fathers and mothers landed on Plymouth rock, bringing their Spartan domestic customs with them, they did not introduce the art of nursing into the New World, for, long before, as we have seen, the Jesuit Fathers of France had pioneered in medicine and the Catholic Sisters had established their mission hospitals. Even before that time the Indians had practised their rude methods of medical and surgical treatment, and in the very dawn of history the Aztecs and Incas had built their hospitals and taken care of their sick.

The organised system of nursing now prevailing in the United States dates, it may be said, from 1871, but, as in England, it was preceded by many tentative efforts that are historically important and significant. Hospitals are the cradles of nursing, and we may properly turn first to the oldest of our hospitals—the Philadelphia, first known as the Philadelphia almshouse and later as " Blockley," and to Bellevue in New York City. The latter, Dr. Carlisle tells us,[1] may lay claim to be the oldest hospital now in existence in the United States. Like many other now great institutions, its origin was of the humblest. Its genealogy runs back into the city of Amsterdam, and to the times when the poor were supported by the church in a modest building which served as a poorhouse. This charity, and a little hospital which was built by the West India Company at the suggestion of its surgeon, were the two roots from which developed the city hospital of Bellevue. The company's hospital dates back to the month of December in 1658, when the village of New Amsterdam only numbered a thousand inhabitants, and was the first one built on United States soil. In 1680 the "old hospital" was sold and a better building provided, and still later the church funds for the poor were increased by an addition from the city fathers. In 1736 a new building was fitted up to serve as a "Publick Workhouse and House of Correction of New York." There were rooms for various kinds of labour, spinning, etc.; quarters for the family of the keeper, and rooms for an infirmary of six beds. This building, the immediate ancestor of Bellevue, stood where the city hall now stands. As time went on it was several times rebuilt and enlarged. The present site of Bellevue on the East River, with a house which

[1] *An Account of Bellevue Hospital, New York*, by Robert Carlisle, M.D., published by the Society of Alumni of Bellevue Hospital, New York, 1893, p. 1.

became the nucleus of the first Bellevue hospital, was purchased by the city with some haste in 1794, a threatened epidemic of yellow fever having caused the city authorities to prepare a "pest-house" for the emergency. The principal building on the domain was a two-story and garret house, and the estate, which was very beautiful, had been named by the owners Bellevue.

For a number of years it was used only when there was yellow fever in the city, being for this purpose placed under the management of the Health Board, but in 1811 more ground was bought around it, and a new almshouse built. The corner-stone was laid July 29, 1811. Delayed by the War of 1812, it was only finished and opened in April, 1816; with the almshouse quarters, a penitentiary, together with wards for the sick and the insane all in the same building with the rooms for the resident physician, the warden, and the attendants. The old grey stone structure fronting the broad arm of the sea called the East River looked dignified and interesting with its extensive green sweep of lawn, adorned with a few fine old trees, but it has had a terrible history. The paupers numbered from sixteen hundred to two thousand, and among them were often as many as two hundred sick. Epidemics, arising from unsanitary conditions and overcrowding, were frequent and severe. Typhus fever, the sinister companion of filth and misery, now all but unknown in America, was then common. The physicians were cruelly

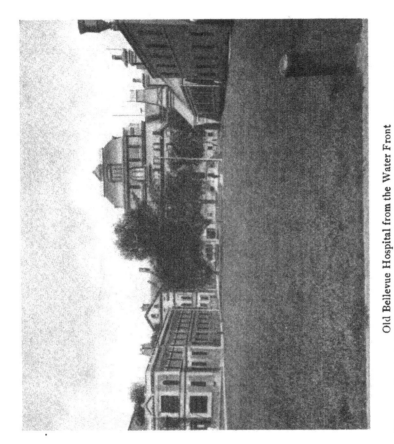

Old Bellevue Hospital from the Water Front

The central main building was the old Almshouse Administration Building, modern wards

overworked, for only three were assigned to supervise the whole household, both sick and well. The nurses (so called) were detailed from the prison, and were appointed in the proportion of one for ten or twenty patients. Political jobbery was rife, and the positions in the hospital were given to political henchmen without the slightest regard to their unfitness for their trust. During many years nothing but horrors existed at Bellevue. In 1826 Dr. Wood complained that the overcrowding was such that men and women ill with small-pox had to be kept in the same ward. In 1832 there was a frightful epidemic of cholera, and the dead lay so thick on the floors that the physicians had to step over their bodies in making their rounds. In 1837 the conditions in general were such as to shock even the aldermen themselves, and a committee of investigation was appointed. The only part of the whole building which was found to be clean and in good order was the female department of the almshouse division, which furnished "a silent rebuke" in its contrast to the rest.[1]

The investigating committee reported that "the condition of Bellevue hospital was such as to excite the most poignant sympathy for its neglected inmates."

Among the specifications they gave were; filth, no ventilation, no clothing, patients with high fever lying naked in bed with only coarse blankets to cover them, wards overcrowded, jail fever rife,

[1] Carlisle, *op. cit.* p. 37.

no supplies, putrefaction and vermin. It was reported, furthermore, that the resident physician with his students (two only excepted), the matron, and the nurses had left the building.[1]

Dr. Benjamin Ogden, a former resident whose administration had been upright, was asked to return, and did so, and succeeded in effecting some reforms in discipline and in solving the problem of supplies.

As a result of this investigation a redistribution of the inmates was decided upon, and, ·in 1836, the male and female prisoners were removed; in 1837 the small-pox cases were provided for in an institution on Blackwell's Island, and thither also the insane patients were removed in 1839; but the almshouse and hospital remained together under the one roof until 1848, when they were separated, and the stone pile of Bellevue began its career as a hospital. This final step in reform was hastened by some forcible letters that had appeared in the *Evening Post* pointing out the maladministration and the high death-rate (about 25 per cent.) of Bellevue, and which were supposed to have been written by Dr. Griscom of the Health Department.[2] This new departure was also consistently supported by the most distinguished members of the medical profession, many of whom, especially Dr. J. R. Wood, had urged a change in the manner of

[1] Carlisle, *op. cit*, p. 39.

[2] Observations on the medical organisation of the hospitals at Bellevue and Blackwell's Island, Oct. 30, Nov. 1, 5, and 6, 1845.

making medical appointments to the hospital. Heretofore these, like the other offices, had been used as political rewards, but in 1847 a new era began with the creation of a Medical Board.

Nor had the profession been altogether indifferent to the disgrace attaching to the system of nursing. At the time of the separation of the almshouse, and previously, when the Medical Board was appointed, the physicians had protested against the internal conditions. In 1857 they had objected to the employment of prisoners and paupers as nurses, and some had asked that Sisters of Charity be placed in the wards.[1]

. An interesting bit of negative testimony as to the status of nursing in those days is furnished by an article written in 1856, describing Bellevue hospital.[2] In this article there is not one word about the nursing or the care of the patients.

In Philadelphia, Blockley also began as an almshouse. It supported and employed the poor, received orphans, the insane, and the sick.[3] Its nursing history is equally terrible as that of Bellevue, and even more of its details have been recorded.

[1] *A Century of Nursing, with Hints toward the Formation of Training Schools for Nurses.* G. P. Putnam's Sons, New York, 1876. p. 14.

[2] " History and Early Organisation of Bellevue," *N. Y. Journ. of Med.*, May, 1856, p. 389.

[3] *History of the Philadelphia Almshouse and Hospital from the Beginning of the 18th to the end of the 19th Century.* Compiled and published by Charles Lawrence. Philadelphia, 1905.

In 1729 the Overseers of the Poor presented a
memorial to the Assembly, asking for a grant of
money for dependent persons, for, although Philadelphia had had an almshouse from 1713, it was
then, and always had been, supported by the
Friends for their own members only.[1] The State
granted the money in 1730, the ground was bought
and the erection of a brick building was begun in
the following year. The historian of Blockley
says, "The Philadelphia hospital is, without
doubt, the oldest hospital in continuous service
in this country." In 1766 the paupers numbered
220, and in 1767 new buildings were put up. During the occupation of Philadelphia by the British
troops the almshouse, like other public buildings,
suffered severely. As soon as the troops entered,
the command was sent to Blockley to turn the
inmates out to make room for them. The Board
of Guardians had the courage to refuse to obey,
but to no avail, for the patients were forcibly put
upon the streets to make room for the king's soldiers.

In 1793 an investigation showing "shocking abuses" is recorded; in the same year also we
come upon the first mention of nurses. The yellow fever raged, and it was "impossible to procure
suitable nurses: only the most depraved creatures
could be hired"; . . . "an abandoned, profli-

[1] It was in the old Quaker almshouse, according to Agnes
Repplier, the brilliant essayist and historian of Philadelphia,
that Evangeline found Gabriel.

gate set of nurses and attendants," who "rioted on the provisions and comforts left for the sick." All the work of the house, nursing included, was supposed to be done by the inmates, and there is no reason to believe that it was of higher grade than that at Bellevue. The treatment of the insane at Blockley was especially heartrending, or, if in other places it was as bad, more meagre details have come down to us. Inconceivable as it sounds, the female lunatics were under the charge of a male keeper, who, assisted by two male paupers, slept among the female insane and took the entire management of the violent cases, even to bathing, or washing, and dressing them. Says the history quoted: "Some of the patients, even in their madness, shrunk from this rude handling and raved with increased fury at their indecent exposure. Revolting to decency as this practice was, it was not without difficulty, and only by degrees, abandoned."[1]

It was also the custom of that inhuman institutionalism to permit the lowest and coarsest of the public rabble to visit the wards for the insane, to laugh, stare, and jeer at them as if they had been wild beasts in cages. But most pitiful, perhaps, of all was their suffering from cold, for in those days there were no central heating plants, and apparently it was assumed that the insane were insensible to degrees of temperature.

Only one short interregnum of peace broke the

[1] *History of the Philadelphia Almshouse*, p. 172.

long and distressing reign of violence, neglect, and cruelty in Blockley.

In 1832 there was a severe epidemic of cholera, and the attendants demanded more wages. To keep them to their duties the wages were increased, but were promptly spent for liquor. An orgy of intoxication ensued, and the helpers, crazed with drink, fought like furies over the beds of the sick, or lay in drunken stupour beside the bodies of the dead. So complete was the demoralisation that the guardians applied to Bishop Kendrick for Sisters of Charity from Emmitsburg. The call was responded to promptly; indeed, the Sisters started two hours after the summons was received. They took in hand the whole desperate situation, at once restored order and disseminated about them an atmosphere of tranquillity and quiet energy. The Sisters remained for some months, and their work was so deeply appreciated by the guardians that the Committee of the House, in a set of resolutions commending their great services, resolved also that they be requested to remain permanently. This, however, Father Hickey, their Superior, negatived, giving his reasons at length. He did not consider Blockley the department of charity in which the Sisters could be most usefully employed, so the guardians were obliged to let them go, with glowing tributes which may well have been heartfelt.[1]

In 1851 the first woman physician was admitted

[1] *History of the Philadelphia Almshouse*, p. 123.

to the service in Blockley, but it is not evident that she was allowed to do anything to mitigate conditions. In 1856 a report giving most horrible details was presented by Dr. Campbell. The institution now comprised small-pox wards, departments for the insane, an asylum for children, a lying-in department, a nursery, a hospital, and almshouses, wherein were congregated the blind, the lame, and the incurables. All these departments were overcrowded, without proper classification, and entirely under the care of the pauper inmates, or paid attendants taken from the same class. The physical conditions of the place, too, owing to the fact that Blockley, like old Bellevue, had always been a paradise for dishonest contractors, were in a shameful state. There was no gas; only small hand-lamps were in use. There was no laundry; the clothing was given out to a small army of washerwomen. In the hospital departments there was not a water-closet, and only one bath-tub, that one being on the men's side.[1] The scandal of the nursing continued until 1884, when it was reformed under Miss Alice Fisher.[2] [The great work done by Miss Fisher, belonging as it does to a later period, will be considered in a later volume.]

The charter of the Pennsylvania hospital was

---

[1] *History of the Philadelphia Almshouse*, 198–202.
[2] See also " History of the Foundation and Development of the First Hospitals in the United States, " *Amer. Journ. of Insanity*, vol. xxiv., 1867–68.

granted in the year 1751. This was the first hospital in the United States in the proper sense of the word, for it was designed solely for the curative care of the sick, and its founders, with an enlightenment unusual indeed at that day, placed the insane in the category of those who were ill and needed treatment. The names most closely connected with the inception and foundation of the Pennsylvania hospital are the honoured ones of Dr. Thomas Bond, who may be regarded as the creator of its plan, and Benjamin Franklin, who did most to realise it. The project of establishing a hospital in Philadelphia had been talked of by the Quakers as early as 1709. There was some slight quarantine provision for strangers, but this was of the crudest nature. There was no care for the insane, who were spoken of in the petition to the Legislature (largely the work of Franklin) as "going at large, a terror to their Neighbours, who are daily apprehensive of the Violences they may commit." [1] The opening of the Pennsylvania hospital inaugurated an era of caring for the insane as patients suffering from mental disease, and giving them appropriate treatment instead of treating them as malefactors. The crudity of earlier care can be gathered from a record dated 1676: "Jan——Complayning to ye Court that his son Erick is bereft of his naturall senses and

---

[1] *History of the Pennsylvania Hospital from 1751 to 1895*, by Thomas Morton, M.D. Authorised by the Board of Managers. Philadelphia, 1897. P. 3.

is turned quyt madd and yt: he being a poore man is not able to maintaine him: Ordered; that three or four persons be hired to build a little block house——for to put in the said madman."[1]

None other of our hospitals possesses so benign an atmosphere of peaceful seclusion, historical association, and dignified traditions as the Pennsylvania. Its ample grounds and quiet situation enhance this feeling, and a certain old-world touch is given by the pedestal on the green lawn, with its inscription which recites the bestowal of the Charter by King George II.

Its early years were checkered, for epidemics of yellow fever and cholera were frequent and terrifying, and times of war brought grave troubles, when wounded soldiers and Hessians were crowded into it without notice or application to the managers. There is no mention of the early nursing arrangements except one allusion to "experienced and trustworthy persons," but the hospital had an interesting experience with women managers in an advisory capacity. In 1824 a "Female Board of Assistants" had been established, and increased in numbers the following year, as the Hospital Board thought that considerable benefit had resulted to the hospital from their disinterested services. But in 1827 a collision occurred between the "Female Board" and the Hospital Board over a question of internal order. The ladies

[1] *History of the Pennsylvania Hospital from 1751 to 1895*, p. 4.

"expressed their disapproval of retaining a certain employee in the hospital in any capacity whatever." History does not relate who this employee was, but it must have been an important one—possibly the matron. The managers refused to accept the judgment of the ladies, and they resigned in a body, whereupon the managers declared the Female Board of Assistants abolished.

Those who know the frequency and ease with which a clever but unreliable woman can deceive the judgment of men, and who also know the superior type of woman that those Quaker dames undoubtedly presented, cannot doubt that they were right and the Hospital Board sadly and totally wrong. In 1864 it was again proposed to have lady visitors appointed to the wards, but only such harmless duties as religious reading aloud and the like were allowed to them. The Pennsylvania hospital established a training school in 1875.

The New York hospital, the next in age, received its charter in 1771. The foundations were laid two years after, but before being finished the structure was burned to the ground, and, when finally completed, was used by the British and Hessian soldiery for a barrack, so that it was not able to receive patients until January, 1791, after it had recovered from the disorganisations of war. The New York, like the Pennsylvania, being a wealthy hospital in which the most prominent and cultured citizens were deeply interested, probably had attendants greatly superior in grade to those

Development of Nursing in America 339

of city hospitals like Bellevue and Blockley. We may believe that they were the best that could be secured, were properly housed and well treated, and held to a conscientious performance of their duties.

The distinction of having made the first attempt to teach its nurse attendants belongs to the New York hospital; andto Dr. Valentine Seaman, one of its medical chiefs, a remarkably broad-minded man, is due the honour of having conceived and initiated the first system of instruction to nurses on the American continent. His services to the cause of education are commemorated by a letter below his portrait in the hospital, in which are the words: "In 1798 he organised in the New York Hospital the first regular Training School for Nurses, from which other schools have since been established and extended their blessings throughout the Community." In a comparative study of the first efforts at nursing reform we must consider this statement as too sweeping, in so far as we accept Miss Nightingale's dictum as to what constitutes a training school, but there is no doubt whatever that Dr. Seaman was, in many of his ideas, far ahead of his time in liberality of view. In connection with the Maternity department of the New York hospital he organised a course of teaching, and gave a series of twenty-four lectures, including outlines of anatomy, physiology, and the care of children, the three concluding ones of which have been preserved in a small volume called *The Midwife's Monitor and Mother's Mirror*, published in 1800 by Isaac Collins. His ideas on midwifery, however, would meet with little medical approbation to-day, for he regarded midwives as indispensable and necessary, and believed they should be thoroughly and carefully taught. In the roll of honour in nursing reform he must stand high with those admirable German professors of medicine who wrote and made propaganda in the latter part of the eighteenth century, and we must always regret that history has preserved so little record of his actual missionary work.

The next attempt to train an intelligent nursing personnel had its origin in Philadelphia among the Friends, whose predominance in that city stamped its early institutions with an enlightened philanthropy. As early as 1786 the Philadelphia Dispensary had been founded for the medical, surgical, and obstetrical service of the poor in their homes, and the originators of the dispensary, in making their public appeals for support, had pointed out the need for such public service with feeling and delicacy. "There are many [thus ran the circular] who cannot, or ought not, go to a hospital." Such persons, they contended, could be attended in their homes without being subjected to the pains of separating from their families; the care given them would be at less cost to the community than that of hospitals, and it would moreover be possible to attend to them in a quiet and refined way, "consistent with those noble feelings

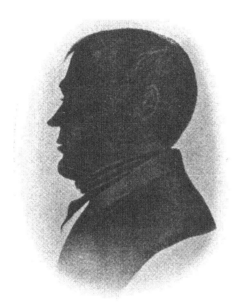

Valentine Seaman, M.D.
Attending Surgeon of the New York Hospital
1796–1817
The first American physician to advocate teaching nurses

which are inseparable from virtuous poverty."
The founders of this charity were active in reliev-
ing the necessities of patients applying to it, but
no records were kept before 1837. In July of that
year a physician was put in charge more especially of the obstetrical service, and thereafter
records were preserved.

This physician was Dr. Joseph Warrington,
whose active wish it had long been to see a
school for the suitable training of women nurses
in connection with a hospital for lying-in women.

He was a man of liberal opinions and high
ideals, and it appears to have been in consequence of an urgent appeal from him that a
number of ladies organised themselves, on March
5, 1839, into a society whose constitution was
opened with this preamble:

Whereas, in our widely extended and densely pop-
ulated city a large number of poor females are subject
to great suffering and risk of life, during and shortly
after the period of parturition, for want of competent
nurses to guard them and their helpless offspring, and
to carry out the directions of the medical attendant
. . . the undersigned, impressed with the importance of this subject, do associate for the purpose of
providing, sustaining, and causing to be instructed
as far as possible, pious and prudent women for this
purpose, and do adopt the following regulations:

I. The Association shall be called the Nurse Society of Philadelphia.

II. The Board of Managers shall consist of twelve

females, who are, or have been, heads of families. [1]

After electing its officers, the board was to take up the city districts, and place a lady visitor in each. The society was to employ, from time to time, as many nurses as would be needed, and to select, for this purpose, females of settled, good habits, quiet and patient dispositions, and with a sense of responsibility. Only those who were well recommended were to be employed and, if unsuitable, they were to be dismissed on the advice of the physician. There was to be a loan closet for the use of the patients, the articles to be in charge of a storekeeper who would distribute them upon an order of the visitor for the district, when they would be carried by the nurses to the patients. The nurses were to hold themselves in readiness to be called by the physician. Each nurse was to spend her whole time with one patient, and was paid two dollars and a half a week by the society. The nurses were supervised, when on duty, by the lady visitor of the district and were taught by the physicians in the lying-in department of the dispensary. The plan of instruction, which was followed from the time of foundation, was arranged by Dr. Warrington, and included lectures, with practice on a manikin. At these

[1] The complete Reports of the society have been consulted and data given are taken almost entirely from them. It is this society that has been already referred to as resembling, and possibly being related to, Mrs. Fry's work in training nurses in England.

lectures both the nurses and young medical practitioners were taught together.[1]

After having served satisfactorily for six cases, they were to receive appropriate certificates, signed by the physician in charge and the lady visitor of the district, and were then eligible for calls to private duty. They worked simply as nurses, not as midwives, and it was the desire of the society not to limit its usefulness to obstetrical cases. Practically, however, these were the only calls. The "Nurse Committee" kept a list of applicants for the position of nurse, made the necessary inquiries, and recommended candidates to the Board of Managers and the physicians. Accepted candidates were called probationers. Between 1839 and 1850 the Nurse Society had employed fifty women, and most of them had an honourable record. Only one was dropped for misconduct and four for intoxication.

In 1849 a Home, the need of which had long been urgently felt, was secured, and opened as a Home and School in 1850. The applicants were now admitted as "pupil-nurses" and were first instructed in cooking in the home kitchen for a few weeks' time. They next received a course of theoretical instruction from the physicians, and were then sent out to cases for two weeks at a time. The committee reported the results of the Home and the better teaching

---

[1] "Training Schools for Nurses," *Penn. Monthly*, Dec., 1874, C. P. Putnam, Boston. Appendix by S.

to be most gratifying, and the applicants of a better grade.   Still the service remained almost solidly obstetrical, though the managers greatly desired to extend it to medical and surgical cases.   Nurses who had received their certificates were now allowed to remain in the Home for a moderate rental, and take private duty calls.   By 1853 the loan closet had been extended by numerous appliances for ordinary sick-nursing, and a resolution was passed by the society reminding the public that nurses would be supplied for medical and surgical cases.   It is not, however, evident from the reports that there was any training given them on these lines, further than some lectures and demonstrations in bandaging.   In 1855 a leaflet appeared signed by Dr. Warrington, Hannah Miller, and Ann Davis, making an earnest plea to young women to enter the nurse's calling. It drew attention to the fact that the demand for nurses was far greater than the supply, as, out of 1656 calls, only 670 could be answered.[1]

To help to bring the work before the public and impress its importance upon the students themselves, it was now agreed that the "certificates of approbation," as the nurses' certificates were called, should be formally presented to them at the annual meeting of the society.

[1] Ann Davis afterward studied medicine, and in 1863 wrote another pamphlet, called *Nursing the Sick and the Training of Nurses*.   This was, however, chiefly addressed to the heads of families, and is of a slight character, though marked with good feeling and common-sense.

The report of 1867 shows steady progress. It gives a list of "graduate nurses" residing in or registering at the Home, and records 252 patients as having received medical and nursing care. There were then thirty-four lady visitors for the districts, some districts having two visitors. The 69th annual report gives a slight historical *résumé* of the work of the society, and refers to the share of Dr. Warrington in its formation in the following words: "One of the primary objects of Dr. Joseph Warrington in founding this society in the year 1828 was to provide, in connection with the hospital for women during confinement, a school in which women would be practically trained in the art of nursing." This reference to Dr. Warrington, and the introduction of this new date, 1828, leads one to suppose that he had had the purpose in mind, and had identified himself with some earlier effort than that related in the reports quoted, and which had, probably, led logically to the establishment of the organised society, although the fact had not been made quite evident in the earliest reports. The 69th report says of the school, "It is the first Nurse Training School in point of time founded in America, and we have the record of but one in Europe of longer standing." The 70th annual report bears on its title-page, after the name, the words, "In active operation since 1828: The First School in America established to Train Women as Nurses."

As a pioneer effort it is certainly most interest-

ing and commendable and affords a valuable study
of co-operation and intelligent thought in advance
of those times. Since the full reform of nursing
has been directed by Miss Nightingale this excellent old charity has not continued to advance
along the whole line. In 1897 it extended its
course to one year, but the nurses were sent out
to private duty after three months' hospital
service. The hours retained the old-fashioned
stamp:—rise at 5.30; wards at 6; breakfast, 7-8;
daily duty, 12½ hours.

The next oldest school in Philadelphia is that
of the Woman's hospital. This entire story is
one of pioneer struggle to break new paths along
the lately won and difficult road of medical education for women, and the nursing shared in
the difficulties of the whole work. The nursing school had been planned and hoped for at
a much earlier date than that of the beginning of actual work, for it was open to pupils in
1861, but none offered themselves until 1863.[1]
It did not advance much before 1872, when
it received an endowment which enabled it to extend its advantages, and little by little it has
brought up its standards to those of the present
day.

Another interesting early nursing foundation,
which has also, and with better reason, been called
the "first training school for nurses in America,"
was that of the New England Hospital for Wo-

[1] "Training Schools for Nurses," *Penn. Monthly, cit.*

men and Children. It also is closely bound up
with the history of the first medical women of our
country, especially with that of Dr. Marie Zakrzewska, who was one of the most brilliant and
original in force and ability. Dr. Zakrzewska was
a German-Pole, highly educated, who was familiar
with the training for nurses then given in the secular school of the Charité hospital in Berlin, where
she had studied midwifery, and later, medicine.
As she was not permitted to take a medical degree
in Germany, she came to America, where Dr.
Elizabeth Blackwell's heroic courage and eminent
ability had recently "hammered at the gates "[1]
of medical education for women.[2] In 1859 Dr.
Zakrzewska was appointed to the chair of obstet-
rics in the New England Female College of Boston,
and it was due to her advice that the trustees
established a small hospital and clinical department in connection with it. The report of 1859–
60 says: "In addition to the work already spoken
of [in the hospital and clinics] we early expressed
our hope to receive and instruct women desiring
to be trained for nurses. This hope we still cher-
ish. We have had, as yet, but one application in
this department."

In the next two years, Dr. Zakrzewska trained
six nurses here, though they did not receive certificates. In the early part of 1862 she withdrew

[1] Phrase used by Oliver Wendell Holmes: *Medical Essays*,
"Scholastic and Bedside Teaching," p. 299.

[2] For interesting details of that struggle see Dr. Blackwell's
book cited, p. 201.

from this position to take one of wider usefulness
offered to her by a group of noble and courageous
pioneers in education who had organised the New
England Hospital for Women and Children and
had asked her to take charge of it.	The honoured
names of Ednah D. Cheney, Lucy Goddard, Louisa
C. Bond, Lucretia French, and many others well
known in New England are bound up closely with
the history of this institution, as well as those of
a few liberal men who believed in opening the
gates.	The incorporation act declared the objects
of the hospital to be :

I.	To provide for women medical aid by compe-
tent physicians of their own sex.	II.	To assist edu-
cated women in the practical study of medicine.	III.
To train nurses for the care of the sick.

The training of nurses was now begun, though
not precisely on the lines of a training school.	Yet
in the period of about ten years before the regular
school was established Dr. Zakrzewska taught
thirty-two nurses, and, as she was a strict disciplinarian, with high standards of practical work and
very thorough in methods, they became "expe-
rienced nurses" of an excellent type.	The annual
report for 1864–65 mentions "the faithful care of
our nurses" and again says:

Each department of the hospital is under the
charge of a head and assistant nurse.	The latter are
often women who, wishing to gain experience for pri-

vate nursing, enter the hospital for a period of six months, during which time they give, in exchange for instruction, their services free of remuneration. . . .

At this present moment, the head nurse of the medical department is a woman of unusual skill and generosity, who serves the hospital from real interest, having twice left very lucrative private nursing in order to take charge of our hospital.

The report for 1867–68 says:

We have again considered the subject of educating nurses, and offer the advantages of the practice of the hospital, with board and washing, and also low wages, after the first month of trial, to those women who wish to acquire skill in this important art. As yet we have had but few applicants who are willing to give the requisite time. We do not feel willing to be responsible for the fitness of a nurse who has been with us for less than six months.

Two years later the report says: "There is great demand for competent nurses. The few who have faithfully served their time with us find more than they can do, and take rank at once as superior, first-class nurses."

In 1872 the hospital moved to the new building at Roxbury, and the modern school of nursing dates from this time. With ampler accommodations, and reinforced by the enthusiasm of Dr. Susan Dimock, who was just back from her studies in Zürich to take the post of resident physician, the managers announced in their report for 1871–72:

In order more fully to carry out our purpose of fit-
ting women thoroughly for the profession of nursing,
we have made the following arrangements: Young
women of suitable acquirements and character will be
admitted to the hospital as school nurses for one year.
This year will be divided into four periods: three
months will be given respectively to the practical
study of nursing in the medical, surgical, and maternity wards, and night nursing. Here the pupil will
aid the head nurse in all the care and work of the ward
under the direction of the attending and resident physicians and medical students. In order to enable
women entirely dependent upon their work for support
to obtain a thorough training, the nurses will be paid
for their work from one to four dollars per week after
the first fortnight, according to the actual value of
their services to the hospital. A course of lectures will
be given to nurses at the hospital by physicians connected with the institution, beginning January 21st.
Other nurses desirous of attending these lectures may
obtain permits from our physicians. Certificates will
be given to such nurses as have satisfactorily passed
a year in practical training in the hospital.

The same report adds:

As long as we were in the old hospital, with space
so inadequate to our needs, we were able to carry out
only partially our plans for training nurses, but finding
the demand so constant for those we have already
trained, and the need of good nurses so great in the
community, we have now determined to use our increased facilities to the utmost, and each year to send
out a small band of trained nurses. At present we

have five in training for the lengthened period of twelve months.

The report of 1872–73 mentions the great success of the new method of training, and of the winter's course of twelve lectures—these being so numerously attended by ladies from outside that it became necessary to regulate admission by ticket. The resident physician's report tells the following pleasing incident:

Last summer the nurses, having heard that the hospital was much in need of money, gave one-fourth of their wages for the rest of the year, saying they would like to do this much for the hospital since it had done so much for them.

The uniform of the early days was perhaps not very strict in uniformity. "A simple calico dress and felt slippers" is the delightfully unsophisticated formula given in the reports.

The first nurse to receive her certificate, and who has since been known by the proud title of "The First Trained Nurse in the United States," was Miss Linda Richards, whose nursing career, still in full activity, has been long and honourable.

Miss Richards writes of those days:

Of the five nurses in our class I first entered the school on the day it was opened, the other four coming within six weeks.[1] Even though the course was

[1] Of this first class of nurses Miss Linda Richards went to Bellevue as night superintendent in October, 1873; remained there a year, and then was offered the position of Sister.

far too short, and the advantages few, we five nurses
of the first class were very happy, very united, and
pretty well instructed. We had no superintendent
of nurses—in our ignorance we did not know that such
an officer was necessary. As I look back I wonder
that we were as well taught as was really the case, and
I sometimes feel that we nurses, eager as we were to
learn, instructed the physicians nearly as much as
they instructed us.

The course of lectures announced for the winter
of 1873–74 was as follows:

Dr. Zakrzewska, 1, "Position and Manners of
Nurses in Families"; Drs. Emily and Augusta Pope,
4, "Physiological Subjects"; Dr. Sewall, 1, "Food
for the Sick"; Dr. Dimock, 2, "Surgical Nursing";
Dr. Morton, 2, "Childbed Nursing"; Dr. Call, 1,
"The Use of Disinfectants to Prevent Contagion";
Dr. Zakrzewska, 1, "General Nursing."

Helen's assistant by the committee, but declining this went to
the Massachusetts General hospital to take the position of
superintendent of nurses which was offered to her at the same
time. Mrs. Wolhaupter, another of the first five, took charge
of the maternity department in the New England hospital
after graduation, then went to Bellevue as head nurse, then
took charge of the Brooklyn Homeopathic Lying-In hospital,
and followed Miss Richards as superintendent of the Massachusetts General training school when the latter left it to
study in England, finally returning to her former post in
Brooklyn. A third graduate, Miss Woods, went to Bellevue
as head nurse, afterwards holding a similar position at the
Massachusetts General for two years, and then became the
first night superintendent of the newly opened Boston City
hospital. The other two devoted themselves to private
nursing.

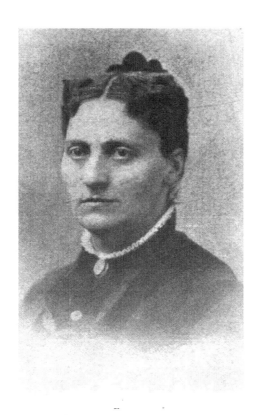

Linda Richards
"The First Trained Nurse in America"
Taken after her graduation

Miss Jammé, who has written an account of this school, of which she was for some years superintendent, says:

At this early period there seems to have been great interest and enthusiasm shown by the pupils, and the doctors in the hospital were especially interested in teaching them. Dr. Zakrzewska taught at the bedside all the simple details of nursing, and all the nurses made rounds every morning and received the orders for their patients. There were no head nurses, no superintendent. Each nurse was given charge of about four patients and was made responsible for their medicines, diet, baths, etc. The physicians were most exacting and critical and demanded very much in the small details for the comfort of the patients. The hospital was very poor: the empty treasury was replenished only week by week by the personal efforts of the directors; doubt and ridicule of the women doctors had to be met bravely, consequently it needed courage to believe in the possibility of the success of the work. The nurses had to be most economical and supplement the efforts of the doctors and directors in every way, to keep the hospital alive. . . . There were only three women in the country who were doing surgical work: Dr. Cleveland in New York, Dr. Elizabeth Kellar in Philadelphia, and Dr. Dimock in Boston. . . . The school continued to grow until in 1882 the course was extended to sixteen months, and it was at this time that a superintendent of nurses was first employed.[1]

[1] "The First Training School in America," by Anna C. Jammé, *Johns Hopkins Hospital Nurses Alumnæ Magazine*, Nov. 1905, pp. 197–201.

The course of training in this school has now been extended to three years, and most of the pioneers have passed away. Dr. Dimock, brilliant and enthusiastic, perished at sea when she was but twenty-eight years of age. Dr. Zakrzewska, full of years and honour, remained up to the end of the century attending and advisory physician of the New England Hospital for Women and Children.[1]

The little town of St. Catherine's, on the other side of the Canadian border, comes into the ranks of the pioneers at this point in building up a hospital and providing training for nurses. This community, the first in Canada to follow the example of Miss Nightingale, began work on these lines in 1864, and owes the development and successful carrying out of its projects largely to the interest of Dr. Mack. Beginning with a little house, which was rented for eight dollars a month, one nurse, and a steward, the hospital grew steadily, and Dr. Mack became successively president of the board, physician of the hospital, and manager and consulting physician. Definite teaching for the nurses took shape in 1873, when through the influence of Dr. Mack Miss Money was sent to England to bring out two trained nurses and five or six probationers. A nurses' home was planned, and in 1874 a defi-

---

[1] Dr. Zakrzewska is the author of an interesting book based on her experiences, entitled *A Practical Illustration of the Right of Women to Labour*. C. H. Dall, Boston, 1860.

nite scheme of instruction and training was in operation. The hospital was called St. Catherine's General and Marine hospital. The nurses were required to bind themselves to serve for three years; for the first six months as probationers, without remuneration, and afterwards with a stipend, board (when not employed outside of the hospital; they were evidently sent to private duty or to other institutions), and uniforms. Every woman entering was required to bring satisfactory evidences of purity of motive, good conduct and character, and of having received the elements of a plain English education. The report of 1875 says: "Every possible opportunity is seized to impart instruction of a practical nature, while teaching will be given in chemistry, sanitary science, popular physiology and anatomy, hygiene, and all such branches of the healing art as a nurse ought to be familiar with."

Protestant sisterhoods have also played some part in the early nursing history of the country. The first impulse toward the formation of sisterhoods within the Protestant Episcopal church came from the Rev. Dr. Muhlenberg, who had visited Kaiserswerth and had become enthusiastic over its spirit and scope of work. He wrote a pamphlet, after his return from Germany, called the *Instruction of Deaconesses in the Evangelical Church*, and it was largely due to his influence and suggestions that the creation of the Sisterhood of the Holy Communion, the first independent community of Protestant Sisters of Charity in the United States, was successfully brought about by the pastor of the church of the Holy Communion in New York City. The sisterhood was established in 1845, thus being coincident with the first English sisterhood; its organisation, however, was not completed until 1852. The Sisters taught, and made the care of the sick one of their objects. They spent four years in nursing the patients of the infirmary supported by the church of the Holy Communion, and, in connection with it, opened a dispensary which has been spoken of as the beginning of the path which led to the founding of St. Luke's hospital; then, when this hospital was opened in 1859 under the auspices of the church, the Sisters were transferred to it and remained in charge until the establishment of the secular nursing school in 1888.

The sisterhood still retains many fields of activity, and professes the care of the sick as a chief interest. The rules of the house, with the exception of a few minor details, were adapted from those of Kaiserswerth, and one of the Sisters of the early period of organisation had gone there for some training. This Sister, as superintendent of St. Luke's hospital later, was active in the movement to prepare nurses for the war of 1861–64 by taking them into the civil hospitals for a short and hurried preparation for the overwhelming exigencies of military hospital service. Excellent and devoted work in this direction was also carried on by a

Protestant Sister in Baltimore, Mrs. Adeline Ty-
lor, who had also had a certain amount of training
at Kaiserswerth, and who, as the head of a community in Baltimore, conducted two large war
hospitals in Chester and Annapolis.[1]

When the appalling outburst of "man's inhu-
manity to man," the Civil War, swept like a storm
over the land, overshadowing, for the time being,
every smaller and less cosmic preoccupation, it
washed away the petty anchors which had kept
the majority of women carefully moored in the
quiet remote little bays of domestic seclusion, and
they floated out upon the stream of public duties.
Abhorrent as is the whole idea of war to those who
see in man nobler possibilities than those of beasts
of prey, it is nevertheless impossible not to recognise the immense opportunities for rearrangement
of social orders which it has given; and in the case
of women it is a striking fact that their modern
movement toward legal and social freedom received an enormous impetus from the dynamic
forces of three epoch-making wars. Thus, the war of
Freedom gave the women of Germany their opening to make their ability felt; out of the Crimean
War emerged the figure of Florence Nightingale,
whose memory and influence will live long after all
the military achievements of that time are forgotten;
and lastly, the Civil War marks the beginning of
all organised concentration of women in this country in public duties.

[1] *A Century of Nursing, cit.*

To give even a partial estimate of the extent
and complexity of the affairs administered by
women during the war is out of the question, and
even the vast proportion of the care of the sick
and wounded can be touched on only in barest
outline.[1]   To tell the story of that war-time nursing is out of our power.   Much of it will probably
never be told, nor will many of its actors be known
to posterity.   The energy and ability of the women
were expressed through the Sanitary Commission,
and this body, which took the place occupied to-
day by Red Cross organisations, received its first
impulse from them, for its historian says: "The
earliest movement that was made for any relief
was begun, it is hardly necessary to say, by
the women of the country."[2]   Two especially
notable figures are associated with its formation: Dr. Elizabeth Blackwell, probably the
most commanding personality among our pioneer physicians, and Miss Louisa Lee Schuyler,
whose mind was worthy of her great ancestor
Alexander Hamilton.   Dr. Blackwell returned
from England, where she had been in intimate relation with Miss Nightingale, full of enthusiasm, in
1861.   She called an informal meeting of women

[1] It is estimated that two thousand women were engaged
in nursing and hospital administration during the Civil
War.
[2] *History of the United States Sanitary Commission.*   By
Charles J. Stillé.   J. B. Lippincott and Co., Philadelphia,
1866.

together at the New York Infirmary for Women and Children, which she had founded some seven years previously. They formed the Ladies' Central Relief Committee, and drafted a letter calling for a mass-meeting at Cooper Union, and there, on April 26, 1861, the proposed Relief Association was enthusiastically endorsed and enlarged, Miss Louisa Schuyler being elected president. There had been some even earlier steps taken. On the 15th of April, the day on which the President's call for troops appeared, the women of Bridgeport, Connecticut, and those of Charleston, South Carolina, had organised societies to provide relief, nursing, and comforts for the volunteers, and a few days afterwards the women of Lowell, Massachusetts, had done the same. On the 19th of April the women of Cleveland, Ohio, had organised with the purpose of assisting the families of volunteers.

The call to the Cooper Union meeting was a stirring document, and was signed by ninety-two women, one of whom was Mrs. Griffin, later, and for many years, the president of the Bellevue training school for nurses. The preliminary meeting at the infirmary had been attended by men also, one of whom, the Rev. Dr. Bellows, assisted in framing the constitution which was adopted for the Women's Central Association of Relief, and which recited, among others, as its objects: "To collect and disseminate information upon the actual and prospective wants of the army; to establish recognised relations with the medical staff and to act as an auxiliary to it; to maintain a central depot of stores and to open a bureau for the examination and registration of nurses." The first overture made by the society to the military officials met with a severe rebuff, and Dr. Bellows, the delegate, was so convinced by the sweeping statements made to him of the full readiness of the army medical department for all emergencies (again, as at Scutari, nothing was wanted) that he returned to the women and reported that he believed their efforts were unnecessary, and would only appear to be foolish. The women, however, disbelieved this statement and refusing to adopt this view continued their preparations. Events soon convinced Dr. Bellows also that he had been too optimistic.

Miss Schuyler and her colleagues early realised the gigantic extent of the task before them, and, largely through their efforts, the Woman's Central Relief Association joined with the Board of Physicians and Surgeons of the Hospitals of New York and the Medical Association for Furnishing Hospital Supplies in making that joint appeal to the President for the creation of a national official commission which resulted in the order issued by the Secretary of War on June 9, 1861, creating the body which was known as the Sanitary Commission. Eight men of eminence and absolute integrity were appointed, Dr. Bellows being chosen president. The Woman's Central Association of Relief now became a branch of the Sanitary Commission, and co-ordinated all of the relief organisations throughout the country, stimulating the formation of branches where they did not exist, and bringing all into one harmonious and magnificent system.[1] Dr. Blackwell was so hampered by masculine jealousy in all she tried to do at that time that, rather than jeopardise the cause to which her heart was. given, she retired from a prominent share in the administrative work of the commission, while none the less actively engaging in its service. The preparation of women as nurses for the wounded soldiers absorbed her attention for a time, and, in co-operation with a committee of women, she selected, trained (as well as the pressure of the emergency would allow), and sent to the front about one hundred nurses. In her own book she says that the most promising of them were sent to Bellevue Hospital for a month.[2] Dr. Blackwell had long been deeply interested in the question of training for nurses, and her intimacy with Miss Nightingale must have accentuated this interest. Her influence and knowledge were continually exerted in behalf of good teaching and a higher standard, but she has been so modest and unassuming about her own work that the full influence of her ideas in the final

[1] See letter from Miss Louisa Schuyler to the 235 Women's Branches, *United States Sanitary Commission* by Katherine P. Wormeley, Boston, 1863, appendix, pp. 271–274.

[2] *Op. cit.*, p. 236.

evolution of trained nursing will perhaps never be quite realised.   In 1859 she and her sister Emily had prepared a statement of their aims and intentions for the New York Infirmary for Women and Children which had been incorporated in 1854 for three purposes: the relief of the sick poor; the training of women physicians; the training of nurses.   In their statement the sisters said: "In this hospital we would also establish a system of instruction for nurses,—its plans to be based on those drawn up by Miss Nightingale for her proposed school in London, . . . with which, though never yet published, we are well acquainted."[1] Long after training schools were an accomplished fact a friend said to Dr. Blackwell: "Thee has had so much to do with the reform of nursing, I think it is too bad thy share in it has not had more recognition." "What does it matter," she answered, "so long as the work itself is done?"

The work of the Sanitary Commission is justly celebrated as a magnificent record of humanitarian work.   Its leaders were all thoroughly acquainted with the sanitary history of the Crimean campaign and with Miss Nightingale's work (it is known, moreover, that they had her counsel and advice), and their purpose from the outset was to prevent useless suffering and to minimise sickness by hy-

[1] *Medicine as a Profession for Women*.   Read at Clinton Hall, Dec. 2, 1859.   Published by Tinson, New York, at the request of the trustees of the infirmary, in 1860.

gienic precautions. Owing to military opposition and jealousy [1] they were not always able to carry out their plans for prevention, though these were always made with far-sighted wisdom. For the care of the sick and wounded soldiers, an admirable system of hospitals was eventually developed under its fostering control, and though the nursing had a thoroughly amateur character throughout the war, it was carried on with unselfish devotion, and many of the nurses, self-taught and disciplined by dire necessity, attained a high degree of practical skill. The most definite landmark in the somewhat formless nursing department of the Civil War was the official appointment of Dorothea Dix as Superintendent of Nurses. This remarkable woman, the female Howard of this country, is too seldom remembered by the present generation.

Dorothea Lynde Dix was born in Maine in 1802. In 1836, while travelling for her health, she visited the family of Mr. Rathbone in Liverpool, the father of workhouse infirmary nursing reform,

[1] Their plans were looked upon as a deep-laid scheme for some selfish purposes, and the Secretary of War at first asked the delegates to state frankly precisely what they wanted, since it was evident they could not want only what they seemed to be asking for. The history mentioned says: "It is humiliating to record the utter inability on the part of our highest American officials to appreciate the best-considered and most widely extended system of mitigating the horrors of war known in history, and especially at a time when the existence of the government was dependent upon the health and efficiency of that army, which the appointment of a sanitary commission was designed to promote." Stillé, *op. cit.*, p. 60.

and in 1841 she began teaching in the prisons of
her native State.   Her attention was drawn to the
condition of the insane, which was then quite as
horrible, in almost all parts of the country, as in
the days of Howard. She determined to investigate
it and for two years made a most searching personal examination of every almshouse and jail
(where the insane were then confined) in Massachusetts. Like Howard, she kept an exact
record of every fact, and when, at the end of her
investigations, she memorialised the Legislature
of Massachusetts, her testimony of what she had
seen was appalling and irrefutable.   Her earliest
supporters were Dr. S. G. Howe and Charles Sum-
ner, and the result of her work in Massachusetts
was the immediate extension of State care for the
insane. For the next twenty years, in every state
of the Union (and that was in the days of rough
travel), she carried on the same close unfaltering
inspection and record-making, and took her accusations and appeals into every Legislature. As
no State hospitals then existed, she became convinced of the necessity of applying the principle
of taxation to this purpose, and the creation of
State hospitals in many states was the direct result
of her conceptions and resolution.   New Jersey
was the field of her first victory in this great piece
of constructive statesmanship, in 1845.

After her wonderful campaign in the states she
conceived the project of persuading Congress to set
aside twelve million acres of the public domain

for the endowment of institutions for the insane, the blind, and other helpless members of society, and she actually pushed this gigantic undertaking successfully through both houses of Congress, and saw her ideal about to be realised, only to be fairly crushed by a disappointment totally unexpected, for the President, Franklin Pierce, small of calibre and mediocre of mind, had the power to undo and prevent great things which he was not capable of creating, and he vetoed the bill.

Miss Dix afterward travelled abroad and carried on investigations into the condition of the insane in a number of foreign countries. Her appointment to the superintendency of the war nursing was in recognition of her vast public services, but she was then nearly sixty years old, worn from her exhausting life-work, and could not adapt herself to the general conditions of a hospital service. She herself said that this was not the part of her life by which she wished to be judged. Her standards were high and inflexible, and she antagonised many of those with whom she was obliged to work. She died in 1887.[1]

[1] See *Life of Dorothea Lynde Dix*, by Francis Tiffany. Houghton, Mifflin & Co., Boston, 1896.

Circular No. 7, issued from the Surgeon-General's office in the War Department, read: "In order to give greater utility to the acts of Miss Dorothy L. Dix as superintendent of women nurses in general hospitals, and to make the employment of such nurses conform more closely to existing laws, . . . Miss Dix has been entrusted by the War Department with the duty of selecting women nurses and assigning them to general or permanent military hospitals. Women

The medical profession first went on record in regard to nursing reform in May, 1869, when, at the New Orleans meeting of the American Medical Association, a report of a Committee on the Training of Nurses, whose chairman was Dr. Samuel Gross, was presented to the meeting.   The committee was a special one, appointed to inquire into the best method of organising and conducting institutions for the training of nurses, and some of its conclusions are of much interest.   The report recited the strange neglect of nursing in the United States; the long-felt need of good nursing; mentioned the fact that the Catholic orders were the only ones who seemed to realise its importance; and said: " It is perhaps fortunate that the mortality occasioned by bad nursing cannot be esti-

nurses are not to be employed in such hospitals without her sanction and approval except in case of urgent need.

Women nurses will be under the control and direction of the medical officer in charge of the hospital to which they are assigned, and may be discharged by him if incompetent, insubordinate, or otherwise unfit for their vocation.   Miss Dix is charged with diligent oversight of women nurses, and with the duty of ascertaining by personal inspection whether or not they are properly performing their duties, and medical officers are enjoined to receive her suggestions and counsel with respect and to carry these into effect if compatible with the hospital service.

As it will be impossible for Miss Dix to supervise in person all the military hospitals she is authorised to delegate her authority. . . .

Women wishing employment as nurses must apply to Miss Dix or to her authorised agents.   Army regulations allow one nurse to every ten patients (beds).   As it is the expressed mated by those most immediately affected by it, as a knowledge of it would entail upon them an immense amount of misery and mental anguish. Nursing in its more exact sense is as much of an art and a science as medicine."

Then followed some statistical description of all the existing Protestant institutions in the Old World, beginning with Kaiserswerth, and including all the London hospitals reformed up to that time. The report mentioned the early American efforts and the vast extent of volunteer nursing of the Civil War, and made the following recommendations:

I. That every large and well-organised hospital should have a school for the training of nurses, not only for the supply of its own necessities, but for pri-

will of the government that a portion of these nurses shall be women, and as Congress has given to the Surgeon-General authority to decide in what number women shall be substituted for men, it is ordered that there shall be one woman nurse to two men nurses. Medical officers are hereby required to organise their respective hospitals accordingly. Medical officers requiring nurses will apply to Miss Dix or her authorised agents.

Sisters of Charity will continue to be employed as at present under special instructions from this office. Signed, Wm. A. Hammond, Surg.-Gen. Miss Dix's requirements for candidates were specified in the next order, Circular No. 8, July 14, 1862.

No candidate for position as nurse was to be considered unless she was between the ages of 35 and 50. Matronly persons of experience and those of superior education and serious disposition were to have the preference. Habits of neatness and order, sobriety and industry were essential.

vate families; the teaching to be furnished by its own medical staff, assisted by the resident physicians.

II.   That, while it is not at all essential to combine religious exercises with nursing, it is believed that such a union would be eminently conducive to the welfare of the sick in all public institutions, and the committee therefore earnestly recommend the establishment of nurses' homes, to be placed under the immediate supervision and direction of Deaconesses or lady superintendents.

III.   That, in order to give thorough scope and efficiency to this scheme, district schools should be formed and placed under the guardianship of the county medical societies of every State and Territory in the Union, the members of which should make it their business to impart instruction in the art and science of nursing, including the elements of hygiene and every other species of information necessary to qualify the student for the important duties of the nurse.

The committee further suggested the importance of forming, in every convenient place, societies of nurses who should have the preference in calls over the uneducated attendants.   This recommendation is an exceedingly interesting one, and well worthy of note as original, since it foreshadowed the actual developments of later years. The report concluded with a summary of the qualities necessary for the nurse to possess, taken, apparently, though without acknowledgment, from the regulations of the Nightingale school, and it was resolved that a copy of the report should be sent to medical societies all over the country.[1]

[1] *Proceedings of the American Medical Association,* New Orleans, May 1869. Reprint, *Med. News,* Philadelphia, 1869, vol. xx., pp. 339, 351. In November of this same year the celebrated scientist Virchow gave similar recommendations to an association of women in Berlin, Germany.

CHAPTER IX

A TRIO OF TRAINING SCHOOLS

THE war came to an end, but the splendid work of the women on the Sanitary Commission and of the nurses in the field could not die away; their aroused energies could not be stifled, nor their fields of activity be again restricted. When they returned from military service it was to take up with moral courage and determination a new campaign for the reformation of civil institutions. The establishment of trained nursing in America came as the result of the war almost as directly as it had done in England. There, Miss Nightingale turned from one work straight to the other; here, the women who were to be the future managers of training schools had their preliminary training in the relief service. The first three schools for nurses established after the war, those from which the steady march of nursing progress in America dates, are monuments to the creative energy of organised women who had learned their power. Two, at least, of them were the work of women's committees, originating with them and not with hospital governors or medical boards, and pushed through in

spite of opposition, doubts, and disapproval from
many quarters.   One and the same year saw this
trio of schools established within the wards of
important general hospitals: Bellevue, opened on
May 1, the New Haven, on October 1, and the
Massachusetts General on November 1, 1873.

In New York State, with its large population of
dependents of all kinds, herded together in bar-
rack-like institutions under the general supervision
of the State Commissioners of Charity, there
was not a woman of enlightened intelligence or
refinement in any position of authority or even of
inspection.   Miss Louisa Schuyler, who had na-
tionalised the work of the Sanitary Commission,
and whose insight grasped the whole problem,
organised the State Charities Aid Association of
New York State, to act as a volunteer, unpaid
body of citizens for the improvement of the public
institutions of charity.   Its form of association
was completed on the 11th of May, 1872, and Miss
Schuyler was elected the first president.   It divided itself into three departments for investigation and active work, dealing with: I—Children.
II—Adult and Able-Bodied Paupers.   III—The
Sick in Hospitals.   The association comprised
both men and women, upon a broad humanitarian
platform, and Miss Schuyler's early reports and
papers are excellent examples of a union of noble
purpose with intellectual and practical ability.
In her first annual report, presented to the Commissioners of Charity, she said, among other things,

in speaking of the visitors to the institutions, that they

represent the best class of our citizens as regards en-lightened views, wise benevolence, experience, wealth, influence, and social position. . . . Ours is neither exclusively man's work nor woman's work. We are men and women working together, supplementing each other's powers. . . .

You will see that we have aimed to place our work upon a foundation as broad as that upon which our own republican form of government rests: to do away with all distinctions of race or sex, of political parti-sanship and sectarian prejudice; to have the work judged by its merits alone, whether it is or is not worthy of support from our citizens.[1]

The Hospitals Committee began work at once, and defined its duties as follows:

I. To inform itself of the number and present con-dition of sick, inebriate, insane, blind, deaf-and-dumb, idiot, and aged paupers in the New York State institu-tions of public charities, and to urge the adoption of such measures as are best adapted to restore the health, alleviate the sufferings, secure the humane care and comfort, and contribute to the happiness of these afflicted and aged people.

II. To collect and impart information in regard to the latest and most approved plans for the con-struction, ventilation and disinfection of hospitals and asylums; to prepare plans of organisation for their kitchens, linen, laundry, and nursing departments; and to acquaint themselves with such hygienic

[1] First Annual Report S. C. A. A., 1873.

and sanitary regulations as are in accordance with the most advanced views of the medical profession.

The first section of the Hospitals Committee appointed to a definite institution was formed on Jan. 9, 1872, to visit the Westchester poorhouse. It consisted of forty-nine members. Its experience was so strikingly like that of the early English groups under Miss Twining and Miss Cobbe that it is well to record it. So long as the ladies were contented to work themselves, and to make no criticism on the management, everything went smoothly. With the full knowledge of the superintendents of the poor they came and went, conducted sewing schools, carried delicacies for the sick, and cared generally for their comfort. But the ladies became aware of many things demanding immediate reform: there was an absence of classification which led to gross immorality, a want of enlightened treatment for the insane, no nursing for the sick, the children were badly fed, badly clothed, badly taken care of, and exposed to the degrading influence of the adult paupers in charge of them. The ladies offered, through the Children's Aid Society, to place the little ones in good homes; the superintendents of the poor refused, wanting them to remain in the county where they could look after them. The condition of the sick was especially pitiable. "It is no exaggeration to say that in most of our county poorhouses no nursing of the sick is ever attempted. . .

Usually the very ill patients are cared for by those in the same room who are less ill. . . . Many patients were in the last stages of pulmonary tuberculosis; in one ward there were several cases of paralysis, epilepsy, one gunshot wound, accident cases, amputation, etc." In one ward the ladies found a terrible case of suffering from carcinoma of the face, and one poor man crushed by a steam shovel and in great agony. They asked the superintendents to employ some one to nurse these sufferers; their request was refused on the ground that there was no appropriation of funds for such expenses. They then begged to be allowed to pay the wages of a competent nurse, to be selected and controlled by the superintendent. This was also refused. "They could not," said the women in their report, "refuse the kindness which death at last brought the sufferers." When the visitors' suggestions for improvements were first made, they were received with civility, but no action was taken. Later they were requested to come only on one day in the week. Finally, when the visitors repeated their petition for better care of the children, and for a nurse for the sick, offering to pay the wages of such attendants until the Board of Supervisors met, the superintendents told them that they had no authority to interfere, that it was desired that they should no longer come as members of an association; they might come as ordinary visitors, but the superintendents personally desired to have no further intercourse with them. Not long after this they were refused admittance.[1]

A perfect example, this, of the reasons why male officials do not want women interfering in their business. But in time, with persistent effort, reforms were set in motion.[2]

The second section, formed on Jan. 26, 1872,

[1] First Annual Report S. C. A. A., 1873.

[2] The State Charities Aid Association stood upon the principle that the taxpayers, supporting as they did all of the public institutions and all of the officials appointed to administer them, had an unquestionable right to inspect these institutions and to see how they were managed.   After their visitors were turned out of the Westchester poorhouse, the S. C. A. A., including, as it did, numbers of public-spirited men, secured legislative enactment largely increasing the powers of the State Board of Charities in the matter of visiting, and then by personal agreement with the board it was arranged that the latter should appoint as its official visitors members of the voluntary society upon the recommendation of the latter. This arrangement lasted for eight years, during which time the foundations of reforms of the most far-reaching character were laid.   The perennial struggle against political corruption and mismanagement of public charitable funds then became too heavy a strain on the moral courage of the board. It first tried to suppress the reports made by the visitors to the S. C. A. A., and so to the public, and finding that this stratagem was resisted it broke off the relationship with the volunteer body.   The S. C. A. A., strong in the support of enlightened public opinion, then asked for legislative authority to continue its inspection of institutions and was actively opposed by the board, but finally secured the recognition it asked.   See *Address from the S. C. A. A. to its Local Visiting Committees throughout the State of New York*, July, 1880 (No. 24 of publications).   Also Nos. 25 and 26, containing Mr. Choate's argument before the Legislature and the final report of the special committee in charge of the bill, June 10, 1881.

was the Bellevue Hospital Visiting Committee, consisting of fifty-three members. The ladies composing it were called together at the invitation of Miss Louisa Schuyler. "Several of them had been members of the Sanitary Commission, and had had experience of hospital work, but the majority had no knowledge of the difficulties of the task before them, and accepted it with all the bravery of ignorance."[1]   Of these ladies, selected, as they were, with care as possessing every possible equipment of ability, character, and social position, many since that time have had a conspicuously important and useful career in the civic and charitable reforms of the city and have been identified with the whole movement of hospital and nursing advance. They now began their work, every member taking certain days on which to visit certain wards.   The chairman, Mrs. Joseph Hobson, was a young married woman, unfamiliar with poverty, sickness, or degradation, and who had never been in a hospital.   On her first visit to Bellevue she wandered bewildered through the long corridors and the series of double wards opening out of one another, wondering how to begin.   A sort of external cleanliness and order prevailed, yet she felt instinctively that things were not right somewhere.   As she explored the rather deserted-looking extent of one

[1] *History of the Establishment of the Bellevue Training School for Nurses*, read at the Waldorf-Astoria, March 6, 1899.

floor, she came upon a young man, who appeared to be a physician, and who was busied about some of the patients. With some embarrassment she went up to him and introduced herself as an official visitor, and said she would be grateful for a few hints as to what to look into. "You want to see things?" said the young man with an inexplicable expression; "well, I can show them to you. Do not appear to be with me, but follow around after me." The young surgeon was no other than Dr. Gill Wylie, who later became so stanch a friend of the training school and loyal supporter of the cause of the training school committee. This now famous specialist was then a young man, fresh from his Southern country home, and held the position of interne, or house-surgeon, with quarters in the hospital. Mrs. Hobson followed him, and watched as he lifted the bed-clothes from a newly-arrived case and proceeded himself to give the patient—a woman—some attempt at a bed-bath.

It must have been such a case as only old Bellevue could show, for the visitor was horror-stricken at the conditions she saw. Dr. Wylie then conducted her to the old bath-rooms (long since demolished), and pointed out the litter of dirty rags on the floor where the "nurse" (a ten-day prisoner from the Island) had her bed. The dinners came up to the wards, and the pieces of fish and potatoes were dumped without dishes on the bare boards of the long tables. Finally they descended to the laundry, for the housewifely eye of the lady had

not failed to rest upon the dull grey sheets and
pillow-cases.   In the laundry was one lone, old,
decrepit man.   He constituted, in fact, the entire
force on duty in the laundry at that time, and for
six weeks he had had no soap, because the appropriation had run out.   Incredible as this may
sound, it was the plain and literal truth.   For six
weeks there had been no soap in the laundry of a
hospital containing some hundreds of patients,
and the laundry staff had dwindled to the one lone
man.[1]

On that day all the horrors of old Bellevue were
doomed to extinction.

A few days after this the committee met to compare notes, and, as one after another of the ladies
arose to read her report and spoke of visits made
to the patients, individual cases in distress helped,
soups and delicacies carried to them, and religious
consolation brought to those desiring it, the young
chairman, unaccustomed to all public duties, grew
hot and quaked with dread and mortification.
She had not talked kindly with a single patient;
she had taken them no beef tea; she had not
inquired whether they would see a clergyman!
Would not her report sound most heartless and
aggressive?   What would the others think of it?
In deep embarrassment she read her itemised
account of all she had seen at Bellevue: the filth
of the patients; the degradation of the attendants;
the inadequacy of all housekeeping details; the

[1] From private sources.

state of the laundry, of the clothes-rooms, of the kitchen. She told of the tea, soup, and coffee made in the same kettles, of the food eaten from the bare boards without plates and even without knives, because it was the opinion of some one in the domestic economy of the place that if the patients had knives they would cut themselves.

There was electricity in the air when she finished, and for a moment there was silence. Then a lady rose and moved that the President should present the report to the Commissioners of Charity and demand an investigation.

That winter the investigation of the hospital conditions was carried on with the utmost thoroughness and conscientiousness. By good fortune one of the Commissioners, General James Bowen, was not of the usual politician type, but a gentleman and personal friend of the visitors. He not only assisted them with official support, but begged them to carry their investigations into the other city institutions. It was no doubt owing to the weight of his personal and civic prestige that the visitors were protected against the antagonism of the petty politicians which, in the Westchester poorhouse and many other institutions, had been freely displayed against them, even when they were women of prominence. Only this one friend on the Board of Commissioners is recorded in the minutes of that institutional invasion, and on the Medical Board only four—Dr. James R. Wood, Dr. Austin Flint, Dr. Stephen Smith, and Dr. James

M. Markoe. To these five men we owe the initia-
tion of reforms in hospital service in New York.
The others were, if not actively in opposition, at
least discouraging. One of the physicians and
even a clergyman who visited Bellevue publicly
expressed the opinion that the hospital was not a
proper place for ladies to visit, and these criticisms
illustrate the character of the stream of disapprobation—social, political, and medical—which the
women had to confront during that momentous
winter.

In a comparatively short time, with the strong
support of General Bowen, the visitors succeeded
in making substantial improvements in the kitchen,
laundry, and supply departments; but when they
came to study a systematic plan for the complete
reorganisation of the whole housekeeping side of
the hospital, one and all became convinced of the
utter hopelessness of any radical or lasting improvement unless there was an entire change in
the system of nursing. As far back as 1848 the
system of convict nursing had been, in theory at
least, discredited, and the hired nurses were supposed to be selected from among poor but repu-
table women of decent habits. This was an ideal
that could be but rarely attained, and when the
visitors began their investigations they found few
such women in the whole building. Almost the
entire staff of female attendants, including the
"scrub-gang" which remained for years after
the training school was opened, was recruited from

the class of petty offenders who had been "sent up," mostly for drunkenness, to the Island, and were called the "ten-day women." If these, in the hospital service, showed any willingness to remain and keep sober, they were retained until their next "spree," and even such accidental mishaps were often overlooked if the "nurses" were at least kindly in their feelings for the sick, and this many of them—unless something happened to arouse their easily excited rage and violence—really were. But even of these there were no night nurses. Three night watchmen guarded the wards at night, and made rounds among the six hundred patients. It is said that they sometimes drugged those who were likely to need attention, and drank the stimulants that had been prescribed.[1]

The visitors accordingly passed a resolution in April, 1872, addressed to the Commissioners of Charity and begging them to consent to consider a plan which the ladies desired to lay before them for establishing a training school for nurses. The Commissioners (through General Bowen's influence) gave a cordial reception to the ladies' letter, and answered it with expressions of approbation. However, they deemed it necessary to refer the plan to the Medical Board for decision. Time went by, but no reply came from the Medical Board. Inquiries were made, and it was found that it had taken no action.

[1] "A New Profession for Women." Franklin H. North. The *Century Magazine*, Nov. 1882, p. 39.

It had already been decided by the committee that a thorough study of training systems already in existence must be made, and Dr. Gill Wylie, still foremost in devotion to the cause, offered to go to Europe at his own expense and bring back a full report of the status of nursing abroad. He made his trip in the summer, returning in the autumn, and brought with him full and interesting accounts of the Nightingale school at St. Thomas's, of the extension of the new system into other English hospitals, of the rise of district nursing and its great possibilities, with a general survey of the nursing conditions in France and Germany, and, most important of all, a long letter of counsel and encouragement from Miss Nightingale, to whom he had immediately communicated his mission.

In view of the silence of the Medical Board, the Bellevue Hospital committee resolved, in September, 1872, to refer the whole matter to the Hospitals Committee of the State Charities Aid Association, and this body prepared a scheme for the establishment of a training school for nurses at Bellevue, and undertook further negotiations with the Medical Board. By the efforts of the four members of the Board who were friendly to the visitors and their plans— Drs. Wood, Flint, Smith, and Markoe—a committee from the Medical Board was finally appointed to receive the communication. Three days later this committee presented the scheme to the full Board, and a unanimous resolution was passed expressing approval of its suggestions, and recommending it to the Commissioners of Charities. The Commissioners in turn considered it, and finally agreed—though with reluctance—to give the committee of ladies six wards in Bellevue for the training of nurses.[1] The victory was now complete. It was an exciting winter in New York society. Little was talked of, in the circles of the members of the State Charities Aid, but the proposed reforms and the projected school for nurses. The report of the Hospitals Committee of the State Charities Aid Association, dated December 23, 1872, or just two days before Christmas, is a notable document and one which ought not to be allowed to fall into oblivion. It gave a most graphic survey of the facts discovered during the visits to the hospitals, emphasised the shameful character of the hospital housekeeping and nursing, noted the advance of nursing under Miss Nightingale and recounted her services to humanity, told of Dr. Wylie's travels and investigations, of the negotiations with the Medical Board and their final consent, and then proceeded to give this inspiring and far-sighted statement of their aims:

In the plan offered for the establishment of the school at Bellevue we ask only for the control and

[1] State Charities Aid Association: *Training School for Nurses to be attached to Bellevue*; report of the Committee on Hospitals. New York, 1877. Called report No. 1 in bound volume.

nursing of six wards: more than this it would be impossible to attempt satisfactorily at first.   In course of time we propose to benefit not only Bellevue, but all the public hospitals, and also to train nurses for the sick in private houses, and for the work among the poor.

As the work advances we hope to establish a college for the training of nurses, which will receive a charter from the State, and become a recognised institution of the country.[1]   Branches of this college would be established in connection with hospitals devoted to particular diseases, such as the Woman's hospital, etc., so that in course of time nurses trained for the treatment of special diseases will be as easily attainable as physicians.   Connected with the college would be a "Home" for nurses, whence they would be supplied with employment and provision made for them when ill or disabled by labour or advanced years. The nurses when trained would receive a diploma or certificate, renewable at fixed periods.   Thus the college would control the nurses during their state of pupilage, and protect the public from imposition, by making it known that a nurse whose diploma or certificate was not in due form had forfeited the confidence of the institution.   .

The work before us is not an inexpensive one.   It should not be regarded merely in the light of a work of benevolence, but as a system of education, calculated to benefit thousands in all ranks of life, and, like the quality of mercy, blessing him that gives and him that takes.

We require at present the sum of $20,000.   A house

[1] The school became incorporated in 1874.

must be had for the Lady Superintendent and nurses: not a mere lodging, but a comfortable home, where, after their daily labours, they may find relaxation and rest, free from the depressing influences of the hospital. Our head nurses, on whom will devolve the task of training the probationers, will be entitled to the high wages they would receive in private houses. To the probationers we shall give moderate wages, on a rising scale, in proportion to their usefulness and term of service.

The money which may now be intrusted to us will be placed in the hands of a committee, chosen from the members of the Bellevue Association—persons of experience, who will devote themselves conscientiously to the work they undertake. The Lady Superintendent will go to England, and make herself acquainted with all the details of her duties, at St. Thomas's hospital and at the Liverpool infirmary. Our head nurses will be chosen with the utmost care, and the physicians and surgeons of Bellevue have offered not only to deliver lectures, but to give personal instruction by the bedside of the patients; and the Commissioners of Charities have testified a most ready willingness to co-operate in our work. Under such auspices we feel confident that we shall achieve the same success that has already been attained in England, if we receive, at the outset, sufficient funds to enable us to work without being constantly trammelled by pecuniary considerations.[1] It will be seen by Dr. Wylie's report that the nurses trained in England are chiefly recruited from the class of upper servants. In

[1] Six weeks after the publication of this report the sum of $23,000 was contributed.

this country, women of that class find plenty of employment at high wages; we propose, therefore, to offer the advantages of our school to women of a higher grade.[1] In this country we have a large class of conscientious and laborious women whose education and early associations would lead them to aspire to some higher and more thoughtful labour than household service or work in shops: such as daughters and widows of clergymen, professional men and farmers throughout New England and the Northern States, who have received the good education of our common schools and academies, and are dependent on their own exertions for support. An American woman, with such an education, and her heart in the work, could be trained to make the best nurse in the world, for the race has ready wit, quick perception, and strong powers of observation. Let her, in addition to these qualities, acquire the habit of obedience and you have all the elements for making a good nurse. To such women we are prepared to offer a career of the widest usefulness: a profession acquired under masters of the highest skill (physicians and surgeons of not only American but of European fame) and an assured means of livelihood. There is an idea prevailing among certain classes that the work of nursing can best be done by persons who receive no pay, but simply a support from the order to which they belong—that the receipt of money gives the stigma of servility to the work. While we would not in any way depreciate the usefulness of those holding these views, we feel that the idea is an erroneous one: that

[1] Women of the class here alluded to are now obtained without difficulty.

such a rule shuts out a vast number whose services would be invaluable.

Why should not Christian women receive proper remuneration for their services as well as Christian men? Does not our Divine Master tell us that "the labourer is worthy of his hire"?

Candidates for this work must not blind themselves to its difficulties. In the wards of a pauper hospital they must come into daily contact with vice and disease in their most repulsive forms; deeply graven on their hearts, and reflected in their lives, must be the words of St. Paul: "Charity suffereth long and is kind; charity envieth not; charity vaunteth not itself, is not puffed up, doth not behave itself unseemly, seeketh not her own, is not easily provoked, thinketh no evil; rejoiceth not in iniquity, but rejoiceth in the truth; beareth all things, believeth all things, endureth all things."

We wish our candidates to be religious women, but we do not require that they should belong to any given sect. To Catholic and Protestant our doors are equally open; we impose no vows; we say to all, in the words of the holy founder of the order of the Sisters of Charity: "Your convent must be the houses of the sick; your cell the chamber of suffering; your chapel the nearest church; your cloister the streets of a city, or the wards of a hospital; the promise of obedience your sole enclosure; your grate the fear of God, and womanly modesty your only veil."

For the Committee on Hospitals,

ELIZABETH HOBSON,
Chairman.

All obstacles being removed, a subcommittee

was appointed to prepare a working plan for the projected school and to deal with all of the preliminary details of its organisation. This committee, which dealt so brilliantly and ably with the responsibility entrusted to it, and achieved a success that has completely revolutionised the care of the sick in the New World, was composed of the following members: Mrs. W. H. Osborn, chairman; Mrs. Robert Woodworth, secretary; Mrs. Wm. Preston Griffin, Mrs. d'Oremieulx, Mrs. Joseph Hobson, Miss Woolsey, Miss Ellen Collins, Miss Julia Gould, Mr. Henry G. Stebbins, treasurer; Dr. W. G. Wylie, Mr. Chandler Robbins. Their years of devoted and untiring service can never be too highly estimated, and their names will claim the gratitude and recognition of future generations.

Miss Nightingale's letter to Dr. Wylie proved to be a strong support to the women in their experiment. Omitting some purely personal details of explanation for not having been able to receive him, the letter ran as follows:

I wish your association God-speed with all my heart and soul in their task of reform, and will gladly, if I can, answer any questions you may think it worth while to ask.

You say "the great difficulty will be to define the instructions, the duties, and position of the nurses in distinction from those of medical men, and you are anxious to get my views in relation to this subject."

Is this a difficulty? A nurse is not a "medical man."

Nor is she a medical woman. (Most carefully do we, in our training, avoid confusion, both practically and theoretically, of letting women suppose that nursing duties and medical duties run into or overlap each other; so much so that, though we often have been asked to allow ladies intending to be "Doctors" to come in as *nurses* to St. Thomas's hospital, in order to ".pick up"—so they phrased it—professional medical knowledge, we have never consented even to admit such applications, in order to avoid even the semblance of encouraging such gross ignorance, and dabbling in matters of life and death, as this implies. You who *are* a "medical man," who know the difference between the professional studies of the medical student, even the idlest, and of the nurse, will readily see this.) Nurses are not "medical men." On the contrary, the nurses are there, and solely there, *to carry out the orders of the medical and surgical staff*, including, of course, the whole practice of cleanliness, fresh air, diet, etc. [The whole organisation of discipline to which the nurses must be subjected is for the sole purpose of enabling the nurses to carry out, intelligently and faithfully, such orders and such duties as constitute the whole practice of nursing. | They are in no sense medical men. Their duties can never clash with the medical duties. Their whole training is to enable them to understand how best to carry out medical and surgical orders, including (as above) the whole art of cleanliness, ventilation, food, etc., and *the reason* why this is to be done *this* way and not *that* way.

And for this very purpose—that is, in order that they may be competent to execute medical directions—to be nurses and not doctors—they *must* be, for discipline and internal management, entirely under a woman, a *trained* superintendent, whose whole business is to see that the nursing duties are performed according to this standard. For this purpose may I say:

1. That the nursing of hospitals, including the carrying out of medical officers' orders, must be done to the satisfaction of the medical officers whose orders regarding the sick are to be carried out. And we may depend upon it that the highly trained intelligent nurse, and cultivated moral woman, will do this better than the ignorant, stupid woman, for ignorance is always headstrong.

2. That all desired changes, reprimands, etc., in the nursing and for the nurses, should be referred by medical officers *to the superintendent.*

That rules which make the matron (superintendent) and nurses responsible to the house surgeons, or medical and surgical staffs, *except* in the sense of carrying out current medical orders, above insisted on, are always found fatal to nursing discipline.

That if the medical officers have fault to find, it is bad policy for them to reprimand the nurses themselves. The medical staff must carry all considerable complaints to the matron: the current complaints, as, for instance, if a patient has been neglected, or an order mistaken, to the ward "Sister," or the head nurse, who must *always* accompany the medical officer in his visits, receive his orders, and be responsible for their being carried out.

(All considerable complaint against a head nurse, or "Sister," to go, of course, to the matron.)

3. All discipline must be, of course, under the matron (superintendent) and ward "Sisters," otherwise nursing is impossible.

And here I should add that, unless there is, so to speak, a hierarchy of women—as thus: matron or superintendent, Sisters or head nurses, assistant or night nurses, wardmaids or scrubbers (or whatever other grades are, locally, considered more appropriate)—discipline becomes impossible. ·

In this hierarchy the higher grade ought always to know the duties of the lower better than the lower grade does itself. And so on to the head. Otherwise, how will they be able to *train?* "Moral influence" alone will not make a good trainer.

Any special questions which you may like to address to me I will do my best to answer as well as I am able.

But I am afraid that, without knowing your special case, I shall be only confusing if I add much more now.

I will, therefore, only now mention, as an instance, that the very day I received your first message (through Mrs. Wardroper) I received a letter from a well-known German physician strikingly exemplifying what we have been saying as to the necessity of hospital nurses being in no way under the medical staff as to *discipline*, but under a matron or "lady superintendent" of their own, who is responsible for the carrying out of medical orders.

You are, doubtless, aware that this is by no means the custom in Germany. (In France the system much more nearly approaches to our own.) In Germany, generally the ward nurse is *immediately*, and for everything under the ward doctor. And this led to consequences so disastrous that, going into the opposite extreme, Kaiserswerth and other German Protestant deaconesses' institutions were formed, where the chaplain and the "Vorsteherin" (female superintendent) were, virtually, masters of the hospital, which is of course absurd.

My friend, then, who has been for forty years medical officer of one of the largest hospitals in Germany, wrote to me that he had succeeded in placing a *matron* over his nurses; then, after one and a half year, she had been so persecuted that she had been compelled to resign; then, that he had remained another year trying to have her replaced; lastly that, failing, he had himself resigned his post of forty years, believing that he could do better work for his reform outside the hospital than *in* it.

It seems extraordinary that this first essential, *viz.*, that women should be, in matters of discipline, under a woman, should need to be advocated at all. But so it is.

And I can add my testimony, as regards another vast hospital in Germany, to the abominable effects of nurses being directly responsible *not* to a matron, but to the economic staff and medical staff of their hospital. And I am told, on the highest authority, that since my time things have only got worse.

But I will not take up your time and my own with more general remarks, which may not prove, after all, applicable to your special case.

But I think I will venture to send you a copy of a paper—the only one I have left. The original was written by order of the (then) Poor-Law Board, for their new workhouse infirmaries, and printed in their reports. So many hospitals then wrote to me to give them a similar sketch for their special use, and it was so utterly impossible for me to write to all, that I abridged and altered my original paper for their use. And this (I fear dirty) copy is the last I have left. Pray excuse it.

Again begging you to command me, if I can be of any use for your great purpose, to which I wish every success and ever-increasing progress, pray believe me, Sir,   Ever your faithful servant,

           FLORENCE NIGHTINGALE.

P. S. You will find in the appendix to the printed paper all the steps of our training at St. Thomas's hospital, under our admirable matron, Mrs. Wardroper; but as she may probably see this letter, I must abstain from praising her, as it were, "to her face," which all noble natures dislike.   F. N.

Fortified by the counsel and encouragement of Miss Nightingale, the appeal to the New York public previously quoted from was issued by the committee, with the gratifying response of funds as mentioned, and the committee agreed to be in readiness to open the training school on the first of May. A house was rented near the hospital as a home for nurses, circulars were issued inviting pupils to apply, and search was made for a superintendent. Time passed and no suitable person for this post was found, and the committee, with much anxiety, saw the first of May approaching. We may borrow from the managers' later account the pretty little anecdote of how this uncertainty was ended:

A member of the committee, in a despondent mood, at this time expressed her anxiety to another, who replied. "I have such faith in this work, and I have prayed so for it, that I shall have that superintendent's bed made, being sure that she will come to occupy it." A few days later the former lady was at her breakfast table when a woman in the garb of a Sister was announced. Her English accent betrayed her nationality as she explained that she had heard we were establishing a training school for nurses in New York, and, as she had had considerable experience in such work, she had come to offer her services. [1]

This was Miss Bowden, known as Sister Helen, of All Saints Sisterhood, of London and Baltimore (for a branch of the community had been established in the latter city, and Sister Helen had been in residence there when the circulars and inquiry for a superintendent had been published), who had been trained in University College hospital, London, where she was distinguished as a fine medical nurse, an excellent teacher, and effective administrator. Having some time at her disposal before returning to England, she had come to New York to propose undertaking the new work. Sister Helen was engaged without delay, and the school opened according to promise on the first of May, in five wards. It is easy to imagine what the difficulties must have been, but since matters turned out well they have been forgotten. The managers' history says:

At the expiration of the first year the house medical staff, who had been friendly from the beginning, ventured to point out to their superiors the improved

[1] *History of the Establishment of the Bellevue Training School for Nurses, cit.*, pp. 5–6.

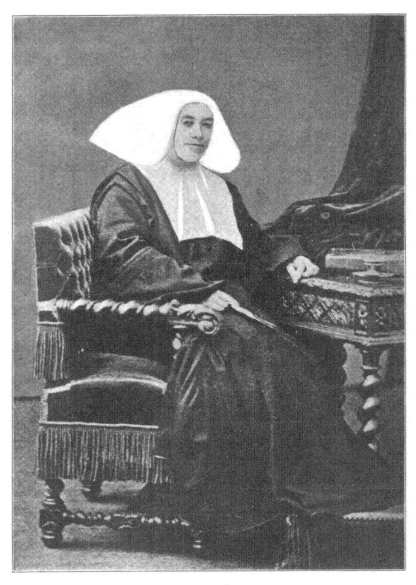

S Helen

Sister Helen of All Saints' First Superintendent of the New York Training School
for Nurses Connected with Bellevue Hospital

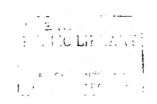

condition of the nursing service under the training
school, and gradually the eyes of these gentlemen
were opened to the fact that their patients recovered
sooner, and the deaths after operations were less frequent, than formerly. The superintendent, Sister
Helen, accustomed to the management of a pauper
hospital in England, and to deal with workhouse authorities, was not daunted by the politics of Bellevue,
so, gradually, during the second year the work assumed permanent shape and was extended to other
wards. The applications from would-be pupils increased; the first pupils became head nurses, and at
the close of the second year the first class
graduated.

During 1874 four more wards were given over to
the school, making nine in charge of the nurses.
The indebtedness of Bellevue, and through it of
the nursing profession generally in the United
States, to Sister Helen can hardly be too warmly
acknowledged, and it can only, indeed, be properly
estimated by looking back upon it from the present time. A strong and dominant character, of
marked executive ability and thorough mistress of
her domain, she laid the firm foundations upon
which the Bellevue school has stood unshaken all
these years. Her first and unvarying position was
to exact respect and consideration for the nurses
from every one in the hospital, as she demanded
deference for herself. A bulky and imposing figure in her religious garb, of heavy and prelate-like
countenance, her chief personal charm was a voice
of unusual sweetness and refinement of enuncia-

tion. A strict disciplinarian, she loved to rule,
but she ruled wisely.   She was not lavish of praise,
even to those she most valued, yet after searching
criticism or severe admonition she knew how to
administer the sweet with the bitter by commenda-
tion, and no faithful efforts escaped her notice.
Of strong and very positive opinions, she was not
without egoism and sometimes failed in tactful
conciliation. A religious woman, and a thoroughly good woman, she was not easily understood, and few reached her innermost confidence,
but those who did so gave her steadfast affection
and loyalty.   She in turn was loyal to her nurses,
protected them, and inspired them with a full
sense of the gravity of their responsibilities. A
certain jealousy is the natural complement of
forceful natures, and this was not absent with
Sister Helen, though it was for her work more
than for herself, unless one might say that her
work was herself.

Fortunately for the school the warden at that
time became a firm friend of Sister Helen and
the nurses and it was his wont to send them
warnings when skirmishes with the enemy
(in the shape of unfriendly politicians) were
likely to be expected.   These worthies, who
had once accepted so indifferently the bad conditions of Bellevue, were now keen to inspect the
nurses' wards and alert to find causes for criticism.   One of the first class of nurses has told of
the rounds they used to make in the bath-rooms

and corners, even wiping the walls with their hands to see if any dust could be found.

Bellevue also owed a debt to the school of the New England hospital, for this pioneer institution sent it two head nurses, Mrs. Wolhaupter and Miss Woods and a night superintendent, Miss Richards, from its first class of graduates. Miss Richards, whose reminiscences cover the whole early field of nursing, came to Bellevue from her *alma mater* on the first of October, when the school was only five months old. After a day or two in the wards she was put in charge at night, with the following instructions from Sister Helen: "You are to see each head nurse before she leaves for the night, and take her orders; you are to send all calls to the physicians, give all medicines, take personal care of all seriously ill patients, instruct the nurses in their duties every hour, and report to each head nurse before going off duty in the morning." The school then had five wards and about one hundred patients. Reports and orders were all verbal and it was through Miss Richards's notes of a case, written to help one of the day nurses in the note-taking required of the pupils by Sister Helen, that the system of written day and night reports and orders came about; for one of the physicians, finding the written record of the night for one patient, was so pleased with it that no time was lost in establishing the rule of written reports throughout.

The managers of the school had from the

outset accepted Miss Nightingale's principles as to the internal organisation and discipline necessary. They say on this point:

The principle which Miss Nightingale insisted upon as fundamental and which excited the greatest opposition among hospital authorities was that all nurses should in matters of discipline be under a woman, who should be responsible to the hospital authorities for the behaviour of her subordinates, and for the faithful performance of their duties; that all complaints should go to her to be investigated, and be by her referred to the supreme authority, whether warden or medical superintendent. This was such an innovation in hospital rule that it created great opposition at first in this country as well as in Europe; but, following the advice of Miss Nightingale, the committee stood firm, carried their point, and as time passed and the school extended, until it controlled all the nursing in the hospital, the rule was accepted without a question, and as other schools were founded the superintendents carried these rules with them, until now no other system is in use in any hospitals in England, nor in civil hospitals in this country.

In other details of form, however, the committee did not aim to follow closely the English model, but developed on their own lines in accordance with the differences in our social structure. Most important of these modifications was the definite and intentional exclusion of the domestic servant class and the determination to offer the training only to those women who had had better educational advantages. This decision, which is set

forth in the above-quoted report of the committee
of which Mrs. Hobson was chairman, is one of the
things for which we have to feel most grateful, for
it has prevented the caste lines which have proved
such practical hindrances and obstacles to progress
in some of the Old-World institutions, set the gene-
eral standard (with some few exceptions) for the
whole country, and supplied our hospitals with a
set of women of fairly similar aims and ideals, who
are enabled to act together with unanimity and
good feeling not otherwise possible.   It is not too
much to say that the comparative homogeneity
of the nursing profession thus attained has facilita-
tated an educational advance which has been of
distinct service to the whole cause of primary education and technical training.   This wise and far-
sighted idea, contemplating not only the reform of
the hospital, but also the opening of new avenues
of self-support to educated women, originated
with Mrs. Hobson, whose whole work on the committee was of an eminently constructive character.
Another variation from the English model was the
shorter course.   As at St. Thomas's, here too the
training was regarded as complete in one year;
that is, instruction was not continued after that
period, but the nurse was only bound by contract
for one year's service after the training year, making practically a two-years' course before she
received her certificate and left the school. A further difference was in the complete exodus of
pupils at the end of their course of training, for our

hospitals did not offer paid positions to head nurses and seniors, but relied almost entirely on the service given in exchange for training; finally, a marked difference from all Continental schools, and from those English ones that had followed St. Thomas's, was in the entire and recognised independence, after training, of the nurse, who then ceased to be under the guardianship of her school except in so far as she might depend upon it for calls to private cases. For this service she paid the school a registry fee, but lived where she pleased and received her earnings herself, in contradistinction to the English nurse, who joined a private staff and received a home and salary, while her earnings went to the school or association or hospital. While each of the American variations had some advantages and some drawbacks, we shall not now enter into them, but leave their consideration for another time.[1]

The discipline and semi-military atmosphere which came so naturally in countries accustomed to nursing orders developed slowly in the early American schools. The idea of a uniform was not liked by the women who first responded to the call to take up hospital nursing, and it was not at once adopted. The members of the committee understood very well the moral effect of uniform, for

[1] From the first the managers had hoped to train nurses for the service of the poor in their homes, and in March, 1876, the first district nurse from Bellevue, supported by one of the managers, joined the Woman's Branch of the City Mission for this service.

they had said in the report already quoted: "A uniform, however simple, is indispensable, and should be rigidly enforced. It is advantageous on the ground of economy as well as neatness, and its effect on a corps of nurses is the same as on a company of soldiers." But the practical difficulty was, how to introduce this idea into the minds of the probationers; for, when all was so experimental and when everything depended on inducing the right class of women to come forward, it was inadvisable to insist upon a uniform in the face of their prejudices against it. In the first class of nurses was a daughter of an old and prominent New York family, on intimate terms with the different members of the committee and comprehending the situation from their point of view. She was also, by good fortune, very beautiful, tall, and dignified. She talked the matter over with some of the committee, and probably also with Sister Helen, and it was arranged that she should have a couple of days' leave of absence. On her return she made her appearance in the wards dressed in the greyish-blue stripe and with apron and cap of white. So charming was she to behold, and so dowdy and insignificant did all the nondescript print dresses look beside her, that prejudice vanished and as rapidly as possible the uniform was adopted, and never again questioned. It would perhaps be too much to claim that it was, in those days, always absolutely uniform, for we seem to gather the hint of an overskirt in the very

charming figure of a nurse sketched from life in
the next decade, and used to illustrate an article
dealing with the new occupation for women. The
dress for winter and summer varied at first, for the
fourth annual report, January, 1877, says on this
point: " The pupils are required to wear the dress
of the institution, *viz.*, a grey stuff dress in winter
and calico in summer, simply made, a white apron
and cap, and brown linen cuffs covering the sleeves
from the wrist to the elbow." The grey stuff dress
for winter was abolished in 1880.

The regeneration of the old hospital was not yet
complete. There remained one department—the
most important of all—where the worst possible
conditions prevailed. This was the maternity
division. As had earlier been the case in King's
College hospital in London, and still earlier in the
Hôtel-Dieu of Paris, the practical management of
this service had not been brought up to the point
of corresponding with the teachings of medical
science. The commonest stupidity of our civilisation is the failure to bring well-known scientific principles into daily practice as hygienic and
sanitary measures, and this discrepancy between
what is taught and what is done existed in
the maternity department of Bellevue. It
had long been known to medical science that
proximity to surgical wards was, for parturient
patients, a most dangerous situation. An extensive literature existed on this subject, of which
Miss Nightingale's work, previously referred to,

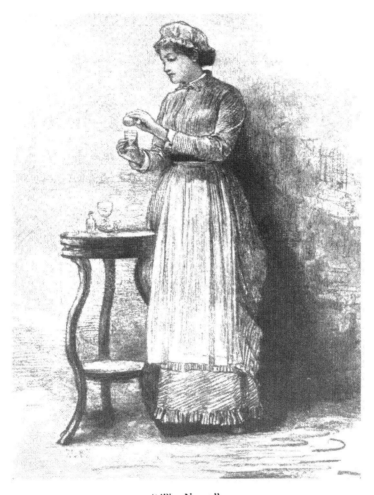

" The Nurse "
Isabel A. Hampton, Bellevue, 1882
Sketched from life for the *Century Magazine*, Nov., 1882, in "A New Profession for
Women "

was one of the most definite and practical. Numerous scientific medical works were extant that pointed out the dangers of surgical poison for the lying-in woman; in fact, the references on this point had previously been enriched by the writings of a distinguished Bellevue physician, who had explicitly stated, in opening his subject, that surgical poison was almost surely fatal to the parturient woman.

Yet, in spite of the teachings and warnings of scientific men, the maternity wards of Bellevue were situated directly above the surgical wards, and communicated freely with the latter by public stairways and corridors. No attempt at all was made to isolate them; on the contrary this service was attached both to the medical and surgical services, so that the same set of house-physicians or surgeons—who were young men just out of the medical school and taking their hospital training—went freely back and forth from one to the other. The study of bacteriology was still elementary, and the rounds from the operating table, the dissection room, the bedsides of patients fresh from the hovels of the city, and the obstetrical wards were carried on without an attempt to separate one from the other. So easy is it for those who are directly absorbed in the scientific and abstract to forget the practical application and care of details.

The managers of the school had the practical results brought to them in a painful way one winter, for puerperal fever spread from Bellevue into the city and entered the homes of some of their own friends. It became epidemic in the wards, and the third annual report of the State Charities Aid Association, March, 1875, states that during the epidemic two out of every five women died.

The managers, naturally enough, were uninformed on the scientific side and did not at first possess a knowledge of the relation between puerperal sepsis and surgical wards. Sister Helen, who needed all her discretion, never told all she knew, but drew the attention of the managers to the forlorn condition of the maternity wards, which were comfortless, unsupervised, and quite lacking in good moral atmosphere, and further mentioned that she heard of many deaths there.

The managers, eager to help the unfortunate patients, and acting on Sister Helen's suggestion, that with a few more nurses added to the staff they might be enabled to care for the maternity ward, went confidently to some of the medical authorities to offer to undertake this extension of the service, when, to their amazement and chagrin, they encountered an outburst of irritated opposition. Their offer appeared to have been looked upon as a criticism, for, incredible as it seems, they were told in plain words that *their meddling in the hospital management had gone far enough, and, as no more of it would be tolerated, it would have to cease.*[1]

Astonished and indignant they returned home,

[1] From private sources.

but not to give up.   By the efforts and through the mediation of Dr. Wood, the matter was carried further, and a time and place appointed for its consideration by a higher body.

At this meeting the ladies did not appear in person, but were represented by their husbands.

It was agreed that the nurses should be placed in the maternity, and in May, 1875, the change was made, the first attempt at negotiations having been made earlier in the year.   The training school report of that year says: "We applied in February to the Medical Board for three lying-in wards at Bellevue.   In May our offer was accepted, and the nurses entered upon the new field of service."

But still the patients continued to die, and in deep discouragement and perplexity one of the managers sat one day in the library of a medical friend, and expressed the disappointment and distress which she felt at having apparently given no better service than the untrained helpers.   They felt, she said, as if they were working in the dark. The medical friend was at that moment hurriedly called away, but as he departed he placed an open book in her hand, saying, "Perhaps this will help you."   It was the treatise before referred to, written by a prominent scientist, whose services had been given to the city poor, and to her amazement she read the opening words enunciating the doctrine of the fatal relationship between surgical and maternity wards.

This was the light that she had felt the need of,

and armed with this declaration, of an indisputable eminence, the courageous woman returned single-handed to the charge, confronted the authorities, and speedily set in motion the forces by which the maternity wards were removed from the precincts of the hospital.[1]   The third annual report of the State Charities Aid Association says on this point: "It was through the representations of our Visiting Committee that these wards were finally closed, and the remaining twenty-five women, already showing symptoms of disease, were removed to the one-story pavilion on Blackwell's Island, and recovered."   Of this transfer of patients Dr. Carlisle says (after discussing the epidemic of sepsis, and remarking that the medical staff, though holding that improvements were needed, did not believe that the wards were at fault), "Nevertheless the opinion of those least capable of judging prevailed, and the lying-in service was taken from Bellevue."[2]

Miss Linda Richards, who was then at Bellevue, writes of those events: "The managers had been very anxious for some time to take the maternity wards, but the doctors said they preferred their old nurses to those in training, and so they had been refused. . . .   After the nurses were finally placed in charge they had the wards for twenty-seven days before they were moved. . . .   The patients were then transferred to rough buildings,

[1] From private sources.
[2] *Op. cit.*, p. 77.

and, strange to say, there was no more fever and only two deaths, though some very sick patients had been transferred."

Still some little time elapsed before the women completed the regeneration of the maternity service. The Island quarters were very satisfactory for those patients who could get there, but there was no provision for emergencies, save a dreary room at the ferryboat landing, where what was possible had been done for emergency patients to ease the trial by having a nurse in attendance. This was a voluntary service on the nurse's part. Finally, the managers, having vainly tried to interest a wealthy private benevolent society devoted to obstetrical relief, but whose funds could be employed only for respectable married women, went to the Grand Jury, and secured the use of the old, dismantled engine-house which has since that day been familiar to all the generations of Bellevue nurses as "The Emergency." The nurses took charge of it on June 13, 1877, and Dr. Wylie, who had been, as usual, a strong friend, was soon able to report that its results surpassed those of any maternity hospital in the country.

The rescue of Bellevue was now effected in all departments, and only needed to be perfected in detail. A recent publication issued by the managers contains the following:

As the work became consolidated in the hospital, its influence began to make itself felt on every side.

The doctors soon discovered that operations never before attempted were possible, in consequence of the care their patients received, and important hygienic improvements were devised and carried out through the united influence of the ladies' committee and the Medical Board upon the Commissioners of Charities.

In 1879 the Sturges Pavilion, in memory of the late Jonathan Sturges, was built for extreme surgical cases by his daughter, Mrs. W. H. Osborn. In 1882 the Marquand Pavilion for women and children was built. In 1883 the Townsend Pavilion was erected for the special treatment of women, and in 1888 a pavilion was built by Miss Dehon also for the treatment of women. In 1891 Miss Lazarus built a pavilion for the special accommodation of graduated nurses who were ill and required hospital treatment, and a fund for its support was given by Mrs. Morris K. Jesup in memory of her sister, Mrs. Theodore Cuyler, who was for many years secretary of the school. Two beautiful chapels were erected for the Protestant and Catholic patients by Mrs. Townsend and Miss Leary. It would be impossible to give in detail an account of the stream of benevolence which through the influence of the training school has been flowing into the hospital during the past twenty-five years, and which has made the institution a benediction to the poor of New York. Not only the hospital, but the whole vicinity has changed its character. The members of the committee were assured that it was not safe for ladies to venture into that part of the city, but they did so fearlessly and were never annoyed; and as time passed the grog-shops diminished, the disreputable buildings disappeared, and now the neighbourhood of the hospital is filled with fine buildings, accommodating the

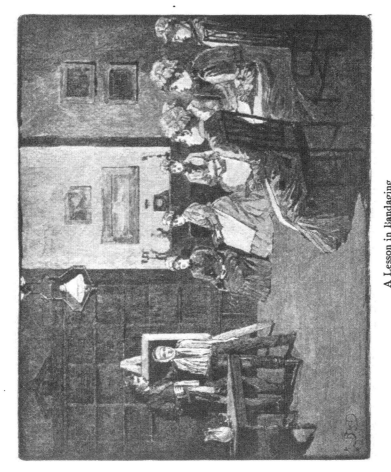

A Lesson in Bandaging

The parlor in the Bellevue Hospital Nurses' Home, in 1882

From "A New Profession for Women." By permission of the *Century Magazine*, New

schools and other institutions which form branches of the hospital."[1]

The general and liberal intelligence displayed by the group of men and women who conducted the reforms at Bellevue is further attested by other records of the State Charities Aid Association. One refers to the maternity ward question. "Our Hospital Committee [says the Third Annual Report], at the request of one of the Commissioners of Charities, has recently been engaged in the preparation of a plan for new maternity wards. But the proposed site is so manifestly unfit that we would here publicly record our protest against it." The site proposed by the hospital, and objected to by the committee, was specified as being too close to the hospital, and just north of the morgue and the dissection rooms. It was ultimately abandoned. The other refers to the hospital as a whole. In 1874 the State Charities Aid Association presented a report recommending the rebuilding of Bellevue on the grounds of its defective ventilation, bad construction, and the existence of pyæmia. The report contained exhaustive statistics and was accompanied by a strong letter from Miss Louisa Schuyler. With good nursing and cleanliness pyæmia soon disappeared, but the structural disadvantages of the hospital have been acknowledged by all subsequent critics, and the building is now (1907) on the eve of being replaced by new structures.

[1] *History of the Establishment, cit.*

In the summer of 1876 the school lost the services of Sister Helen, who, with impaired health and other obligations before her, returned to England. She had placed the school on a firm basis, made it indispensable to the hospital, and had begun to send out trained women to extend the new system and teaching. Her pupils were ready and able to teach nursing, but none of them, probably, would have been able to cope with the undercurrents of opposition and enmity that still sought every opportunity of undermining the authority of the superintendent of nurses, as Sister Helen, from her great experience, was able to do. Only those who have met corrupt political influence in hospitals know what this enmity is. Her successor, Miss Eliza Perkins, though not a nurse, and of a character unlike Sister Helen's, nevertheless possessed the skill and ability needed for the position, and she was selected as the head of the school. Sister Helen grounded her thoroughly in all the principles of discipline, order of seniority, division of authority and responsibility, and general nursing ethics, as well as the etiquette involved in the successful administration of a hospital training course; and admirably did Miss Perkins apply them during her fifteen years of rule.

Sister Helen sailed for England leaving behind her the following letter of farewell for the nurses for whom she had done so much and by whom she was so greatly esteemed:

THE TRAINING SCHOOL,

314 East 26th St., May 1st, 1876.

TO THE MEMBERS OF THE TRAINING SCHOOL.

Dear Friends and Fellow-Workers:—I had quite intended to have a little talk with you this evening and wish you all good-bye, but I am stupidly weak and may not be able to bear it.   So I will write you a loving farewell instead.

May God bless you all, and prosper you in your work, and give you the grace of perseverance.   So far you have done nobly.   To-day completes our first three years.   I look back on the past with great thankfulness for what has been achieved.   Three years ago we commenced what was by many thought to be a doubtful undertaking.   Now the training school is a flourishing institution, standing well with the public and valued by those best able to judge,—the medical staff at Bellevue and the employers of our private nurses. I endeavoured to establish the work on a right foundation.   The ladies of the committe have done all in their power to advance it.   But all this would have been of no avail but for the earnest, self-sacrificing work of the nurses.   May the spirit long live.

Now I feel I have only to thank those most who have been with us longest.   A few more words and I am done.   I thank you lovingly for the affectionate sympathy you have shown me during my illness, the way you have done your duty with little trouble to Miss Van Rensselaer and have let me alone.   Once more good-bye and God bless you.

I hope when you read this you will not say, "Sister speaks as if we were never to see her again." Only remember parting is certain, meeting always doubt ful, especially when one is in ill-health and about to cross the Atlantic.

SISTER HELEN OF ALL SAINTS.[1]

The Massachusetts General Hospital of Boston was the next of the trio of general hospitals to open a school for nurses. The "History of the Boston Training School" published as a part of the annual report in 1904, says:

It is to the Woman's Educational Association we owe the suggestion of a need in Boston of a training school for nurses. The matter came up for discussion at a meeting held in April, 1873, and the first practical steps were taken toward the founding of a system now so well recognised not only as a means of education for women, but as a necessity to meet the demands of the community.

The Second Annual Report of the Woman's Educational Association gives more fully the very first steps:

A meeting was called as early as June, 1872, to consider the subject, and it was made a special object of discussion in two or three meetings during the next autumn. In the winter of 1873 a member of the committee heard of the excellent school for nurses which had been established in New York. She made a visit there, and satisfied herself that the plan was a wise one and would succeed. The report induced the committee to believe that they had really found what they

---

[1] Sister Helen later gave distinguished service in the colonial wars of England. After one such campaign she returned to her home and died in the closing years of the century.

had been so long seeking. They called a parlour meeting in order to consider the subject more fully and to interest persons outside of the association in the plan. This meeting brought out the expression of so much interest and so much sympathy with the movement that, though the difficulties of the undertaking were seen to be great, the committee reported in favour of it at the regular meeting of April 10, and recommended that it should be committed to the charge of twelve ladies and gentlemen, who should organise it and carry it on independently of this association. In consequence of this action a circular was sent out summoning a meeting of all those who were interested either for or against the training of nurses.

The meeting was held in May, 1873, and was large and representative. There were those who, without knowing how such a revolution was to be brought about, were eager for the day when this new order of being, a trained nurse, was to be had for the asking and pay; for it must be remembered that it was not only the quality, but the quantity, that was lacking, and, literally speaking, the whole of a long day sometimes had to be spent in looking for a reliable nurse. There were not many physicians present: a few came to watch proceedings, some to speak—not unfriendly words, though rather anxious ones. Dr. Susan Dimock gave encouragement with most delightful voice and manner. The upshot of it all was that a committee was formed, and then the work began . . . first to decide upon a plan, to ask for the co-operation of physicians, and to raise money. . . . A letter was sent to the trustees of the Massachusetts General hospital asking their permission to establish the training school in connection with that hospital. The answer seeming favourable to the plan, a conference was arranged.[1]

The trustees responded with, on the whole, gratifying readiness, though they held off a little warily from the possibility of interference with their authority. They proposed placing two wards in the care of the training school committee, but under the following conditions: that the relation between hospital and school should continue during the pleasure of the trustees; that the school should take on as pupils such nurses then employed in the wards as the trustees wished to retain; that the nurses and pupils of the school should not attend the patients of the hospital without previous instruction in moving and caring for bed-patients; that nurses should agree to remain for at least two years, but that the trustees reserved the right to discharge them from service in the wards for sufficient cause; that the superintendent, nurses, pupils, and all persons employed by the school should be under the medical jurisdiction of the physicians and surgeons (and, of course, subject to the rules of the trustees), and that "no instruction of or interference with said persons within the hospital shall be permitted without consent of such physicians and surgeons"; that wages should be paid by the hospital and not by the school, and that the duties of the superintendent should not conflict with those of the matron.

[1] " Early History of the Boston Training School," by Mrs. Curtis and Miss Denny, members of the original board. The *Amer. Journ. of Nursing*, February, 1902, p. 332.

The training school committee, finding these regulations leaned a little too far in favour of the trustees, offered to accept the responsibility for the wards and the nursing provided the trustees were willing to modify some of their conditions—among others, that the school also have the right to terminate the connection with the hospital, not less than two months' notice being required in either case; that the director of the school also should have the right to discharge any nurse or pupil, and that the word "interference" should not be held to apply to the rules and discipline which (subject to the regulations of the hospital) the directors might judge necessary for the good government of the school, nor any visits of directors made to inform themselves of the condition of the school.

These modifications were evidently agreed to by the trustees, for the training school committee now set to work in earnest, raised the money, rented a house for the nurses, and undertook to be ready by the 1st of November to take charge of the wards. Short as was the time allowed, the committee met its obligations to the day, and with a superintendent, two head nurses, and four pupils, took charge of its two wards on the 1st of November.

The hospital, in its interior, and its former nursing service, was very different from Bellevue. The Massachusetts General stood with such institutions as the New York and Pennsylvania hospitals, and all of its arrangements were equal to the best known at that time. It was clean, bright, pleasant, and the comfort of the patients was considered in every way. It was already historically important as the scene of the first major operation performed under the influence of ether, for it was there that Morton had demonstrated, on October 16, 1846, the discovery of anæsthesia, having previously experimented upon himself. The Massachusetts General was noted for the dignity and refinement of its operation-room work, and for white linen coverings of especial purity and fineness. The women who had worked there as nurses were of a highly estimable type, good, conscientious, and faithful. An account of the early days in the hospital by one of its matrons makes this fact very clear, even if there were not other testimony.[1]

The conditions were not very comfortable for the nurses. Miss Sturtevant had entered the hospital as assistant nurse at seven and a half dollars a week in 1862. The nurses slept in little rooms between the wards, two in one bed, which was folded out of the way by day, for the room then became a passage, or consulting-room, or even a place for dressings and minor operations. The hours on duty were from five in the morning to half-past nine in the evening, with an occasional

[1] " Personal Recollections of Hospital Life before the Days of Training Schools," by G. L. Sturtevant. *The Trained Nurse*, December, 1895, pp. 287–291.

hour off.   The nurses had a dark and dingy dining-room, with pewter tumblers and other fittings to match.   There was no lucrative private duty to look to, as nursing was considered to be an occupation only suitable for elderly females.   Nevertheless, many excellent women served conscientiously in the hospital for years at a time.   There were eleven head nurses and about sixteen assistants, besides "night watchers."   The way the work was arranged was very crude and was, indeed, inherited from earlier centuries.   For instance, all soiled linen was first washed by the nurses in the ward bath-rooms before being sent to the laundry. Miss Richards has described the curious rotation of service—how each nurse had a round of duty from ward-work and the care of patients to a turn at the washtubs, and how tenaciously this custom was clung to.   Nothing, however, could better illustrate the different character of the old nursing system and the new than the story which is related by this same veteran pioneer:

In one of the large hospitals where I was organising a training school n those early days, before I had really taken hold of the work, but was finding my bearings before making changes, I was making rounds one morning when, upon entering a ward, I saw at a glance that a man in a bed near the door was dying. The nurse stood near, in full view of the man's face, quietly doing her morning dusting, and doing it well.

I stepped to the bedside, examined the patient's pulse, wiped the dampness from his face, and then, going back to the nurse, who was still dusting, I inquired, "How long has this man been in this condition?" She looked up with a very blank expression on her face and asked, "What condition?" I said, "Do you not know that the man is dying?" She answered with surprise, "Why, no." I instructed her to send for the doctor at once, place screens around the bed, and to stay with the patient as long as he lived, and passed on. Later in the day, when I made rounds again, the nurse came to me and said, "Miss Richards, would you mind telling me how you knew that man was dying?" I asked her how long she had been in that ward, and she replied two years. Then I said to her: "You have been in this ward all that time, with patients coming and going and with some dying: will you tell me how you can have been here so long and not know when a man is dying? I will tell you how I know: by caring for my patients, by carefully watching them and observing the changes from day to day and from hour to hour, by being interested in each one as a human being entrusted to my care." This will give some idea of the quality of the nursing before training schools were organised.[1]

The first superintendent of nurses was Mrs. Billings, who had had experience as a hospital nurse during the Civil War. Sister Helen of Bellevue was appealed to to give Mrs. Billings some insight into training school management, and with some reluctance, based on the shortness of the time allowed her, consented to give her two months'

[1] "Thirty Years of Progress," by Linda Richards. *American Journal of Nursing*, January, 1904, pp. 263–267.

experience.   Mrs. Billings, however, only held her position a few months, and was succeeded by Mrs. Mary von Olnhausen, a woman of highly original and picturesque characteristics, who had served as a sort of free lance through our own civil and the Franco-Prussian wars, and who has left an entertaining account of her dramatic career.[1]

Though Mrs. von Olnhausen proved to be too impuls've and individualistic to be a successful head, not having had the kind of training necessary for the enforcement of discipline, the training school committee did not lose courage, although the success of their experiment hung for a time wavering in the balance.

The medical staff from the beginning had not wanted the school.   They preferred their old-fashioned nursing system and the old untrained nurses, and when the wards under the new arrangement did not run smoothly the school was considered to be the whole cause of trouble.   Finally the trustees told the training school committee that if they could place a graduate nurse in charge the school would be given another year's trial, but if, at the end of that time, it had not yet been proved to be of real value to the hospital, it would be given up.   At th's critical juncture Miss Linda Richards was put in charge, and from her advent date the real progress and success of the

[1] *Adventures of an Army Nurse*, by Mary von Olnhausen, edited by James Phinney Munroe. Little, Brown & Co., Boston, 1903.

new system.   Her own recollections of that time
are full of interest.   She says:

On the one hand the committee, a body of brave men
and women, fought for the school, and on the other
the physicians, with two exceptions, were against it.
Between the two stood the trustees.   I fully realised
that, if I failed to prove that educated and trained
nurses were superior to uneducated, untrained ones a
death-blow would be given to the school in that hospital and serious injury would be sustained by the
movement generally.

In order to make a record for the cause Miss
Richards took charge of all special night duty and
gave her personal attention to all serious cases, in
addition to carrying out her general duties of supervision and teaching as superintendent.   She
writes:

I was blessed with an extraordinary amount of
strength, could endure hardship well, and possessed
a hopeful disposition, so I was able to do plenty of
work of a sufficiently good quality to prove the supe-
riority of the new over the old.   My first happy day
there was at the end of three months, when the superintendent of the hospital told me that the trustees
had voted to give the school another ward, and added:
"The school is safe.   Before another year comes round
you will have the nursing of the entire hospital in
charge."   It so proved, and gradually the medical
staff came to feel that trained nurses were valuable;
one by one they became firm friends of the school, and
at the end of my first year the trustees adopted the

school as a part of the hospital, with a committee of its own. We had a small but comfortable home, and felt that we stood upon firm ground.

Miss Richards stayed there two and a half years, and then went to England to study training school methods there. She continues:

For the last year and a half the wheels ran very smoothly indeed. I have never worked with a more loyal, helpful committee, and but for their help and support those first months would have been very hard to live through. They were not happy at their best. I seldom look back upon them. I seemed to meet hostility on all sides. We were living down a strong prejudice. We suffered, but we conquered, and I am glad that I fought that fight."

From here, having placed the school on a firm foundation, Miss Richards went to St. Thomas's hospital, England, where she was permitted to spend eight weeks in visiting wards, assisting with work or not, as she chose, and witnessing operations. Her experiences there were very interesting. She met many of the women who were notable in nursing work, and tells the following little anecdote of Miss Nightingale:

I had been in the "home" less than a week when an invitation came from Miss Nightingale for me to visit her in her London home. Shall I ever forget the excitement that invitation caused? Miss Crossland told me Miss Nightingale would ask my opinion of the different nurses, both ladies and others, and I could see that there was a little anxiety felt concerning the answers I might give. I went on the appointed day and must say I did not feel quite at my ease as the maid took me to Miss Nightingale's room, but one look into those kind, clear-blue eyes and the hearty grasp of the little hand quite set me at ease, and before I knew it I was talking as freely to her, who had done more than any woman living to alleviate suffering, as I would have to a life-long friend. Miss Nightingale was lying upon the bed (I have never seen her in any other position, though I afterwards had the very great pleasure and honour of visiting her a few days in her beautiful country home). She was dressed in black and on her head she wore a very becoming cap. . . . Miss Nightingale said, "I am very glad to see you and talk of the training school work in America." She asked me much in detail, and carefully wrote all down. When I returned to the hospital the questions were numerous: "What did Miss Nightingale say?" "What did she want to know?" But had she asked me for criticism, which she did not, I could have found none, and as I look back to-day I can think of none. . .

I went from Edinburgh for a few days with Miss Nightingale and received from her words of encouragement which have lasted all these years. In one of her letters to me just as I was leaving England she bade me and our profession Godspeed, saying, "Outstrip us, that we in turn may outstrip you again."[1]

Miss Linda Richards has had a rarely extensive and useful career as a nurse. On her return from England in 1878 she organised the training school of the Boston City hospital. In 1885 she was sent by the American Board of Missions to Tokio, Ja-

[1] "Recollections of a Pioneer Nurse," by Linda Richards. *American Journal of Nursing*, January, 1903, pp. 248, 252.

pan, where she organised a school to train Japanese nurses.   On her return she organised the school of the Methodist hospital, Philadelphia, and in 1893 was called to her *alma mater* as superintendent.   Miss Richards has been continually called from one hospital to another, either to organise a new school, or to build up one that was undeveloped.   In this way she has given service at the Homeopathic hospital of Brooklyn, the Hartford hospital, the University hospital, Philadelphia, and then began a series of regenerative services in hospitals for the insane, beginning with that at Taunton, Massachusetts.   Her success in creating a new ideal and developing improved systems of nursing in these hospitals has been so distinguished that here too she has been called from one post to another to organise and teach.

The Connecticut Training School, opened in New Haven, was the last of the distinguished trio, though it had obtained its charter before the Bellevue school had one.   A notable feature in the inception of this school is the prominent part taken by men in bringing about the new style of nursing, though in New Haven, too, as well as in other places, the activity of the women during the Civil War had permeated all society with new standards. The management of the hospitals throughout Connecticut was largely in the hands of the General Hospital Society of Connecticut, a dignified and weighty body that, in 1876, celebrated its semi-centennial.   This society first considered the subject of training. Its own records are very brief,[1] but we shall quote Mrs. Francis Bacon's history of the foundation of the Connecticut Training School,[2] omitting only her preamble.

The great need for nurses seems to have impressed the gentlemen of the Hospital Society as early as 1872, a year before we had thought of the matter, and at their annual meeting, May the 9th of that year, they discussed the subject and appointed a committee, "consisting of Drs. White, Jewett, and Daggett, to inquire and report on the practicability of making the hospital available as a training school for nurses."

Before the committee had time to report to the Hospital Society in the spring of 1873, Mr. Charles Thompson, of this city, who in his own family had suffered from the ignorance of the old-fashioned nurse, and who was familiar with the European system of training schools, called upon Dr. Francis Bacon, accompanied by his and our friend Dr. William L. Bradley, for the purpose of consulting him as to the desirableness of attempting to establish a school for nurses in New Haven.

So that from two different directions simultaneously a movement was being made which resulted in the founding of this school.

Mr. Thompson's interest was gratefully appreciated, and the result of his conversation with Drs. Bradley and Bacon was that he was asked to draw up a plan

[1] See *The Semi-Centennial History of the General Hospital Society of Connecticut*, by P. A. Jewett, M.D. New Haven, 1876.

[2] Read at the graduating exercises, 1895. Reprinted in *The Trained Nurse*, October, 1895, pp. 187–193.

embodying his ideas as to the training of nurses, and this plan was submitted to the committee above mentioned; and following this, at the next meeting of the General Hospital Society, this paper was read, which Dr. Bishop has kindly copied from the proceedings of the society, April 17, 1873:

"The committee to whom was referred the subject of a training school for nurses would respectfully report:

"1st. That in their opinion it is not expedient for the Hospital Society to undertake the direct organisation and management of a training school for nurses.

"2nd. They are highly gratified to learn that arrangements are in progress for the organisation of a training school for nurses by a society devoted to that special object.   They, therefore, recommend the adoption of the following resolutions:

"*Resolved*, That this society feels deeply impressed with the importance of encouraging in every suitable manner the special education and training of nurses for service in hospitals and in private families, and for attendance upon the sick poor; therefore,

"*Resolved*, That if a society is organised for the training of nurses, the directors of the General Hospital Society of Connecticut are hereby authorised and advised, under suitable regulations, to afford to said society such facilities for the instruction of nurses as can be given at the hospital, consistent with the proper management of and general interests of the hospital.

"(Signed),

"M. C. WHITE, D. L. DAGGETT, P. A. JEWETT, } *Committee.*"

It was a very fortunate coincidence that just at the moment when the Hospital Society, after a year's consideration, had decided against organising or managing a training school, we, without collusion, should have offered to do this work for the institution.

This report of the hospital committee to the Hospital Society is the first definite and official action taken upon the subject of training nurses in New Haven. It is the little seed from which we have in twenty-one years branched out into full usefulness.

Acting upon the encouragement thus received, and inspired by Mr. Thompson, thirty or forty ladies and gentlemen associated themselves for the organisation of the Connecticut Training School. A pamphlet explaining the plan and setting forth its advantages was printed at Mr. Thompson's expense, and the cooperation of all good citizens was asked, packages of the pamphlets and circulars were mailed to every prominent physician and clergyman in the State, and many cordial endorsements were received.

. . . After a careful study of the English hospital school methods, a plan was drawn up for the organisation of this school and for its connection with the hospital, a series of resolutions were proposed for the consideration of the directors of the hospital, and, armed with all this, Dr. Bacon presented to the directors at their next meeting the proposal that the new organisation should assume the charge of the nursing at this hospital. . . .

These resolutions are the ones which, printed and framed, hung for years in the hospital office, and they give our status with regard to the hospital, define our relations with each other, and they have been extensively borrowed by other training schools.

Here we were then, fairly launched, but without a penny of money or a single pupil, and now the hard work, which for twenty-one years the school committee has carried on, commenced. The ladies at once set themselves to the work of finding pupils and securing a superintendent. Circulars in large type and bright colours were distributed at the railroad stations and mailed to rural post-offices, with the request that the postmaster would pin them up in some conspicuous place.

Ladies' missionary associations in eighteen towns were asked to make the plan known and to put up, in places where they would attract attention, the advertising circulars. Articles were written to all the leading newspapers of the State, and were extensively copied in the smaller rural journals. Nearly all the applications came from young women who had read in obscure villages the articles copied from papers in larger towns.

While all efforts were being made to interest young women and secure pupils, Mr. Thompson devoted himself to raising money, and but for his generosity we could not have begun the school. In September, 1873, he authorised us to draw upon him for $1,000, and under certain conditions for $2,500. In March, 1874, through the kindness of Dr. Moses C. White, Mrs. Gill, of West Haven, left us a tract of land which will later become valuable, and through Mr. Thompson's further efforts $10,000 to $12,000 were contributed by many generous friends as an endowment.

May 21, 1873, the full school committee held its first formal meeting for the appointment of a superintendent of nursing. Many hospitals had been visited

and inquiries' made, and at last the only training
school in existence in this country [this statement
overlooks the New England hospital for Women and
Children], the Woman's hospital of Philadelphia,
referred to above, sent us our first superintendent.
Answers began to come in from applicants for admission, and out of twenty-one, six, the number to which
the hospital limited us at first, were finally selected.
Two of these failed, through sickness, at the last moment, and on October 6, 1873, our first four pupils
arrived late in the evening, and in a dreary storm.
The new wards to the south were not free from the
workmen, but small sleeping rooms were assigned to us
on the top floor, and comfortably furnished. The
diet kitchen, in the basement, had been fitted up at
the expense of the training school, floor laid, stove
and kitchen utensils supplied, and our four nurses
and their superintendent found themselves at once
plunged into hard work. The north ward was full of
typhoid fever, ten cases, six men and four women, and
wards 1 and 2, E and W., were opened and filled during the first week. The committee's journal reads:
"Our nurses for the first five weeks did very hard work.
The fever cases were severe, some of the patients entirely delirious, throwing themselves out of bed, or
getting up and dragging their sheets and blankets out
into the entry, if the nurses had to cross from the
men's to the women's ward. The four nurses in turn
sat up night after night and did duty during the day
in the other wards, or diet kitchen, where the special
diet for thirty was cooked and distributed to all parts
of the hospital *by the nurses who cooked it.*" The journal adds: "All the men nurses, on the arrival of the
young women, at once set themselves to take their

ease and to shirk all concern with distributing the diet or returning the dishes.''

The school at last engaged and paid three women from the city to help in the stress of work. On the 1st of October, 1873, there were seventy-two patients in the hospital, but by December 31 the average for the quarter had risen to 110. Not until a year later had we permission to raise the number of pupils to eight, and it was May, 1875, before we were allowed nine in consequence of the night service.

Hard as the work has often been in later years, no class of nurses ever had such demands made upon its endurance as this pioneer class of pupils met and struggled through. All the typhoid fever cases recovered, and it was a proud moment for the school when the value of the work done was fully appreciated and acknowledged by Dr. Moses C. White, the attending physician. "I have never before," he said, "had a case of fever in the hospital without a black crust tongue," no appearance of which had he found since our nurses took hold. Through Dr. White's efforts little improvements were added, and at the request of our superintendent he secured additional closets in the north ward entries. Our nurses, who have more closets than they know what to do with, may think what such a statement as this in the committee's journal implied: "The new closets being put up, the miscellaneous packing of slices of bread, old clothes, bedding, oil lamps, rags, etc. (which had always been stowed in the *same* closet) was put an end to." I mention these little details that our nurses may more fully appreciate the comfort which has surrounded them, in contrast to the difficulties faced by the first brave four. Everything, as I have said, was in a transition state. The nurses were crowded, as their numbers increased, into the three small rooms in the top floor of the new building—four in a room—and the clothes-horse screens which divided their beds one from another were the first screens of the kind used in the hospital.

The first superintendent of nursing was asked to take her dinner at the table with fourteen men patients in the basement, and later the pupils' meals were served in their own diet kitchen, and very poor ones they were, too. . . .

The ladies' committee, too, was new to the business before it and learned by experience the needs of the school.   One of the first things to do was to abate the trailing skirts and jewelry of the newly arrived pupils, whose ideas were crude as to the proper dress for a trained nurse.   I remember one morning I was met by the head nurse with the despairing question: "What *shall* I do with Miss ———? She appeared at breakfast with all her long hair curled down her back." Caps were immediately introduced, and no one needs now to be told that bushy hair is out of place in a sick-room. All the irregularities were slowly corrected; comfort came out of confusion. The surgeons, assured of good nursing, undertook operations never before attempted in a hospital. And on March 26, six months after we began, the Hospital Society, which had ordered an inquiry made as to our work, directed the secretary, Dr. C. A. Lindsley, to inform us in writing as follows: "In regard to the work undertaken by the school in the care of the sick and disabled, we find for it many general commendations.   The physicians and surgeons report a decided improvement in the nursing, and speak strongly of the good already accomplished." By the end of the first year nearly one hundred applications for admission to the school had been made, and we had all the pupils we were allowed to receive, though a majority of the young women withdrew their names on learning that hard work was required. For it came to be slowly understood by outsiders that heart and soul and mind and strength must be put into this work if it were to be well done. There was the same lack of understanding during our Civil War, and among the enthusiasts who wished to be forwarded to the front came a young New York woman to the nursing committee one day, and stated her requirements in taking up the service for the wounded. They included a daily bath on the battle-field, and when common-sense was talked to her, and her services were declined, she left greatly disturbed, and saying that, though she could not work, she thought she might be allowed to soothe and sympathise.

By the end of our second year we were able to send out our first graduates to private families. Six of them nursed thirty-seven cases with entire satisfaction to the patients. By the fourth year we began to furnish superintendents of nursing to other hospitals, and to nurse the poor free of charge in New Haven. Fifty charity visits were made that year. By the sixth year we felt strong enough to publish our own hand-book of nursing. By the seventh the seventeen pupils had quite outgrown their quarters in the mansard story, and Mrs. Noah Porter, the president of our board, appealed at our annual meeting, January, 1881, for funds to build a dormitory. So complete was the public confidence in us that the entire amount ($12,000) needed for the building was raised at once, and Professor Eaton and Dr. Bacon, who had been appointed by the hospital directors for this service, staked out the site on the hospital grounds, and by October 26, 1882, our pleasant building was opened, Mr. R. S. Fellow and Dr. Shew, of the Middletown hospital, having selected for us the furniture from a factory in New Hampshire at a cost of about $1,000 more. We were in clear water now, and little remains to tell you except a story of continual prosperity. . . .

In concluding this sketch of the early days of our first three schools for nurses we cannot do better than quote from a pamphlet written by one of the Bellevue Hospital committee [1] which is full of practical wisdom and foresight. After a broad historical review and study of methods of institutional management it points out the anachronism of having the governing boards for mixed institutions composed entirely of men, and says:

The most thorough way to secure oneness of organisation and purpose would be to add to the hospital board a certain number of ladies, and to make the school of nursing committee one of the regular sub-committees of the board. . . . Hitherto the movement toward improving the nursing service of public hospitals has come from outside persons as a rule: it has not originated with the governing bodies. As nursing is work which peculiarly requires feminine supervision, the majority of the members of school committees hitherto have been women. . . . If hospital governors object to extraneous authority . . . .

[1] *A Century of Nursing, with Hints toward the Organisation of a Training School.* (The author was Mrs. Hobson.) 1876.

why should they not invite the school committee to become members of their board . . . . under their own control as are their other committees? . . .

In the case of a large public hospital, *i. e.*, a tax-payers' hospital, the outside committee has its advantages. If its members find themselves unreasonably obstructed, they have the remedy of the English ministry: they can "go to the country."

A great deal would depend upon the character of the hospital and its own form of government. Any plan of organisation is the best which will keep all discussion of questions of general policy and of the mutual relations that are involved aboveboard and open, and that will leave neither opportunity nor necessity for attempt on the part of any one to carry points by indirect or personal influence. . . . Better the treaties which the Paris administration makes with its Sisterhoods than any effort to diplomatise one's way into a hospital and shuffle along there without a full, clear, written agreement on the points in advance, so far as they can be foreseen, between the committee of the school and the governing bodies of the hospital. . .

As the object of the hospital is the nursing of the sick, the superintendent of the school becomes the most important female officer. She should, therefore, if possible, be the matron as well as the nursing head for the whole hospital; in which case she would require an assistant to whom she could delegate certain classes of housekeeping duties. . . .

Too frequent changes among head nurses are undesirable from a disciplinary point of view. It would be an advantage to a school to be able to retain and pay adequately a certain number of skilled trainers for head nurses of wards or groups of wards. . . .

Committees would do well to start on the plan with the idea that careful didactic and technical instruction must be a part of their plan and that they will need a school outfit: classroom, blackboard, textbook, and manikins; the cost of which should be considered an essential original outlay, and not left to any after chance.

American schools pay their pupils monthly wages, but these, if paid at all, ought to be moderate. Schools should not compete with each other on the basis of numbers or high wages, but on that of the quality of nurses they turn out, and the best pupils are sure to value instruction more if they are not paid for acquiring it. Those schools will probably prove to be the most successful where the pupils can be brought to feel that they are studying a profession, or learning a trade, under the ordinary conditions imposed on men and women who are preparing themselves for any business in life.

It is a question whether a nursing school should class itself with charities. If money appeals to the public must be made, why should they not be made on the higher ground that colleges take?

Why should there not be endowed tutorships and free scholarships for nurses in Bellevue and Baltimore? . . .

In concluding this brief sketch the writer urges all women engaged in hospitals and training schools to bear in mind that their greatest success will lie in keeping the standard of their work, as to the character and tone of the direction, and the quality of the instruction given, at its highest possible point. Schools should be practically normal schools, whose graduates should feel that wherever they go they must carry the spirit of the school with them and that training can go on in every hospital ward where a competent head nurse is found.

Doubtless there will be obstacles to encounter, but these should only nerve to steadier effort, for it is well to remember that any obstacle either thoughtlessly or maliciously thrust in the way of women of culture who undertake offices of charity in public institutions is a blow direct, not so much against them, as against the helpless and suffering classes of society of whom they are the natural guardians and consolers.

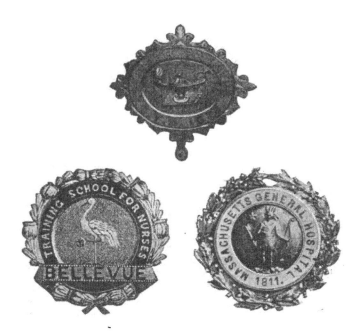

BIBLIOGRAPHY.

The grouping according to subject is to facilitate study or courses of reading. Some of the footnote references are repeated here, while others are new. No attempt has been made to give a full list of magazine articles. Many books on nursing, as well as text-books, belonging more especially to the last twenty-five years, will be listed in another volume.

GENERAL NURSING HISTORY.

* *Offentliche Krankenpflege im Mittelalter.* Dr. Victor Fossel. Reprint from *Mittheilungen des Vereines der "Ärzte in Steiermark."* Nos. 4 & 5, 1900. Graz, Austria.

The Historical Development of Modern Nursing. A. Jacobi, M.D. *Popular Science Monthly,* xxiii., 773–787.

* *A Century of Nursing.* Reports of *State Charities Aid.* New York. 1876.

Die Geschichte Christlicher Krankenpflege und Pflegerschaften. Dr. Henrich Haeser, Berlin, 1857.

* *Christian Charity in the Ancient Church.* Gerhard Uhlhorn, Stuttgart, 1882.

Handbuch der Krankenversorgung und Krankenpflege. Liebe, Jacobsohn und Meyer, Berlin, 1899. August Hirschwald. In 3 vols.

* *Considérations sur les Infirmières des Hôpitaux, Thèse présentée et publiquement soutenue à la Faculté de Médecine de Montpellier.* Dr Anna Hamilton, Imprimerie Centrale du Midi, Montpellier, 1900.

* *Les Gardes-Malades Congréganistes, Mercenaires, Professionnelles, Amateurs.* Drs. Anna Hamilton and Felix Regnault. Vigot Freres, Paris, 1901.

* *The Evolution of the Trained Nurse.* Ethel Gordon Fenwick. *The Outlook.* Jan. 6, 1900.

* *The History of Nursing in the British Empire.* By Sarah Tooley. Bousfield, London, 1906.

* *Recollections of a Nurse.* By E. D. London, Macmillan & Co., 1889.

RELIGIOUS NURSING ORDERS.

* *Sisterhoods in the Church of England.* Margaret Goodman. London, Smith, Elder & Co., 1864.

* *Handbook to Christian and Ecclesiastical Rome.* M. A. R. Tuker and Hope Malleson. Macmillan. New York and London, 1900.

* *The Military Religious Orders of the Middle Ages.* F. C. Woodhouse, M.A. London, 1879.

* *Deaconesses.* Rev. J. S. Howson. Longmans, 1862.

* *Sisters of Charity, Catholic and Protestant, at Home and Abroad.* By Mrs. Jameson. London, Longmans, Brown, Green and Longmans, 1855.

* *Hospitals and Sisterhoods.* Mary Stanley. 2nd edition. London, John Murray, 1855.

* *Sisterhoods and Deaconesses at Home and Abroad.* Henry C. Potter, D.D. New York, E. P. Dutton & Co., 1873.

* *Deaconesses in Europe.* Jane M. Bancroft, Ph.D. New York, Hunt & Eaton, 1890.

* *Deaconesses, Ancient and Modern.* Rev. Henry Wheeler. New York, Hunt & Eaton, 1889.

* *The Deaconess: Her Vocation.* Bishop Thoburn. New York, Hunt & Eaton, 1893.

* *Deaconesses, Biblical, Early Church, European, American.* Lucy Rider Meyer. Cincinnati, Cranston & Stowe, 1889.

* *Woman's Work in the Church.* John Malcolm Ludlow. London, 1865.

KAISERSWERTH BIBLIOGRAPHY.

* *Kaiserswerth and the Protestant Deaconesses.* By Miss Sewell. *Macmillan's Magazine*, January, 1870.

Jahresberichte über die Diakonissen Anstalt zu Kaiserswerht am Rhein. Kaiserswerth.

* *Mutter Fliedner. Zum Gedächtniss.* Kaiserswerth. 1892.

Pastorin Friederike Fliedner; die erste Vorsteherin der Diakonissen Anstalt. Reprint from monthly magazine published at Kaiserswerth, called *Armen-und-Kranken-Freund*, 1871.

An Account of the Institution for Deaconesses. By Florence Nightingale. London, 1851.

* *Life of Pastor Fliedner.* Trans. from the German by permission of his family, by Catherine Winkworth. London, 1867.

* *Das Diakonissen Mutterhaus und seine Töchterhäuser.* Dr. Julius Disselhoff, Kaiserswerth. 1893.

* *Kaiserswerth. Zur Erineerung an den Besuch der Diakonissen Anstalt in Kaiserswerth.*

* *Jubilate. Denkschrift zur Jubelfeier.* Julius Disselhoff, Kaiserswerth, 1886.

* *Jahrbuch für Christliche Unterhaltung.* Kaiserswerth, 1894. Lives of Friederike and Caroline Fliedner.

* *Theodor Fliedner. Kurzer Abriss seines Lebens und Wirkens.* Georg Fliedner. Kaiserswerth, 1886–92.

Theodor Fliedner, der Begrunder von Kaiserswerth. Fritz Fliedner, 1886.

Gertrud Reichart. Armen und Kranken Freund, 1869.

Kollektenreise nach Holland und England. Th. Fliedner. Essen, Bädeker, 1831.

Das Erste Jahr-Zehnt der Diakonissen Anstalt. Kaiserswerth, 1836–37.

Kurze Entstehungsgeschichte der ersten evangel. Liebesanstalt zu Kaiserswerth. Armen und Kranken Freund, 1856; also separate leaflet.

Haus-Ordnung und Dienstanweisungen für die Diakonissen Anstalt zu Kaiserswerth. Th. Fliedner. Kaiserswerth, 1845.

* *Life of Agnes Elizabeth Jones*, by her sister. (Contains much detail of the life at Kaiserswerth, where she spent a year. Appendix A was first published in the *Dublin University Magazine*, April, 1859, as an article called "Kaiserswerth, the Training School of Florence Nightingale."

* *A Pilgrimage to Kaiserswerth.* L. L. Dock in *Short Studies on Nursing Subjects.* New York, 1900.

NIGHTINGALE BIBLIOGRAPHY.

Experience of a Civilian in Eastern Military Hospitals. Peter Pincoffs, M.D. Williams & Norgate, London, 1857.

Excellent account of Miss Nightingale in the chapter called "The Providence of the Barrack Hospital."

The Seat of War in the East. William Simpson. Day & Sons, London, 1902. Reprinted from ed. of 1855. A good chapter on Miss Nightingale.

The Illustrated History of the War with Russia. E. H. Nolan, Ph.D., LL.D. J. S. Virtue, London, 1857. Excellent account of Miss Nightingale in chapter called "Scutari and its Hospitals."

The Invasion of the Crimea. Kinglake. 1880. Vol. 6, chap. xi. An excellent and fascinating chapter on Miss N. and her work called "The Care of the Sick and the Wounded."

* *Scutari and its Hospitals.* Rev. Sydney G. Osborne. Dickenson Bros., London, 1855.

The Story of Florence Nightingale. W. J. Wintle. *Sunday-School Union,* London. No date. Good and detailed account of her early life.

* *Florence Nightingale.* Eliza F. Pollard. S. W. Partridge Co., London, 1902. The most complete and full as to detail, quiet and authoritative in tone.

Fights for the Flag. Contains life of Miss Nightingale called "The Lady with the Lamp." W. H. Fitchett. Geo. Bell & Sons, London, 1898.

* *Great Men and Famous Women.* Vol. iii. Life of Miss Nightingale, by Lizzie Aldridge. Selmar Hess, New York.

* *Notable Women.* Contains life of Miss Nightingale. Ellen C. Clayton. Dean & Son, London. No date.

* *The Life of Florence Nightingale.* Sarah Tooley. Bousfield Co., London, 1906.

* *Life of Sidney Herbert, Lord Herbert of Lea.* By Lord Stanmore. Murray, London, 1907. In 2 vols. Contains portions of Miss Nightingale's letters not heretofore published.

MISS NIGHTINGALE'S WRITINGS.

1851. *The Protestant Deaconesses of Kaiserswerth.* A pamphlet describing the Kaiserswerth institutions and training. A long quotation from it in Appendix, Note A, *Hospitals and Sisterhoods,* by Miss Stanley.

1857. *Statements Exhibiting the Voluntary Contributions.* Being a report giving complete statistics and record of all the voluntary contributions which had passed through her hands during the war. Harrison, St. Martin's Lane.

1857–1860. *An Exhaustive and Confidential Report on the Workings of the Army Medical Department in the Crimea.* Used in the reorganisation of that service. Never printed.

* 1858. *Notes on Matters Affecting the Health, Efficiency, and Hospital Administration of the British Army.*

* 1859. *Notes on Hospitals.* First presented to the Engl. Nat. Asso. for the promotion of Social Science.

1859. Enlarged and revised edition of same. Longmans, Green & Co.

* 1860. *Notes on Nursing; What it Is and What it Is Not.* In many editions. D. Appleton, New York.

* 1861. *Notes on Nursing for the Labouring Classes.* A modified edition of *Notes on Nursing*, with special reference to the care of babies, and a new chapter addressed to the older sisters (little mothers).

1862. *Army Sanitary Administration and its Reform under the late Lord Herbert.* Read at London meeting of the Congrès de Bienfaisance, June, 1862.

1863. *The Sanitary State of the Army in India.* Observations on the evidence contained in the statistical reports submitted to her by the Royal Commission on the same. Reprinted by order from the report of the Royal Commission. Edw. Stanford, 6 Charing Cross, 1863.

1863. *How People may Live and not Die in India.* Read at the Edinburgh meeting of the Nat. Soc. Sci. Cong., in 1863. Reprint as pamphlet.

* 1865. *An Introduction to an Account of the Origin and Organisation of the Liverpool School and Home for Nurses.*

* 1867. Suggestions for the Improvement of the Nursing Service of Hospitals and on the Methods of Training Nurses for the Sick Poor. Written by request of the Poor Law Board after the Poor Act of 1867; in their reports and in *Blue Book*, "Metropolitan Workhouses."

* 1868. *Una and the Lion.* An introduction to the Memorial of Agnes E. Jones, by her sister. First appeared in *Good Words*, June, 1868.

* 1871. *Lying-in Hospitals; with a Proposal for Organising an Institute for Training Midwives and Midwifery Nurses.* Longmans, Green & Co., 1871.

1873. *Life or Death in India.* Read at the Norwich meeting of the Nat. Asso. for the Promotion of Soc. Sci., 1873. Published as pamphlet with an appendix on irrigation, called "Life or Death by Irrigation."

* 1873. *"A Sub-Note of Interrogation."* *Fraser's Magazine*, May, 1873.

1876. A letter to the *Times*, April 14. Reprinted as pamphlet called *Trained Nursing for the Sick Poor: a Home for Nurses in connection with the National Society for Providing Trained Nursing for the Sick Poor.* Expresses her views on district nursing.

1891. Article on *Hospitals and Nursing, Chambers's Encyclopedia.*

* 1892. *The Reform of Sick-Nursing, and the Late Mrs. Wardroper*, Brit. Med. Journal, Dec. 31.

* 1893. *Rural Hygiene: Health Teachings in Towns and Villages.* Read at the Conference of Women Workers, Leeds, November, 1893.

* 1893. *Sick-Nursing and Health-Nursing.* Written for and read at the Nursing Section of the Congress of Charities and Correction in Chicago, World's Fair, 1893.

1894. *Village Sanitation in India.* Read before the Tropical Section, 8th Internat. Cong. Hygiene and Demography, Budapest, September, 1894.

1894. Two articles in *Quain's Dictionary of Medicine.* "Nurses: Training of," "Nursing the Sick." 1894. In later editions of Quain these articles have been entirely garbled by a medical editor and their individuality is quite lost.

GENERAL BIOGRAPHY.

Amalie Sieveking. In German—*Denkwürdigkeiten aus dem Leben von.* M. E. Vorwort von Dr. Wichern. Hamburg, 1860. In French—*Mémoires authentiques*, etc. Paris and Geneva, 1860.

* *Mutter Fliedner. Zum Gedachtniss.* Kaiserswerth. 1892.

Life and Works of Deaconess Harriet Monsel. Rev. T. T. Carter. London.

Makrina, das Hochgebild einer Christlicher Jungfrau. Hamburg. Ag. des Rauhen Hauses, 1864.

* "Friederike Fliedner, the First Superintendent of the Deaconess Institution at Kaiserswerth." The *British Journal of Nursing*, May 26, 1906, *et seq.* Trans. by L. Metta Saunders.

* The same in German, in *Kaiserswerth Bibliography*.

* *Memorials of Agnes Elizabeth Jones*, by her sister. James Nisbet & Co., London, 1885. (12th edition.)

* *Sister Dora.* By Margaret Lonsdale. Boston, Roberts Bros., 1880. From the 6th English edition.

Olympia. An account of in *Die Alte Kirche:* part 9, *das vierte Jahrhundert.* By Friedrich and Paul Böhringer. Contents, Johannes Chrysostomus und Olympias. Stuttgart, 1876. Published by Meyer & Zeller.

Fabiola and the Roman Matrons. An account of in *St. Jerome; la Société Chrétienne à Rome et l'emigration romaine en Terre Sainte.* Thierry (Amedée), Paris, 1867.

* On similar lines, *The Makers of Modern Rome*, by Mrs. Oliphant, New York and London, Book I; *Honourable Women not a Few*, Macmillan Co., 1896.

Histoire de Sainte Hildegarde. Le R. P. Jacques Renard. Paris. 1865.

* *Histoire de Mlle. Le Gras (Louise de Marillac).* By the Countess de Richemont. 4th ed. Paris, Ch. Poussielgue, 1894.

* *La vie de Mademoiselle Le Gras.* By Monsieur Gobillon Paris. 1676.

* *Vie de Mademoiselle Mance and History of the Hôtel Dieu of Ville Marie* (Montreal). Published by the Sisters of the Hôtel Dieu de Ville Marie. 1854. In 2 vols.

* *Memoirs of Edward and Catherine Stanley* (containing a biographical notice of Mary Stanley). Edited by Arthur Penrhyn Stanley, D.D. 3d edition. John Murray, London. 1880.

* *Life of Dorothea Lynde Dix.* By Francis Tiffany. Boston and New York, Houghton, Mifflin & Co., 1892.

EARLY TEXT-BOOKS ON NURSING

Von der Wartung der Kranken. Unzer, 1769.

Unterricht für Krankenwärter. Franz May, Mannheim, 1784.

Manuel pour les gardes malades. Carrère, Strassburg, 1787.

Unterricht für Personen welche Kranken warten. J. G. Pfähler. Riga, 1793.

Die Kunst der Kranken zu pflegen. Anselm Martin, München, 1832.

Anleitung zur Krankenwartung. Dieffenbach, Berlin, 1832.

* *The Domestic Management of the Sick-Room.* Anthony Todd Thomson, M.D., F.L.S. 1st American from 2nd English ed. London, Lee Bros., 1845. 1st English ed. 1841.

* *The Nurse's Guide.* By J. Warrington, M.D. Philadelphia, Thomas, Cowperthwaite & Co., 1839.

* *The Young Mother's Guide and Nurse's Manual.* By Richard S. Kissam, M.D. 2nd ed. Hartford, 1837.

* *Friendly Cautions to the Heads of Families, etc., with Ample Directions to Nurses who Attend the Sick.* 3d ed. By Robert Wallace Johnson, M.D. 1st American ed. Philadelphia, 1804.

* *The Good Nurse; or hints on the management of the Sick and Lying-in Chamber and the Nursery.* No author named. London, 1825. Dedicated to Miss Priscilla Wakefield.

* *The Good Samaritan, or Complete English Physician.* By Dr. Lobb, member of the Royal College of Physicians in London, and other eminent Practitioners. London. No date.

* *The Practice of the British and French Hospitals. A Select Body of useful and elegant Medicines for the several disorders incident to the Human Body, etc.* London, 1773.

* *The Science and Art of Nursing the Sick.* By Æneas Munro, M.D. Glasgow, James Maclehose, 1873.

* *Accidents: Popular Directions for their Immediate Treatment.* By Henry Wheaton Rivers, M.D. Boston, Thomas H. Webb & Co., 1845.

* *The Nurse.* No author given. London, Houlston and Stoneman. No date. (About 1830?)

* *An Essay upon Nursing and the Management of Children.* By W. Cadogan, late physician to the Foundling Hospital. 9th ed. London, 1769.

* *Hints for the Nursery, or the Young Mother's Guide.* By Mrs. C. A. Hopkinson.. Boston, Little, Brown & Co., 1863.

* *First Helps in Accidents and in Sickness.* Published with the recommendation of the Highest Medical Authority. Boston, Alexander Moore; New York, Lee, Shepard & Dillingham. 1871.

* *Till the Doctor Comes.* By George H. Hope, M.D. New York, G. P. Putnam's Sons, 1871.

* *Handbook for Hospital Sisters.* By Florence S. Lees. Isbister & Co., London, 1874.

* *Bellevue Manual*, 1887. Called "A Manual of Nursing." Compiled from suggestions of Dr. Emily Blackwell, and material from a manual by Miss Zepherina Veitch and Domville, M.D. Also much from Miss Nightingale and Florence Lees. Compiled by Victoria White, revised by Dr. Mary Putnam Jacobi. G. P. Putnam's Sons, New York.

Connecticut Manual, New Haven. 1878.

Charity Hospital Manual. New York. By Dr. Frankel. 1878.

UNITED STATES—GENERAL OUTLINES OF HISTORY

* "Miss Linda Richards." By one of her Pupils. *American Journal of Nursing*, October, 1900, p. 12 *et seq.*

* "How Trained Nursing began in America. By Linda Richards. *American Journal of Nursing.* November, 1901, p. 88.

* "The Reform in Nursing in Bellevue Hospital." By L. L. Dock. *American Journal of Nursing*, November, 1901, p. 89 *et seq.*

* "Early History of the Boston Training School." By Miss Curtis and Miss Denny. *American Journal of Nursing*, February, 1902, p. 331 *et seq.*

* "Recollections of a Pioneer Nurse." By Linda Richards. *American Journal of Nursing*, January, 1903, p. 245, *et seq.*

* "A New Profession for Women." *Century Magazine*, July, 1882.

* "History of the Establishment of Bellevue." By the Managers. Read at the Waldorf-Astoria, March 6, 1899, on the 25th anniversary of the School.

* *Reports of the New York State Charities Aid Association:* Report of Committee on Hospitals, No. 1, 1872. Report of Special Committee in regard to building New Bellevue, No. 4.

"Training Schools for Nurses." By Chas. P. Putnam, Boston. *Penn Monthly*, December, 1874.

* *An Account of Bellevue Hospital.* Robert Carlisle, M.D. New York, 1893.

Appendix to the Life of Elizabeth Agnes Jones. By her sister. From the second London edition. (Contains in appendix an account of American nursing.)

* "The Organisation of Training Schools in America." By Louise Darche. *Chicago World's Fair Papers*, p. 518.

For the convenience of students, material that may be found in the reference library of the Johns Hopkins Training School for Nurses has been marked with an asterisk. The greater part of the footnote references is also to be found there.

MISCELLANEOUS

(Found only in French libraries)

Histoire de Saint Césaire, by the abbé J. M. Trichaud, Arles, 1853. Contains rules of the nuns of Arles.

L'ancien Hôpital d'Aubrac, by the abbé Bousquet, Montpellier, 1841.

Histoire de Saint Radegonde, by the abbé Briand, Poitiers; also a large edition illustrated.

L'Hôtel-Dieu de Beaune, 1445–1880, by the abbé E. Bavard, Beaune, 1881. Illustrated.

La vie de Mlle. de Meleun (Melun), by George and Louis Josse, Paris, 1687.

Histoire de Sainte Chantal, by the abbé Bougaud, Paris, 1863.

Les Sœurs Hospitalières, by Dr. Armand Despres, Paris, 1886.

INDEX

A

Abelard's instructions to Heloise, i, 156

Air cushions and rings, invention of, i, 255

Alexandria, early hospital work at, i, 120–121

American Medical Association, report of Committee on Training of Nurses, ii, 366–369

Ancient Rome, charities of, i, 90–91; good-will of gods in cure of disease, i, 84; organised medical service, i, 87–89

Angers, organisation and training of Sisters at, i, 426–427

Animals, habits in illness, i, 9–11; mutual aid instinct, i, 1–6

Anne of Austria as a nurse, i, 349

Appliances, hospital and nursing, i, 233–256

Arabians and hospital work, i, 246–249

Army medical service, origin of, ii, 313,

Association of Charity, establishment of, i, 407

Assyrians and Babylonians, disease theory of, i, 58; medical records of, i, 56; regulations for the practice of surgery, i, 56–57

B

Athelstane, founder of first hospital in England, i, 450

Augustinian Sisters at Hôtel-Dieu, Paris, i, 294–334; in Canada, i, 369–383; in England, i, 448–457; origin of, i, 294

Babylonians and Assyrians, disease theory of, i, 58; medical records of, i, 56; regulations for the practice of surgery, i, 56–57

Barber-surgeons, origin of, i, 477

Basil, bishop of Cesarea, work of, i, 123–125

Basilias, establishment of, i, 123

Bath-tubs, need of, urged by Dr. John Gregorie, i, 470

Beaune, description of hospital at, i, 269–270

Beds, canopied, objection to, i, 253, 255

—iron, introduction of, i, 242; objections to, i, 255

—jointed, first use of, i, 253

—wooden, in use during eighteenth century, i, 251

Bed-screens, portable, invention of, i, 253

Bedsores, early treatment of, i, 253

Bed-warmers, early use of, i, 252, 255

447

29

Meals, serving of, in early hospitals, i, 255

Mediæval nursing orders, i, 336–354

Mediæval surgery and medical treatment, i, 447–498

Medical books, early, i, 488–490

Medicine, instruction in, in connection with monasteries, i, 152; practice of, by ancient Romans, i, 83–92; practice of, by ancient Greeks, i, 67–82; practice of, by early Egyptians, i, 47–55; practice of, by monastic orders, i, 153

Medicine-man, development of, i, 14–15, 20–21

Men as nurses, i, 101

Mexico, old Spanish hospitals in, i, 402

Middlesex Hospital, England, economies of, i, 474; extracts from minutes, i, 475–476; regulations, i, 473–474

Monasticism, first example of, i, 136; rise of, 144–170; rules governing, i, 144

Monastic orders and the practice of medicine, i, 153

More, Hannah, influence of life on development of reforms, i, 531

"Mother of the Poor" (Mme. de Lamoignon), i. 409

Mothers as nurses, Florence Nightingale on, ii, 216–263

Municipal control of English hospitals, i, 460–461

Münster, Friederike, *See* Fliedner, Friederike

N

Nantes, installation of Sisters at, i, 429

Napoleonic war, influence on nursing reform, i, 540

National Nursing Associa tion England, organisation of, ii, 299–300

Nazeau, Marguerite, one of the first Sisters of Charity, i, 421

Neale, Rev. Dr., founder of St. Margaret's Sisterhood, ii, 96

New England Hospital for Women and Children, beginning of nursing work, ii, 346–349; establishment of training school, ii, 349; extract from account of, ii, 353; extracts from early reports, ii, 348–351; requirements for admission to training school, ii, 350

New York Hospital, establishment of, ii, 338; establishment of training school, ii, 339

Nightingale, Florence, at Kaiserswerth, ii, 29, 31, 112; at Scutari, ii, 120–143; comments on, from Kinglake. ii, 131–133; co-workers of ii, 287–311; descriptions of, ii, 127–131; education of, ii, 105; extracts from writings of, ii, 208–223, 224–237, 241–259, 260–286, 388–393; memorial of, Mrs. Wardroper by, ii, 190–194; note on, from Julia Ward Howe's *Reminiscences.* ii, 110; note on, from Caroline Fox's *Memoirs*, ii, 105–106; on "children's epidemics," ii, 215; on conditions of the British Army, ii, 224–231; on dangers in the nursing profession, ii, 272–277; on discipline of nurses, ii, 264; on essentials of a good training school, ii, 265–267; on essentials of health, ii, 213–214; on friendly visiting, ii, 237; on future of nursing, ii, 278–280; on health and nursing the well, ii, 269–271: on home

St. Francis of Assisi, work of, i, 211–214
St. John Chrysostom, hospital at Constantinople founded by, i, 127
St. John the Almoner, Hospital of, origin of, i, 174–175; rule regarding reception of patients, i, 184
St. John's House, London, connection with Charing Cross Hospital, ii, 94; connection with King's College Hospital, ii, 90–91; difficulties with King's College, ii, 93–94; founding of, ii, 80; organisation of, ii, 82; and the Crimean War, ii, 86–89
St. Thomas's Hospital, duties of matron, i, 463; duties of nurses, i, 464, 466–467; duties of the Sister, i, 466; Nightingale School for nurses established, ii, 181; origin, i, 462
St. Vincent de Paul, character of, i, 405; division of poor by, i, 410; first organised charity by, i, 406; opposition of, to monastic vows among Sisters, i, 422; rescue and relief of galley-slaves by, i, 411; rules to Sisters, i, 422; work for the welfare of children, i, 436
St. Vincent de Paul, Order of, at Angers, i, 426; at Mans, i, 430; at Nantes, i, 429; first vows of Sisters, i, 430; growth and activity of, i, 437; introduction of, into United States, i, 439; present activity in Rome, i, 345; rules of, i, 422–425, 431
San Bernardino, work, i, 244
Sanitary Commission, creation of, at the opening of the Civil War, ii, 360; work of, ii, 362–363

Sanitation in India, Florence Nightingale on, ii, 232–237; of early hospitals, i, 249–253
Saracens, hospitals of, i, 246
Sarrazin, naturalist and physician, i, 392
Savages, nursing among, i, 21–25
Schuyler, Louisa, work of, ii, 358–360, 371
Scurvy, treatment by Indians, i, 362
Scutari hospital, conditions during the Crimean War, ii, 121–124, 138–141
Secular orders, rise of, i, 257–280
Servant-nurses at Hôtel-Dieu, Lyons, i, 283–284; at Hôtel-Dieu, Paris, i, 328 in England, i, 502–503
Sieveking, Amalie, establishment of friendly visiting by, i, 546–548; first nursing work of, i, 545
Sisterhoods. See Nursing orders
Sisterhoods, Protestant, in connection with nursing, ii, 355–357
Sisters of Charity (see also Nursing orders), at Angers, i, 426; at Mans, i, 430; at Nantes, i, 429; first step toward founding of, i, 416; nursing duties restricted, i, 438; opposition to, i, 429; original home of, i, 420
South, Dr. J. F., opposition of, to the Nightingale school for nurses, ii, 177–181
Soyer, Alexis, description of Florence Nightingale, ii, 128–129
Spanish hospitals in America, i, 402–403
Spiritual care of patients, correspondence with early English hospitals, i, 509

Women, activity of, during
Napoleonic war, i. 540;
as physicians and sur-
geons during the Middle
Ages, i, 97; as physicians
and surgeons in fiction, i,
347; as teachers of medi-
cine, i, 162; at head of early
monastic nursing, i, 147–
150; in charitable and nursing work in the seventeenth
century, i, 467; value of,
in hospital work as shown
at Kaiserswerth, ii, 45;
work of, during the Civil
War, ii, 358–363; workers
of the early church, i, 95–
117

Women's Central Relief Association, organisation and
work of, ii, 359–361

Work among fallen women,
i, 162

Workhouse infirmaries, introduction of nursing into,
ii, 294

Workhouse reform by Agnes
Jones, ii, 297–298; by Louisa
Twining, ii, 287–288, 290

Wylie, Dr. Gill, account of
visit to St. Thomas's Hospital, ii, 202–203; assistance of, in nursing reform
at Bellevue Hospital, ii,
377

X

Xenodochium, or home for
strangers, establishment of,
i, 119, 123; work and scope
of i, 121–122

AKLK

ary